HANDBOOK

of CRITICAL CARE AND EMERGENCY ULTRASOUND

NOTICE

Medicine is an ever-changing science. As new research and clinical experience broaden our knowledge, changes in treatment and drug therapy are required. The authors and the publisher of this work have checked with sources believed to be reliable in their efforts to provide information that is complete and generally in accord with the standards accepted at the time of publication. However, in view of the possibility of human error or changes in medical sciences, neither the authors nor the publisher nor any other party who has been involved in the preparation or publication of this work warrants that the information contained herein is in every respect accurate or complete, and they disclaim all responsibility for any errors or omissions or for the results obtained from use of the information contained in this work. Readers are encouraged to confirm the information contained herein with other sources. For example and in particular, readers are advised to check the product information sheet included in the package of each drug they plan to administer to be certain that the information contained in this work is accurate and that changes have not been made in the recommended dose or in the contraindications for administration. This recommendation is of particular importance in connection with new or infrequently used drugs.

HANDBOOK of CRITICAL CARE AND EMERGENCY ULTRASOUND

Kristin A. Carmody, MD, RDMS, RDCS
Director of Emergency Ultrasound
Boston Medical Center
Assistant Professor of Emergency Medicine
Boston University School of Medicine
Boston, Massachusetts

Christopher L. Moore, MD, RDMS, RDCS
Director of Emergency Ultrasound
Assistant Professor of Emergency Medicine
Yale University School of Medicine
New Haven, Connecticut

David Feller-Kopman, MD
Director, Bronchoscopy and Interventional Pulmonology
Associate Professor of Medicine
Johns Hopkins Hospital
Baltimore, Maryland

Mc
Graw
Hill **Medical**

New York   Chicago   San Francisco   Lisbon   London   Madrid   Mexico City
Milan   New Delhi   San Juan   Seoul   Singapore   Sydney   Toronto

The **McGraw·Hill** Companies

Handbook of Critical Care and Emergency Ultrasound

1 2 3 4 5 6 7 8 9 0   CTP/CTP   15 14 13 12 11

ISBN 978-0-07-160489-5
MHID 0-07-160489-8

This book was set in Times by Glyph International.
The editors were Brian Belval and Christine Diedrich.
The production supervisor was Catherine Saggese.
Project management was provided by Anupriya Tyagi, Glyph International.
The cover designer was LaShae V. Ortiz.
China Translation and Printing Services, Ltd. was printer and binder.

Library of Congress Cataloging-in-Publication Data

Handbook of critical care and emergency ultrasound / [edited by]
 Kristin Carmody, Christopher L. Moore, David Feller-Kopman.
   p. ; cm.
 Includes bibliographical references and index.
 ISBN 978-0-07-160489-5 (softcover : alk. paper)
 1. Critical care medicine.   2. Ultrasonic imaging.   I. Carmody,
Kristin.   II. Moore, Christopher L.   III. Feller-Kopman, David J.
 [DNLM: 1. Ultrasonography—methods.   2. Critical
Care.   3. Emergency Medical Services—methods.   4. Emergency
Treatment—methods.   WN 208]
 RC86.7.H362   2011
 616.02'8—dc22

                                                    2011003738

McGraw-Hill books are available at special quantity discounts to use as pre-
miums and sales promotions, or for use in corporate training programs. To
contact a representative please e-mail us at bulksales@mcgraw-hill.com.

We dedicate this book to all the patients who entrust us with their care and in whom ultrasound can help us arrive at better therapeutic decisions and perform safer procedures.

CONTENTS

Kenton Anderson, MD
Director of Emergency Ultrasound
Wilford Hall Medical Center
San Antonio, Texas

J. Scott Bomann, DO, RDMS, RDCS
Director of Emergency Ultrasound
Department of Emergency Medicine
Wellington Hospital
Wellington, New Zealand

Kristin A. Carmody, MD, RDMS, RDCS
Director of Emergency Ultrasound
Boston Medical Center
Assistant Professor of Emergency
    Medicine
Boston University School of Medicine
Boston, Massachusetts

Peter Doelken, MD
Division of Pulmonary, Critical Care,
    Allergy and Sleep Medicine
Associate Professor of Medicine
Medical University of South Carolina
Charleston, South Carolina

David Feller-Kopman, MD
Director, Bronchoscopy and
    Interventional Pulmonology
Associate Professor of Medicine
Johns Hopkins Hospital
Baltimore, Maryland

Puncho Gurung, MD
Division of Pulmonary, Critical Care,
    Allergy and Sleep Medicine
Medical University of South Carolina
Charleston, South Carolina

Beatrice Hoffmann, MD, PhD, RDMS
Assistant Professor
Director of Emergency Ultrasound
Johns Hopkins Medical Institutions
Department of Emergency Medicine
Baltimore, Maryland

Calvin Huang, MD
Fellow in Research, Fellow in
    Ultrasound
Department of Emergency Medicine
Massachusetts General Hospital
Boston, Massachusetts

James Q. Hwang, MD, RDMS, RDCS, FACEP
Staff Physician, Kaiser Permanente
South San Francisco, California

Adolfo E. Kaplan, MD
Volunteer Professor
Department of Family Medicine
McAllen Family Medicine Residency
    Program
McAllen, Texas

Frederick Korley, MD
The Robert E. Meyerhoff Assistant
    Professor
Department of Emergency Medicine
The Johns Hopkins University
Baltimore, Maryland

Pierre Kory, MPA, MD
Assistant Professor of Medicine
Albert Einstein College of Medicine
Division of Pulmonary, Critical Care,
    and Sleep Medicine
Beth Israel Medical Center
New York, New York

Yiju Teresa Liu, MD, RDMS
Emergency Ultrasound Fellowship
    Director
Assistant Professor of Emergency
    Medicine
The George Washington University
Washington, DC

Fernando A. Lopez, MD
Director of Emergency Ultrasound
Assistant Professor
Department of Surgery
Division of Emergency Medicine
Duke University Medical Center
Durham, North Carolina

William Manson, MD, RDMS, RDCS
Director of Emergency Ultrasound
Assistant Professor
Department of Emergency Medicine
Emory University School of Medicine
Atlanta, Georgia

Joshua Markowitz, MD, RDMS
Assistant Professor
Jefferson Medical College
Associate Director of Emergency
  Ultrasound Albert Einstein Medical
  Center Department of Emergency
  Medicine
Philadelphia, Pennsylvania

Paul H. Mayo, MD
Director MICU
Long Island Jewish Medical Center
Professor of Clinical Medicine
Albert Einstein College of Medicine

Martin L. Mayse, MD
Assistant Professor of Medicine and
  Surgery
Director of Interventional Pulmonology
Washington University in St. Louis
Division of Pulmonary and Critical Care
  Medicine
St. Louis, Missouri

Cynthia Moon, MD
Director of Emergency Ultrasound
Division of Emergency Services
Methodist Hospitals
Gary, Indiana

**Christopher L. Moore, MD, RDMS,
RDCS**
Director of Emergency Ultrasound
Assistant Professor of Emergency
  Medicine
Yale University School of Medicine
New Haven, Connecticut

**Michael R. Osborne, MD, RDMS,
RDCS**
Associate Professor of Emergency
  Medicine
University of Kentucky College of
  Medicine
Department of Emergency Medicine
Lexington, Kentucky

Nova Panebianco, MD, MPH
Associate Director of Emergency
  Ultrasound
Assistant Professor of Emergency
  Medicine
University of Pennsylvania
Philadelphia, Pennsylvania

Cori McClure Poffenberger, MD
Director, Adult Emergency Department
Harbor-UCLA Medical Center
Assistant Clinical Professor of Medicine
David Geffen School of Medicine at
  UCLA

Richard C. Redman, MD
Division of Pulmonary, Allergy, and
  Critical Care Medicine
Duke University Medical Center
Durham, North Carolina

Scott L. Shofer, MD, PHD
Interventional Pulmonology Program
Assistant Professor of Medicine
Division of Pulmonary, Allergy, and
  Critical Care Medicine
Duke University Medical Center
Durham, North Carolina

Edward Tham, MD
Clinical Instructor
Department of Emergency Medicine
Eastern Virginia Medical School
Norfolk, Virginia

Jonathan S. Thierman, MD, PHD
Department of Emergency Medicine
Johns Hopkins Hospital
1830 East Monument Street
Baltimore, Maryland

Momen M. Wahidi, MD, MBA
Director of Interventional Pulmonology
  and Bronchoscopy
Associate Professor of Medicine
Division of Pulmonary, Allergy, and
  Critical Care Medicine
Duke University Medical Center
Durham, North Carolina

Over the last several decades, the technological advances in ultrasound have been staggering. Ultrasound is now widely available as an affordable, safe, portable, versatile, and high-quality imaging tool for diagnostic and procedural guidance across a wide variety of specialties.

However, ultrasound remains a user-dependent technology. This technology can only be effective when used by people who understand what it can do as well as its limitations.

The uses of ultrasound in the critical care and emergency setting share many aspects—both critical care and emergency medicine involve the care of patients with a broad array of potentially life-threatening conditions that can be diagnosed using ultrasound and aided with ultrasound-guided procedures.

The purpose of this manual is to serve as an easily accessible, practical guide for point-of-care ultrasound use in both the critical care and emergency department setting. We hope that emergency and critical care providers will be stimulated to learn more, deepen their knowledge of sonography, and broaden their use of ultrasound to improve the care of their patients.

1 Critical Care and Emergency Ultrasound

Kristin Carmody

INTRODUCTION

Ultrasound has long been accepted as a safe and accurate imaging modality. Over the last several decades, advances in the equipment, training, and applications of ultrasound have expanded its use as a point-of-care tool. Increasing evidence supports the use of bedside ultrasound as advantageous to both the clinician and the patient, particularly in the critical care and emergency setting.

HISTORY

Ultrasound first became available for clinical care in the 1960s and began to be used widely by various specialties by the 1970s. Early ultrasound machines were bulky, expensive, complex, and time consuming to use. In the late 1980s, advances in ultrasound equipment made point-of-care ultrasound (POC US) more feasible. Machines became more compact and portable, allowing them to be taken to the bedside easily. This equipment has continued to develop with improved imaging, better displays, easier image transmission and storage, and less expensive equipment.

Initial reports of POC US use emerged in the 1970s from Europe. These studies described the use of ultrasound in detecting free fluid by surgeons in acute trauma. In 1988, David Plummer, an emergency physician from the United States, described how bedside echocardiography could save lives in patients with penetrating trauma. In 1993, the FAST acronym was coined at an international consensus conference, initially standing for "focused abdominal sonography in trauma" and later expanded to "focused assessment with sonography in trauma." The FAST exam allowed expeditious diagnosis of hemoperitoneum, hemothorax, and hemopericardium in trauma patients. The FAST exam is widely used and has been incorporated into the ATLS (Advanced Trauma Life Support) protocol.

Emergency medicine as a specialty was a relatively early adopter of POC US. In 1994, the Society for Academic Emergency Medicine (SAEM) published a "model curriculum" for bedside ultrasound training in residency. In 2001, the American College of Emergency Physicians (ACEP) published their "Emergency Ultrasound Guidelines," including recommendations on the scope of practice, indications to perform bedside exams, the credentialing process, quality assurance measures, documentation procedures, and the appropriate practices and standards that emergency physicians should adhere to. These guidelines were updated in 2008 to reflect the advancing technology and new applications that have since emerged.

POC US has been used in the critical care setting for decades, particularly to guide procedures such as central venous access. Ultrasound-guided central venous access was listed by the Agency for Healthcare Research and Quality (AHRQ) as one of the top ways to reduce medical errors, based largely on data from the critical care setting. More recently, interest in the use of POC US for focused diagnostic and additional procedural applications in critical care has increased. Organizations such as the Society of Critical Care Medicine (SCCM) have endorsed the benefits and have developed recommended training guidelines for the use of ultrasound in the intensive care unit. Recently, the Accreditation Council for Graduate Medical Education (ACGME) has required ultrasound training as part of critical care fellowships.

While there are certain differences, it has been increasingly recognized that POC US applications in critical care and emergency settings share many similarities. This book is intended to provide up-to-date, clinically useful information on how to use this tool.

PHILOSOPHY

The core philosophy of bedside POC US is that it is a focused goal-directed examination (or set of focused exams) intended to answer specific binary questions or guide a procedure with direct impact on the care of the patient. POC US should be integrated with the history and physical examination of the patient.

The focus of acute POC US is different from exams done by consultative services, such as radiology, gynecology, or cardiology. These other specialties typically perform comprehensive organ-based ultrasound. Bedside POC US exams are focused, limited, and goal-directed. They are typically intended to answer a simple "yes" or "no" question: "Is there an aortic aneurysm present in this elderly patient with abdominal pain?" or "Is there an intrauterine pregnancy in a young woman presenting with pain and hypotension?" These exemplify patients who may have life-threatening conditions and the use of timely ultrasound can accelerate their treatment and improve the prognosis.

While consultant-performed ultrasound may be indicated in certain situations, there are many advantages to bedside POC US. Consultant-performed ultrasound typically involves transport of a patient out of the care area, where an examination is often performed by a sonographer, with images transmitted and interpreted by another individual. Any step of this process may be delayed or not easily available. Removing the patient from the care area consumes time and resources, and may be dangerous in patients with life-threatening conditions. Ultrasound at the bedside can be repeated as many times as needed to monitor a patient's response to treatment. In many situations, bedside ultrasound may obviate the need for additional studies, particularly those that may be invasive (such as diagnostic peritoneal lavage), or imaging involving ionizing radiation.

Another advantage of POC US is that several goal-directed questions may be answered during a single POC examination. This is particularly helpful when a presenting sign or symptom could have several potentially serious etiologies. The fact that POC US may easily transition between cardiac and general applications also allow examinations that often could not be done without involving two separate consultants. The FAST exam is a good early example of this, combining focused views of the abdomen, pelvis, thorax, and heart as part of an integrated examination. Other such examinations may combine several focused applications in trying to determine the etiology of unexplained hypotension, dyspnea, or chest pain.

In addition to its diagnostic capabilities, ultrasound provides an invaluable adjunct for many (most) invasive bedside procedures. This includes highly invasive procedures, such as pericardiocentesis, thoracentesis, paracentesis, and central line placement, but also encompasses tasks such as difficult peripheral line placement. Ultrasound guidance for procedures has been shown to increase success rate, decrease complications, and may expedite the care of unstable patients.

SCOPE

ACEP provides a useful paradigm for categorizing POC US depending on its intended use. These include resuscitative, diagnostic, symptom or sign-based, procedural guidance, and therapeutic monitoring.

- *Resuscitative ultrasound:* Used in such situations as cardiac arrest to confirm the presence or absence of cardiac activity.
- *Diagnostic ultrasound:* Used to diagnose an emergent condition at the bedside.
- *Symptom- or sign-based ultrasound:* Uses specific algorithms that delineate which organ systems should be examined based on the patient's primary complaint. For example, how to proceed in case of a patient who presents with undifferentiated hypotension or shortness of breath.
- *Procedural guidance ultrasound:* Is used for invasive procedures where the evidence is enough to support its use. This is intended to limit the risks associated with the event. For example, in central line placement, the use of ultrasound guidance has a higher rate of first-time success and has lower patient complications compared to the blind technique.
- *Therapeutic treatment or monitoring ultrasound:* Is used to ascertain whether a specific intervention is successful. For instance, in a patient with hypotension with evidence of a collapsed inferior vena cava by ultrasound, monitoring the changes that occur after the administration of intravenous fluids helps to guide the physician in further treatment choices.

Based on the categories of bedside ultrasound described above, the 2008 ACEP guidelines include 11 examinations that are considered core emergency ultrasound applications, and most of which are applicable in the critical care setting. The following core exams were chosen by ACEP as representing applications that can be consistently applied with benefit in the emergency setting:

1. Trauma (FAST)
2. Intrauterine pregnancy
3. AAA (abdominal aortic aneurysm)
4. Cardiac
5. Biliary
6. Urinary tract
7. DVT (deep venous thrombosis)
8. Soft tissue/musculoskeletal
9. Thoracic
10. Ocular
11. Procedural guidance

The specific approach and techniques used for each of these applications is discussed fully in subsequent chapters. There are also new and emerging applications that are still being investigated, but have gained attention recently. These include:

- Advanced echocardiography
- Trans-esophageal echocardiography
- Bowel (intussusception, appendicitis, pyloric stenosis, diverticulitis, small bowel obstruction)
- Adnexal pathology
- Testicular ultrasound
- Transcranial Doppler
- Contrast studies

APPROACH TO BEDSIDE, GOAL-DIRECTED, PHYSICIAN-PERFORMED ULTRASOUND

Critical care and emergency settings are extremely busy and physicians are expected to handle many patients at once. This suggests and emphasizes the importance of performing bedside ultrasound only on ideal patients. The approach to using bedside ultrasound in the critical care and emergency patient is shaped by the philosophy and scope discussed above. Bedside ultrasound should be used only in *defined clinical situations*. The following guidelines should help the physician decide which patients will benefit from a bedside exam.

1. Will the bedside ultrasound answer a "yes" or "no" question?
   - Is there a AAA (abdominal aortic aneurysm)?
   - Is there an IUP (intrauterine pregnancy)?
   - Is there free fluid in a trauma patient?
   - Is there a pericardial effusion?

   These are examples of questions that can be answered quickly at the bedside and are not intended to be all-inclusive. If the question being asked is more complex, a complete study may need to be performed. For example, a bedside ultrasound performed on a patient who presents with vaginal bleeding, who is not pregnant, would be of little utility to the emergency physician. This exam would not answer a "yes" or "no" question, therefore, it is outside the scope of emergent bedside ultrasound.

2. Will the bedside ultrasound be limited and goal-directed?
   If there is suspicion for a particular disease, the ultrasound exam should be limited to specific organ systems that can be evaluated expeditiously. For instance, in a patient with RUQ (right upper quadrant) pain which the clinician is suspecting acute cholecystitis, the gallbladder should be examined, and perhaps the adjacent kidney and lower thorax if there is no biliary pathology. However, the exam may not (and generally should not) include a comprehensive evaluation of the liver or pancreas. The exam should be clearly defined and goal-directed, "Does the patient have acute cholecystitis or not?" It should impact the clinical decision-making process of the physician who is performing the exam. A comprehensive exam is not indicated, nor is it within the scope of critical care or emergency ultrasound practice recommendations. If the diagnosis cannot be made quickly, the patient may require a more comprehensive ultrasound or other exam, not best suited to the bedside.

3. Is ultrasound the modality of choice to confirm the suspected diagnosis?
   If an ultrasound is the test that would be ordered by the treating physician to confirm or rule out a disease process, then an initial ultrasound should be performed at the bedside. If a bedside test indicates pertinent findings, the proper consultative services can be notified earlier and patient care accelerated instead of waiting for a radiology-performed examination. Alternately, if bedside ultrasound does not reveal any evidence of pathology, an alternate modality such as computed tomography may be better suited to reveal pathology.

4. Bedside ultrasound in unstable patients
   Ultrasound is the perfect modality to evaluate an unstable patient who has no definitive diagnosis. For example, patients who present with hypotension, hypoxia, tachycardia, or altered mental status who cannot give a good history, have unreliable physical examinations, and cannot be safely transported out of the department can be evaluated at the bedside. "Does the unstable trauma patient have a hemoperitoneum or hemopericardium?" "Does the young women who is pregnant and hypotensive have an empty uterus and free fluid indicative of a ruptured ectopic?" "Does the hypoxic and tachycardic patient

have signs of right ventricular strain on their echocardiography?" "Does the hypotensive elderly patient with abdominal pain have a ruptured aneurysm?" These are examples of patients who benefit immediately from a quick bedside ultrasound examination.

5. Bedside ultrasound for procedural guidance
   Using real-time ultrasound guidance to perform an invasive procedure is now the standard of care in many situations. The advantages of visualizing the needle as it approaches the structure of interest has obvious benefits, including higher rates of first-time success, faster times for completing the procedure, avoidance of other vital structures, and improved patient comfort. The many procedures that ultrasound guidance are now used for include: pericardiocentesis, thoracentesis, paracentesis, central lines, nerve blocks, joint aspirations, peripheral intravenous lines, and more applications to come.

6. Integration of bedside ultrasound into specific algorithms
   There are many patients who present to the critical care or emergency setting who do not have a clear diagnosis. Ultrasound can help narrow down the differential within minutes of the patient's presentation. There are specific algorithms to follow based on a patient's main complaint. For example, in the patient who presents with undifferentiated abdominal pain, a quick bedside ultrasound can be used to rule out free fluid, a AAA, acute cholecystitis, or hydronephrosis.

For the patient who presents with hypotension, an ultrasound can be used to evaluate for free fluid and a AAA. A quick assessment of volume status can be ascertained by evaluating the inferior vena cava and performing focused echocardiography to rule out cardiac dysfunction and effusion.

For the patient who presents with shortness of breath or chest pain, the lungs can be evaluated for effusions or interstitial edema, the heart can be looked at for function and effusion and also signs of right ventricular strain.

If the treating physician is able to formulate possible differential diagnoses based on the patients' complaints, a quick focused ultrasound following these algorithms may help point toward the correct diagnosis and hasten treatment.

There are always risks to performing any bedside ultrasound exam and relying on real-time physician interpretations. The most experienced physician present should make any decisions in clinical care that are based on a bedside ultrasound. The advantages of using bedside ultrasound to guide patient care must be balanced against the necessity for specialized training. Most professional organizations, such as ACEP, provide recommended guidelines for proficiency training and teaching techniques for students, residents, and faculty. Finally, if there is any doubt related to the findings of a bedside ultrasound, the most experienced clinician should be notified. In this case, additional confirmatory studies may be needed and the appropriate specialty services should be consulted.

CONCLUSION

The application and scope of physician-performed bedside ultrasound continues to expand. Physicians are now using ultrasound to investigate patient symptoms and organ systems that were once thought to be unattainable using this modality. The newer technology, portable machines, increasing availability, and improved storage and documentation procedures has made the use of ultrasound an integral part of diverse specialties. It has now become the standard of care for many procedures performed in emergency departments and intensive care units. In addition to its diagnostic capabilities and its assistance with procedural guidance, ultrasound offers a noninvasive method to monitor therapeutic interventions.

With appropriate understanding, training, and practice, POC US offers a readily available, noninvasive, reproducible modality that can expedite and improve care in the critical care and emergency settings.

Additional Reading

American College of Emergency Physicians Policy Statement, Emergency Ultrasound Guidelines. http://www.acep.org. Accessed Oct 2008:1-38.

Joseph AP. Emergency ultrasound: the scope of practice. *Ultrasound.* 2007:15(4):229-235.

Kendall JL, Hoffenberg SR, Smith RS. History of emergency and critical care ultrasound. *Crit Care Med.* 2007:35(5):S126-S130.

Kirkpatrick AW, Sustic A, Blaivas M. Introduction to the use of ultrasound in critical care medicine. *Crit Care Med.* 2007:35(5):S123-S125.

Neri L, Storti E, Lichtenstein D. Toward an ultrasound curriculum for critical care medicine. *Crit Care Med.* 2007:35(5):S290-S304.

2 Ultrasound Basics

David Feller-Kopman

ULTRASOUND PHYSICS

Ultrasound (US) uses the transmission and reflection of mechanical waves to generate an image. US frequency (f) is the number of wavelengths per second and is measured in hertz (Hz) (Fig. 2-1). As humans can hear sound in the 20–20,000 Hz range, US is defined as sound with a frequency >20,000 Hz, or 20 kilohertz (kHz). Diagnostic sonography for most medical applications uses frequencies of 2–20 megahertz (MHz).

US frequency is independent of the medium through which the sound is traveling and is a property of the crystals in the US transducer. Modern transducers now often include a range of frequencies ("broadband") and/or allow for frequency adjustment. Propagation speed (c) describes how fast the US travels through a given medium. Unlike frequency, the propagation speed depends on the medium through which the sound travels. The wave velocity in fluid or tissue is approximately 1540 m/s (although it does vary slightly depending on the type of tissue) as compared to the propagation speed through air at a velocity of approximately 330 m/s. The relationship of frequency, wavelength, and propagation speed is described by the equation $c = f\,\lambda$. Because frequency is constant, wavelength varies directly with propagation speed (ie, $f = c/\lambda$). Thus, when propagation speed increases, wavelength increases, and vice versa. The change in the speed of sound at tissue interfaces results in a change of wavelength, which is responsible for determining image contrast, and resolution.

The power of an US wave refers to the amount of energy passing through the tissue in a unit of time and is expressed in watts. In the majority of compact US units, the power is fixed, though it may be adjusted on more sophisticated machines. If using one of these units, one should always use the lowest power that will produce the desired imaging as higher powers (>1 W) can result in cellular and tissue damage. This principle is commonly referred to as ALARA (**A**s **L**ow **A**s **R**easonably **A**chievable).

GENERATING THE ULTRASOUND IMAGE

Transducers convert one form of energy into another. Piezoelectric transducers convert electrical energy into mechanical energy by inducing vibration of the ferroelectric materials in the transducer head. These vibrations are transmitted through the tissue, echo back at boundaries of tissue that have different acoustic impedance, and are then converted back to an electrical signal. The transducer thus acts as an US transmitter and receiver. When the boundary between two tissues has high acoustic impedance, most of the US is reflected back to the transducer. If two materials have the same acoustic impedance, their boundary will not produce an echo. Typically, only a small fraction of the US pulse is reflected back, with the majority of the pulse continuing along the beam line, but can also be scattered or refracted.

As an US pulse (or echo) propagates through tissue, the energy contained within the beam progressively diminishes, or becomes attenuated. Attenuation

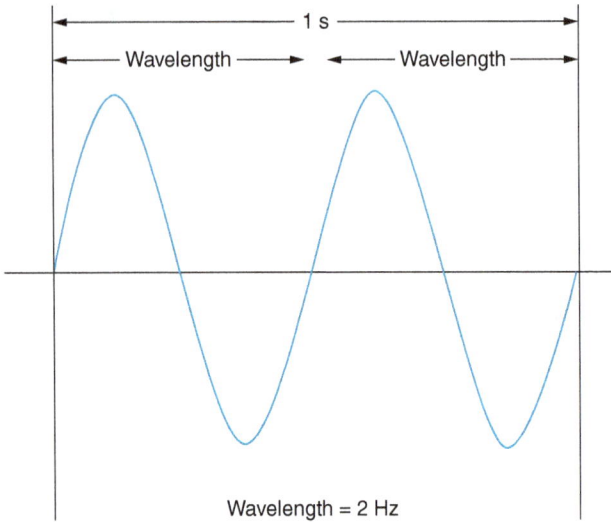

FIGURE 2-1 Hertz is equal to the number of wavelengths per second.

results from absorption of energy, with the energy lost as heat, as well as from scattering of the US beam. The amount of attenuation depends on the frequency, as well as the medium through which the US beam travels. In soft tissue, US energy is absorbed and scattered, and the amount of attenuation is directly proportional to the frequency. Though liquids do not significantly absorb or scatter US energy, attenuation does occur, and is proportional to the square of the frequency. Therefore, to image structures deep in the body, lower frequency transducers are required. Higher frequency waves, however, have better axial resolution, or the ability to distinguish two objects along the beam axis. Lateral resolution depends on the beam width as well as the focal zone (see later) of the transducer. The ideal transducer would be of sufficient frequency to penetrate to the desired depth without significant attenuation, yet have a frequency high enough to provide the best resolution (Fig. 2-2).

APPEARANCE OF ULTRASOUND IMAGES ON THE SCREEN

The received echo signal is displayed visually in either a brightness mode (B-mode) (Fig. 2-3, top) or a motion mode (M-mode) (Fig. 2-3, bottom). M-mode displays the motion (Y-axis) of the echo reflection over time (X-axis) on a single line of the B-mode image and is used for precise measurements of size and distances, especially with rapidly moving structures such as cardiac valves or fetal heart rate. In both B- and M-modes, it is the amplitude (measured in decibels) of the returning echo signal that determines the brightness on the screen, and the amount of reflected echo is a function of the density and nature of the target, as well as the angle at which the sound wave is reflected. The B-mode image is produced by sweeping the US pulse perpendicular to the axis of the US beam, and as this occurs at rates of 20–40 frames per second, it is seen as a continuous image by the human eye.

Echogenicity refers to the ability of the tissue to reflect the pulsed echo. This is primarily determined by the density and acoustic impedance of the tissue. By convention, tissues such as the liver and kidney are said to be isoechoic. Tissues that

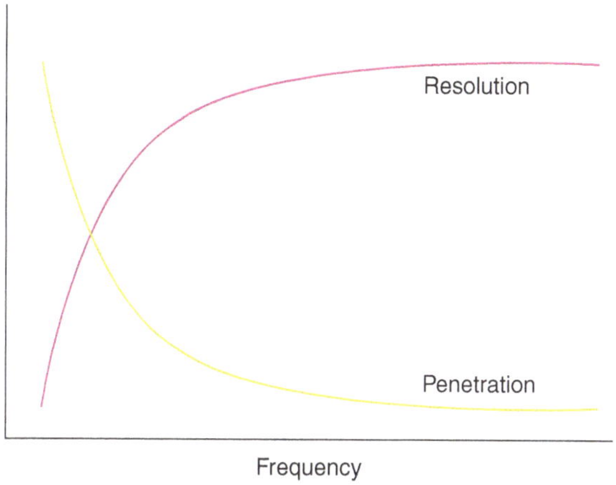

FIGURE 2-2 The relationship of frequency to penetration and resolution.

reflect more US waves back to the transducer are hyperechoic, whereas fat, blood, and fluid tend to absorb more of the US energy and are hypoechoic. The gray scale of B-mode imaging is the range of echo strength on the black–white continuum. Bone is a significant absorber and scatterer of US energy (see later). Since air reflects nearly 99% of the US waves, the US transducer needs to be coupled to the tissue with gel or other fluid in order for the waves to penetrate more deeply. Even with coupling, however, it is very difficult to image beyond the periosteum (the internal components of bone) or air-filled structures such as the lung.

The image seen on the US screen can be made to appear more white or black by adjusting the gain or the amplitude of the received echo. This is analogous to

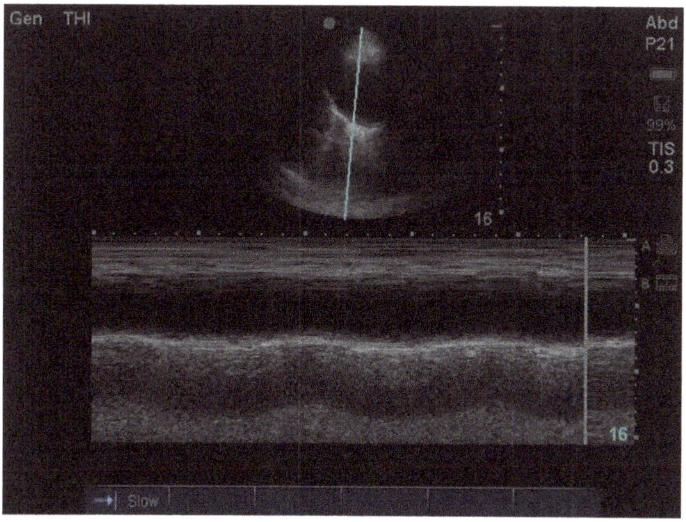

FIGURE 2-3 Top image: brightness (B) mode. Bottom image: motion (M) mode.

adjusting the volume on a radio receiver—the received signal is amplified prior to being transmitted to the speaker. The only other way to increase the brightness of an image is to increase the power out of the unit. Time-gain compensation refers to the ability to adjust the gain at varying depths such that despite the fact that the echoes from deeper structures undergo more attenuation, they appear equally bright.

All frequencies have associated harmonics or integral multiples of the fundamental frequency. For example, a second harmonic has twice the frequency as the first harmonic (fundamental frequency). As US waves travel through tissue, they become slightly distorted due to frequency components made up of higher-order harmonics. Since the harmonics are of higher frequencies than the fundamental, they are subject to more attenuation. Tissue harmonic imaging (THI) is used to improve lateral resolution by minimizing the reflections and scattering created by superficial structures with the fundamental frequency.

DOPPLER

The Doppler effect describes the changes in frequency and wavelength as perceived by an observer moving relative to a sound source. As the sound source moves closer to the receiver, the wavelengths become compressed. Likewise, as the sound source moves farther from the receiver, the wavelengths lengthen. Because wavelength is inversely proportional to frequency (when velocity is constant), the observer will detect a perceived frequency which is different from that emitted by the source when the relative velocity is zero.

There are several US modes that utilize the Doppler effect, including continuous-wave (CW), pulsed-wave (PW), color-flow, and power Doppler US. CW Doppler uses the continuous generation and sensing of the reflected echo and is primarily used for looking at high velocity movement, such as flow through stenotic heart valves. PW Doppler uses the standard pulse-echo mechanism and is able to analyze the Doppler characteristics at a given region of flow. Due to the intermittent nature of transmission and receiving, there is a velocity limitation beyond which the US will misinterpret velocity and direction of flow. This velocity limitation is defined as the Nyquist limit which is equal to ½ the pulse repetition frequency (PRF). PRF is the number of pulses the transmitter emits per second. When the Nyquist limit is reached, aliasing will occur when using PW Doppler. The term aliasing is used to describe an apparent reversal of direction that is caused by a relatively low sampling rate. On a PW Doppler tracing, this will appear as the tip or peak of the wave being truncated and appearing on the other side of the baseline. If high velocities are suspected, CW Doppler is the mode of choice.

Color-flow Doppler produces an image that shows both the relative velocity and direction of flow. By convention, flow moving toward the transducer is colored red-orange and flow moving away from the transducer is colored blue. This is important to remember, as the novice ultrasonographer may interpret red to mean arterial blood and blue as venous blood, when in fact the colors are purely dependent on the direction of flow relative to the transducer. It is also important to remember that if the movement of the target is perpendicular to the US beam, it will not give rise to any Doppler frequency shift. Power Doppler, on the other hand, solely relates information about velocity, and not the direction of flow. An advantage of power Doppler is that it is more sensitive than color-flow Doppler for detecting slower flow rates and smaller vessels.

BASIC INSTRUMENTATION

All US units have an electrical source, a piezoelectric transducer, and a computer processor that will turn the energy from the received echo into a visible picture. There are several types of US transducers, including simple single-element disc transducers, annular, linear, sector, phased-arrays, and radial probes. The differences in these probes lie in the way the beam is focused, the beam pattern, and the ability to electronically steer the beam.

Each of these transducers generates an "A-line," that is, one beam or pulse that is directed in the axial plane of the US. The B-mode image is produced by sweeping the A-lines along the transducer to produce a footprint that is square/rectangular, trapezoidal, or circular, depending on the probe. As mentioned earlier, the amplitude of the echo determines the brightness of the pixel, and the position of the pixel on the screen is determined by the depth from which the returning echo originates.

All transducers, aside from radial probes, have an identifier on them that corresponds to a mark on the screen so the operator can correlate what they are seeing to the orientation of the probe. The sophistication of the computer processors has allowed many functions (such as power and focus) to be preset, or set automatically depending on which transducer is being used.

US units have several knobs, buttons, and dials, and a recently coined term, knobology, describes the understanding of what these controls do. It is important to learn the knobology of the unit you will be using and at a minimum, be able to enter pertinent patient data (name, medical record number), store movies/still images, as well as control depth, contrast, and gain. Many units are also able to provide basic measurements such as distance or more complex measurements such as gestational age, volume, and cardiac output.

IMPORTANT ULTRASOUND ARTIFACTS

Much of what is seen on B-mode imaging relies on the accurate interpretation of US artifacts. As mentioned earlier, fluid does not significantly attenuate US energy. As such, structures that are deep to a fluid-filled space may exhibit relative acoustic enhancement (Fig. 2-4) and appear brighter than one would expect based solely on tissue characteristics and depth. Acoustic shadowing is the effect opposite to enhancement, and is seen when an intervening structure strongly attenuates the US energy (Fig. 2-5). This is classically described for rib shadows, gallstones, and more solid tumors.

When a strong echo is obtained, as is the case with bone, air, the diaphragm, or a needle, the reflector can continue to give rise to the echo even as the US transducer sweeps the beam laterally. This generates a long, curved, hyperechoic line called a side lobe artifact. These artifacts have a radius of curvature that corresponds to the distance between the transducer and the strong reflector. A mirror image artifact also results from the US beam, encountering a strong reflector such as the diaphragm, and produces a false image equal in distance, and deep to the reflector, that disappears with subtle changes in transducer positioning (Fig. 2-6).

A refraction artifact occurs when sound waves travel through materials with different acoustic transmission speeds. This is most commonly seen at the border between a fluid filled structure and solid organ such as at the edge of the gallbladder or urinary bladder. A dark area or "shadow" will be seen extending downward from this border and is known as "edge artifact" or "lateral cystic shadowing". It is important to not to mistake this artifact for a shadowing gallstone (see Chap. 11).

Reverberation artifact occurs when sound waves are reflected back and forth at close intervals. A reverberation artifact is commonly seen when ultrasound encounters either air or a metallic object, creating a tapering and repeating hyperechoic line distal to the hyperechoic structure. The artifact seen is commonly referred to as a "comet tail" or "ring down" artifact. In the case of air, a "dirty" comet tail is present, with somewhat more irregular tapering lines. Metallic objects such as a needle, guidewire, or foreign body will create more regularly spaced tapering lines and can be helpful in procedural guidance in locating the needle tip.

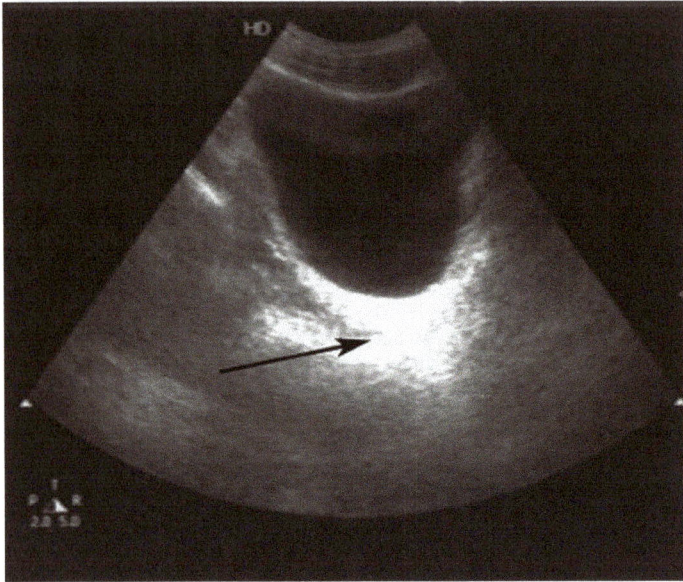

FIGURE 2-4 Acoustic enhancement increasing the signal off the posterior wall of the bladder (black arrow).

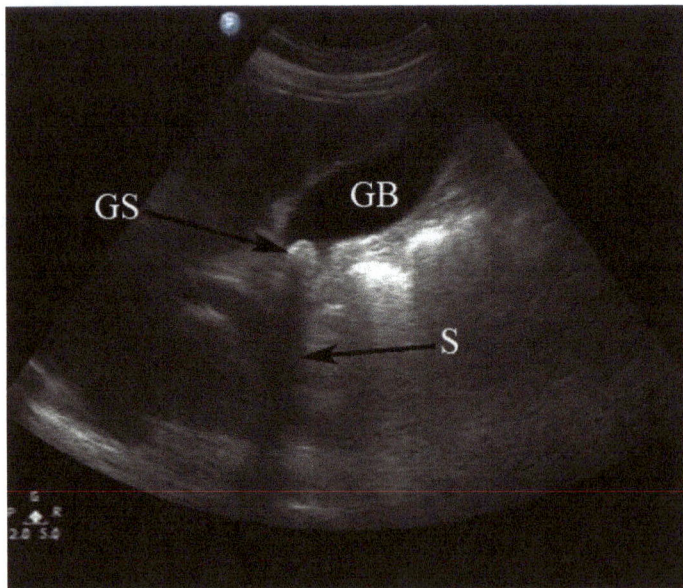

FIGURE 2-5 Acoustic shadowing (S) due to a gallstone (GS) blocking the ultrasound beam. GB: gallbladder.

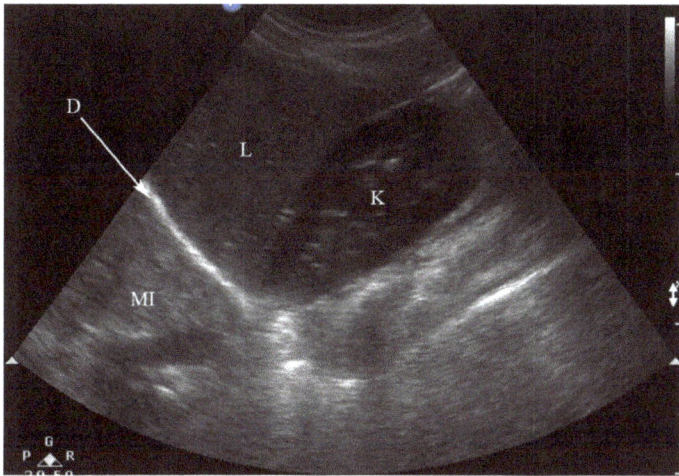

FIGURE 2-6 Image illustrating "mirror image artifact." There is a mirror image (MI) of the liver (L) above the diaphragm (D) in the thoracic space. This tells the sonographer that there is no fluid within the pleural space. K: kidney.

Two common reverberation artifacts seen when performing thoracic US are "A" and "B" lines. "A" lines are hyperechoic horizontal lines that may be seen between rib shadows and are equally spaced with a distance equal to the skin-pleural distance (Fig. 2-7). "B" lines, or comet-tail artifacts, originate from the pleural surface, and spread vertically to the edge of the screen without fading (Fig. 2-8). "B" lines erase "A" lines and move with respiration.

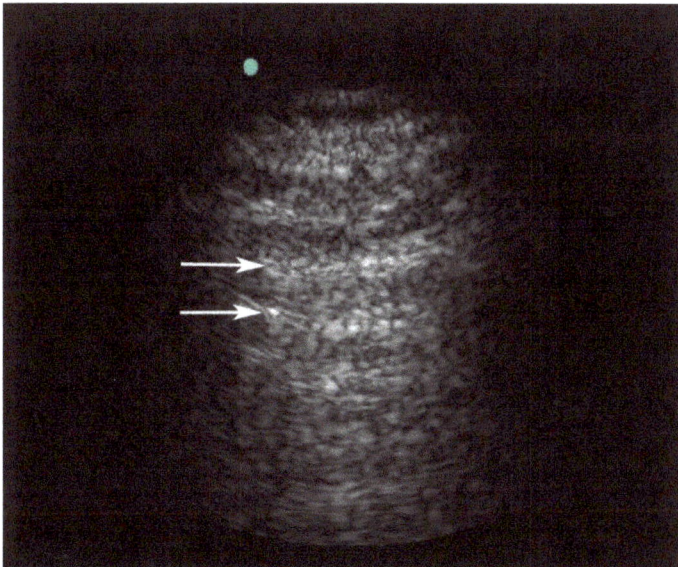

FIGURE 2-7 "A" lines from the pleural line illustrating reverberation artifacts (arrows).

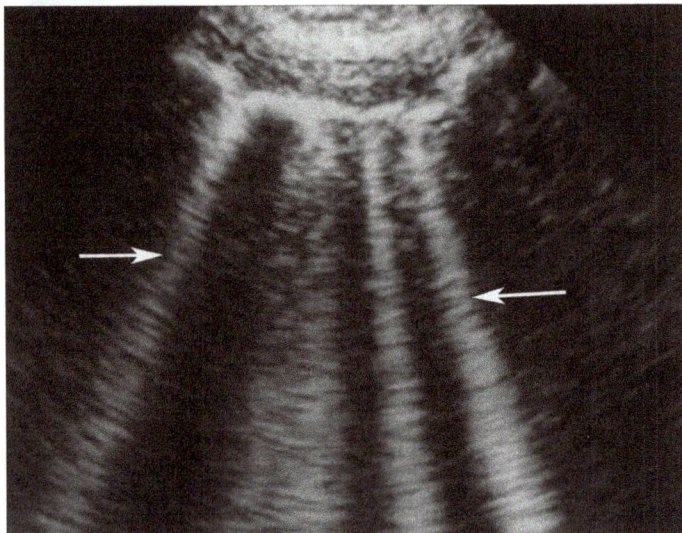

FIGURE 2-8 "B" lines (also known as comet-tail artifacts) (arrows).

Finally, though not truly an artifact, the operator should be aware of poor image quality due to inadequate coupling gel, or anatomic limitations such as obesity or surgical dressings. One may need to position the patient in a way to bring the target closest to the transducer, and scan in multiple planes in order to obtain a satisfactory image.

CONCLUSION

Prior to incorporating the use of ultrasound into ones daily practice, it is essential to understand the basic physics and principles of ultrasound imaging, including the way an image is formed and manipulated. An understanding of Doppler imaging as well as interpretation of artifacts is equally important. Some "golden rules" of ultrasound imaging include "1) Never make an interpretation on a single image...2) Because a feature is displayed it is not necessarily real...3) Because a feature is not displayed it is not necessarily not there." (see Kossoff 2000.) It is only through practice and repeated imaging that one develops the skills necessary to utilize the benefits of ultrasound imaging.

Additional Reading

Aldrich JE. Basic physics of ultrasound imaging. *Crit Care Med.* 2007 May;35(suppl 5):S131-S137.

Kossoff G. Basic physics and imaging characteristics of ultrasound. *World J Surg.* 2000 Feb;24(2):134-142.

Lawrence JP. Physics and instrumentation of ultrasound. *Crit Care Med.* 2007 Aug;35(suppl 8):S314-S322.

Scanlan KA. Sonographic artifacts and their origins. *Am J Roentgenol.* 1991 June;156(6):1267-1272.

Smith RS, Fry WR. Ultrasound instrumentation. *Surg Clin North Am.* 2004 Aug;84(4):953-971.

3 Ultrasound Orientation

Christopher L. Moore

INTRODUCTION

Ultrasound orientation is essential to understand what is being seen in point-of-care ultrasound. There are two key aspects: how the indicator is oriented relative to the screen and how the probe and indicator are placed and oriented relative to the patient. As described in Chap. 2, the conventional ultrasound image is a two-dimensional plane composed of frames made up of scan lines that are updated many times a second to create a moving image.

Ultrasound orientation can be challenging because it involves understanding how a two-dimensional plane may cut through a three-dimensional object in any of the three standard planes (sagittal, transverse, or coronal), as well as any oblique orientation between those planes. However, one of the great advantages of ultrasound is the ability to obtain images from a variety of different approaches, and a thorough understanding of orientation will allow you to take advantage of this.

INDICATOR-TO-SCREEN ORIENTATION

There are two rules for indicator-to-screen orientation in standard emergency ultrasound imaging, which uses the same convention as general radiology imaging:

1. The top of the screen is closer to the probe. Bottom of the screen shows structures farther away from the probe.
2. The left side of the screen, as it is viewed, corresponds to the side of the probe marked with an indicator.

Imaging performed by cardiology specialists uses a different and opposite convention for rule 2, which will be discussed in more depth later.

The "indicator" may differ widely between manufacturers, and is typically a bump or a groove. It is important to verify your orientation prior to beginning any exam. This should be done by placing a small amount of gel on the side of the probe where you believe the indicator to be, and confirming that the side with the gel corresponds to the left of the screen as it is viewed (Figs. 3-1a and b).

INDICATOR-TO-PATIENT ORIENTATION

Once the indicator-to-screen orientation is understood and verified, the probe is placed on the patient and images are viewed on the screen.

The top of the screen will show structures closer to where the probe is placed, with the bottom of the screen showing structures farther away from the probe face. The left of the screen will show structures toward where the indicator is directed.

Another way to think about this is to think of holding the probe in front of you, with the indicator on your left. In this way you are looking through the plane of the ultrasound, with the left side of the screen being on your left.

When you are located on the right side of the patient, a sagittal plane will be obtained by directing the indicator to your left (toward the patient's head), and

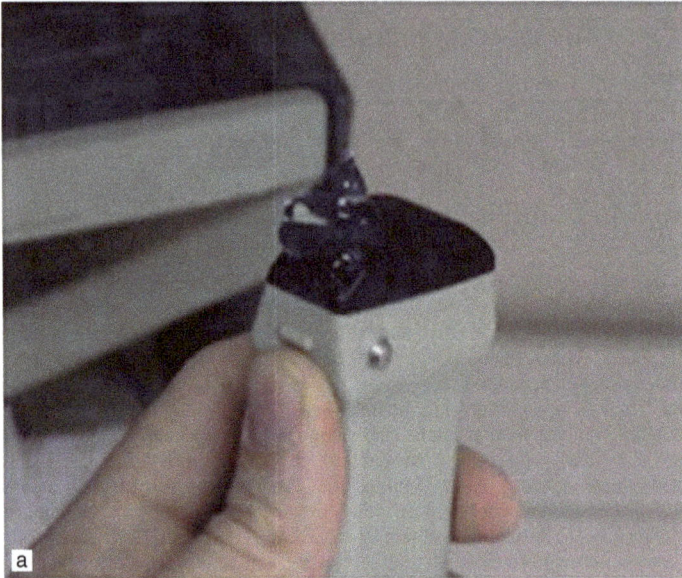

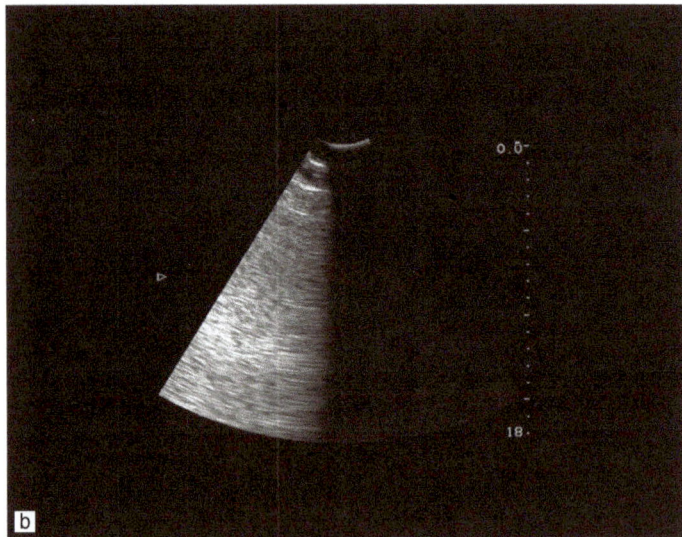

FIGURE 3-1 (*a*) Shows a thumb placed on the indicator, with gel placed on the face of the probe on that side. (*b*) Shows what should be seen on the screen in general imaging orientation.

this will be the left of the screen. For a transverse plane, think of yourself as looking up from the patient's feet, with right-sided structures on the left of the screen.

Most of emergency ultrasound can be performed in this orientation, with the indicator (screen left) being toward the patient's right, patient's head, or in the 90° arc between these directions.

ANATOMIC PLANES

There are three standard anatomic planes (Fig. 3-2):

- Transverse (or axial)
- Sagittal (or longitudinal)
- Coronal (or frontal)

TRANSVERSE PLANE

The transverse or axial plane is obtained by placing the probe on the anterior surface of the patient (typically the abdomen or pelvis) with the indicator directed to the patient's right (your left looking up from the feet) (Fig. 3-3a).

In this orientation, anterior structures will be toward the top of the screen and posterior structures toward the bottom. Right-sided structures will be on the left of the screen as it is viewed, and left-sided structures on the right of the screen (Fig. 3-3b).

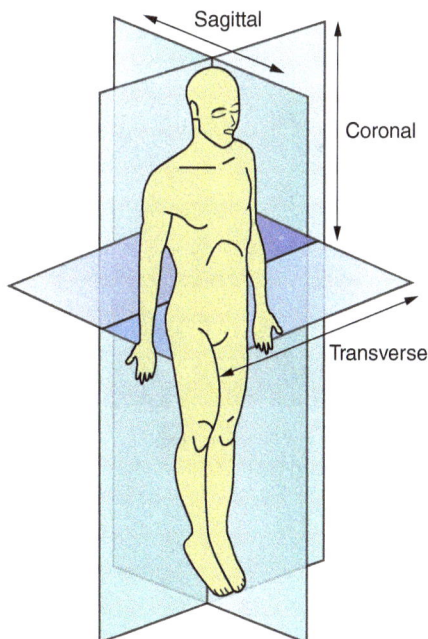

FIGURE 3-2 Anatomic planes. Sagittal (longitudinal), transverse (axial), and coronal (frontal).

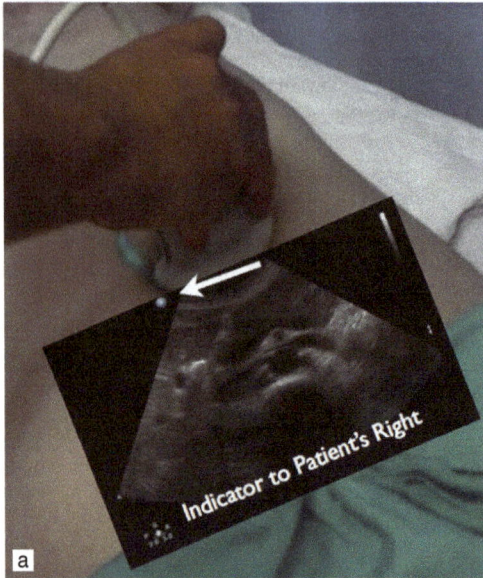

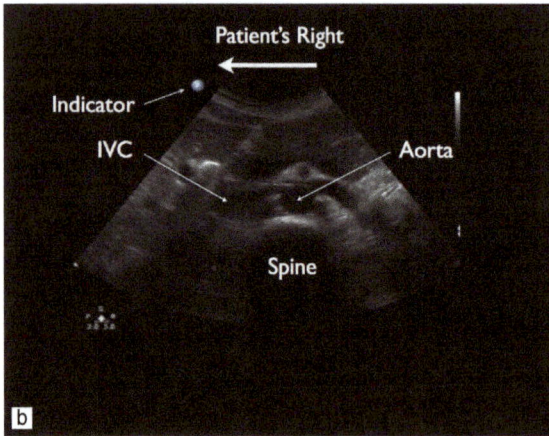

FIGURE 3-3 (*a*) For a transverse view of the aorta, the probe is placed between the umbilicus and xiphoid process with the indicator toward the right. (*b*) The image can be thought of as looking upward from the patient's feet, similar to a CT scan.

SAGITTAL PLANE

The sagittal plane is obtained by placing the probe on the anterior of the patient with the indicator toward the patient's head (your left if you are on the right side of the bed). This view can be obtained by rotating a transverse view 90° clockwise (Fig. 3-4*a*).

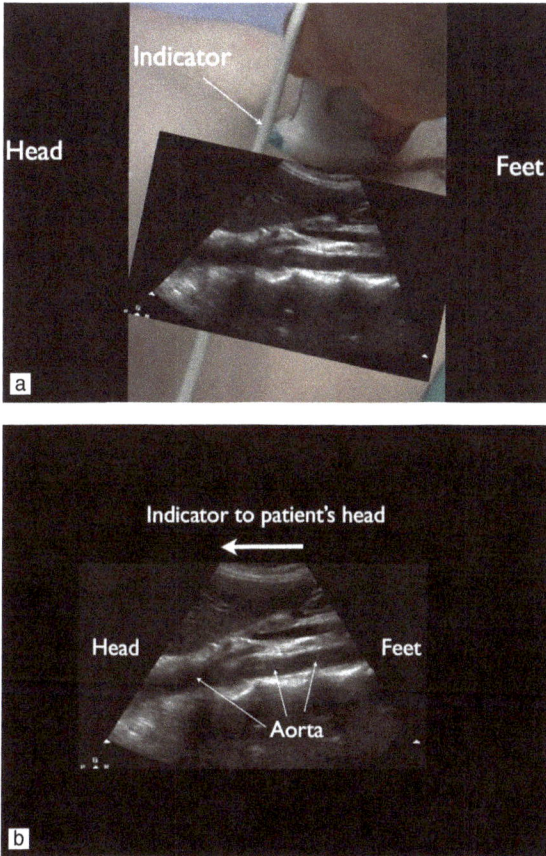

FIGURE 3-4 (*a*) Shows the probe placed on the anterior abdomen with the indicator toward the head. Again, this can be thought of as looking through the plane of the ultrasound with the indicator on your left as you stand on the right side of the patient. (*b*) Shows how the image would appear on the screen (with structures labeled).

Anterior structures are again at the top of the screen and posterior structures at the bottom. The patient's head (cephalad) is to screen left and feet (caudal) to screen right (Fig. 3-4*b*).

CORONAL PLANE

The coronal plane is obtained by placing the probe on the right or left flank with the indicator to the patient's head (Fig. 3-5*a* and *b*). If the probe is on the right, the top of the screen will be right and the bottom left (Fig. 3-5*c*); if the probe is on the left, the top of the screen will be left and the bottom right (Fig. 3-5*d*). In both the cases, the indicator should be directed to the patient's head and thus cephalad structures will be screen left and caudal structures will be screen right.

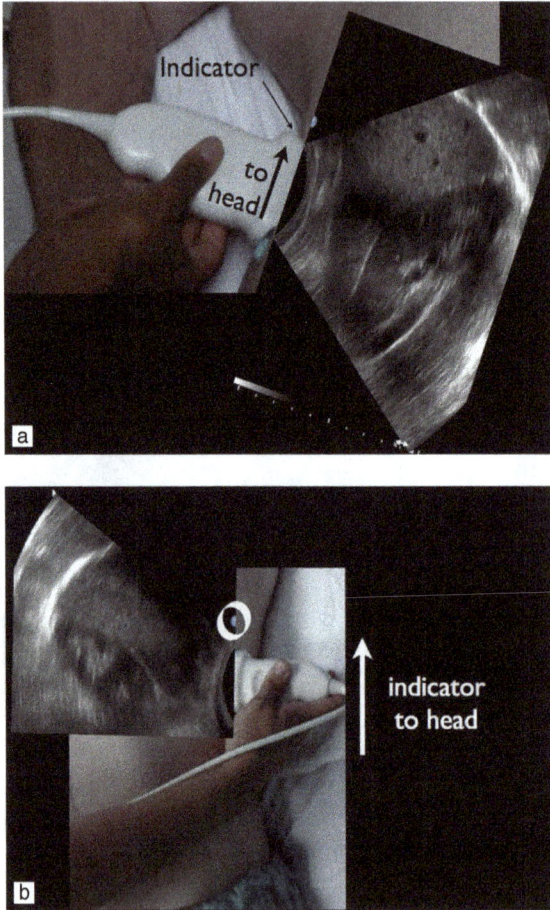

FIGURE 3-5 (*a*) Shows how the probe is placed for a coronal view of the right flank. (*b*) Shows probe placement for a coronal view of the left flank. In both the cases, the indicator is directed toward the head (left of screen as it is viewed). The resulting images are shown in (*c*) and (*d*). Note the similarities in the appearance, with the diaphragm to screen left in both images, but the top of the screen being either right or left flank.

This plane is most commonly used to image the hepatorenal and splenorenal spaces, including the kidneys and lower thoraces.

ADJUSTING THE PROBE—OBLIQUE PLANES

Once the probe is placed on the patient, the probe may be adjusted in several ways to direct the plane on the body and obtain an optimal image. In certain cases, the best images are obtained by combining these maneuvers to obtain an

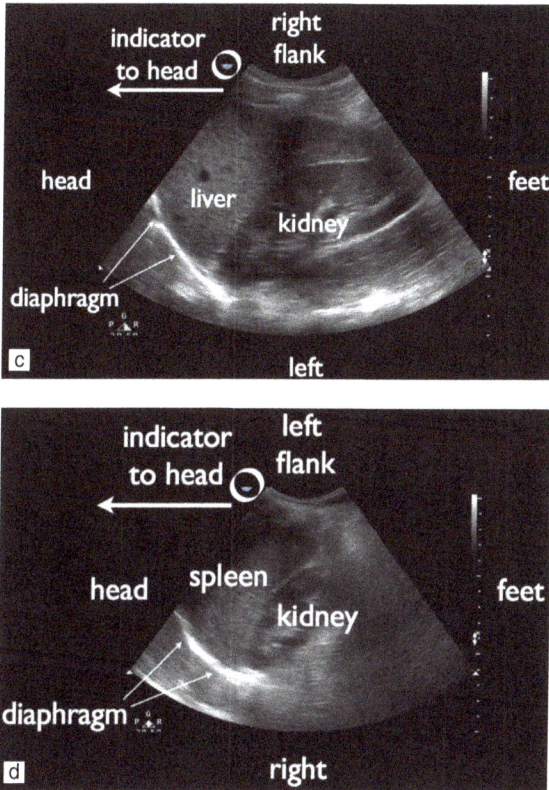

FIGURE 3-5 (*Continued*)

oblique plane. This is particularly true when trying to image between ribs and in cardiac imaging (echocardiography).

There are three basic maneuvers:

- *Angling or tilting the probe:* Keeping the probe in the same place, tilt the plane of the probe inferiorly, superiorly, or angle it to the left or right. When the plane of the image is fanned, it is angled orthogonally to the axis of the plane, fanning through the image (ie, tilted inferiorly/superiorly in the transverse plane or angled left/right in a sagittal plane). This is a very effective way to image entirely through a three-dimensional object using a two-dimensional plane. Once an image is obtained, the view should be maximized using this maneuver prior to sliding or moving the probe.
- *Sliding or moving the probe:* Keeping the same angle and indicator direction, move the probe to the left, right, up, or down. This also includes gentle but firm pressure to view deeper objects, particularly in the abdomen or pelvis.
- *Rotating or turning the probe:* Keeping the probe in the same place and the plane at the same angle to the body, rotate the indicator clockwise or counter-clockwise (ie, from a transverse to a sagittal orientation). Most rotation of the probe will take place in the 90° arc between sagittal and transverse.

SPECIAL CASE: INTERNAL JUGULAR CENTRAL LINE

When inserting an internal jugular line, the clinician is at the head of the bed, looking toward the patient's feet—opposite of looking from the feet upward.

In keeping with the orientation principle of looking through the plane of the ultrasound with the indicator on your left, the indicator should now be toward the patient's left, opposite of how it is normally oriented. This way, the movement of the needle will correspond to the correct side of the screen; that is, in a transverse plane (short-axis view of the vessel), moving the needle to the right will also move to the right on the screen.

SPECIAL CASE: CARDIAC IMAGING

Cardiac ultrasound (echocardiography or echo) presents particular orientation challenges. In addition to being a complex three-dimensional structure in an oblique orientation, the indicator-to-screen orientation convention adopted by cardiology is opposite of other ultrasound imaging—the indicator corresponds to the right side of the screen as it is viewed rather than the left.

Both conventions are internally consistent, but can create confusion when scanning the heart as part of an integrated examination (such as the FAST exam) or switching between general and cardiac imaging. This commonly occurs in emergency and critical care applications.

It is the recommendation of this book that in point-of-care ultrasound clinicians keep a consistent orientation throughout all examinations, including cardiac ultrasound.

It may be helpful to create a preset on the machine named "ED ECHO" or "CC ECHO" in which cardiac imaging is optimized, but the indicator corresponds to the left of the screen.

SPECIAL CASE: TRANSVAGINAL IMAGING

Sonography of the pelvis may be confusing, particularly when imaged from an intravaginal approach. Some sonographers of the pelvis invert rule 1 (described earlier), displaying the structures nearest the probe at the bottom of the screen. This makes intuitive sense for the pelvis, but inverts the screen relative to other examinations and will not be used in this book.

It is important to get oriented prior to beginning the exam. The indicator should correspond to the left side of the screen, and the thumb placed on the indicator prior to insertion.

The indicator (thumb) may then be directed superiorly for a sagittal plane, or to the patient's right for a coronal plane.

While the plane with the indicator to the patient's right is coronal (parallel to the bed in a supine patient), it is analogous to the transverse plane that is obtained in transabdominal imaging, with right-sided structures on the left of the screen.

KEY POINTS

- Orientation is essential to understanding ultrasound.
- The top of the screen shows structures closer to the probe, the bottom of the screen structures farther away.
- By convention, in general imaging the indicator on the probe corresponds to the left of the screen as it is viewed. An opposite convention is used in cardiology, but will not be used in this book.
- The indicator is generally directed toward the patient's head or patient's right. When imaging from the right side of the patient, this corresponds to the left of the sonographer, looking up from the feet for a transverse view or across the patient for a sagittal view.

- Certain types of imaging and procedures may require special considerations for orientation.

Additional Reading

Moore C. Current issues with emergency cardiac ultrasound probe and image conventions. *Acad Emerg Med.* 2008;15:278-284.

4 Probe Selection, Machine Controls, and Equipment

Joshua Markowitz

INTRODUCTION

A basic understanding of physics and orientation is essential for understanding ultrasound. However, when standing in front of the ultrasound machine, you need to make some concrete decisions about what probe to use, and what buttons to press, in order to obtain a good image—sometimes known as *knobology*.

This chapter covers the basics of probes and probe selection as well as the buttons found on typical ultrasound machines. While these controls are fairly standard, there are variations from machine to machine and the users will need to spend some time familiarizing themselves with the actual equipment they have—preferably before entering the patient's room. Some additional equipment and logistical concerns have also been discussed.

PROBE SELECTION

Probes are generally described by the size and shape of their face ("footprint"). Selecting the right probe for the situation is essential to get good images, although there may be times where more than one probe may be appropriate for a given exam. There are three basic types of probe used in emergency and critical care point-of-care ultrasound: linear, curvilinear, and phased array. Linear (also sometimes called vascular) probes are generally high frequency, better for imaging superficial structures and vessels, and are also often called a vascular probe. Curvilinear probes may have a wider footprint and lower frequency for transabdominal imaging, or in a tighter array (wider field of view) and higher frequency for endocavitary imaging. A phased array probe generates an image from an electronically steered beam in a close array, generating an image that comes from a point and is good for getting between ribs such as in cardiac ultrasound.

Both curvilinear and phased array probes generate sector or "pie-shaped" images, narrower in the near field and wider in the far field, while linear probes typically generate rectangular images on the screen.

STRAIGHT LINEAR ARRAY PROBE

The straight linear array probe (Fig. 4-1*a*) is designed for superficial imaging. The crystals are aligned in a linear fashion within a flat head and produce sound waves in a straight line. The image produced is rectangular in shape (Fig. 4-1*b*). This probe has higher frequencies (5–13 MHz), which provides better resolution and less penetration. Therefore, this probe is ideal for imaging superficial structures and in ultrasound-guided procedures.

- Vascular access (central and peripheral)
- Evaluate for deep venous thrombosis
- Skin and soft tissue for abscess, foreign body
- Musculoskeletal—tendons, bones, muscles

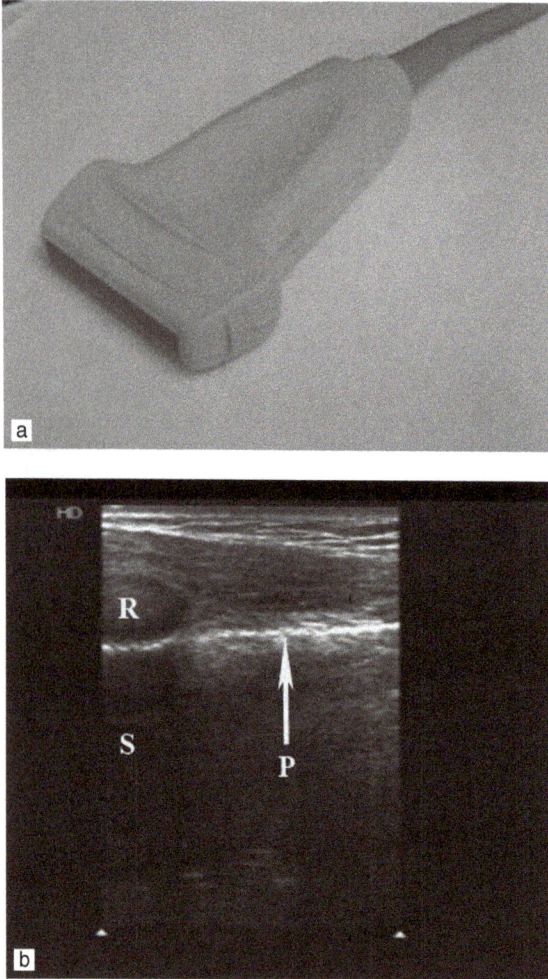

FIGURE 4-1 Straight linear array probe (*a*). Lung imaging using the straight linear array probe (*b*). Note the rectangular shape produced by the probe. R: rib, P: pleural line, S: rib shadow.

- Testicular
- Appendicitis in thin patients
- Evaluation of the pleural line for pneumothorax, interstitial fluid
- Ocular ultrasound
- Other procedures (arthrocentesis, paracentesis, thoracentesis, nerve blocks, etc)

CURVILINEAR ARRAY PROBE

The curvilinear array or convex probe (Fig. 4-2*a*) is used for scanning deeper structures. The crystals are aligned along a curved surface and cause a fanning

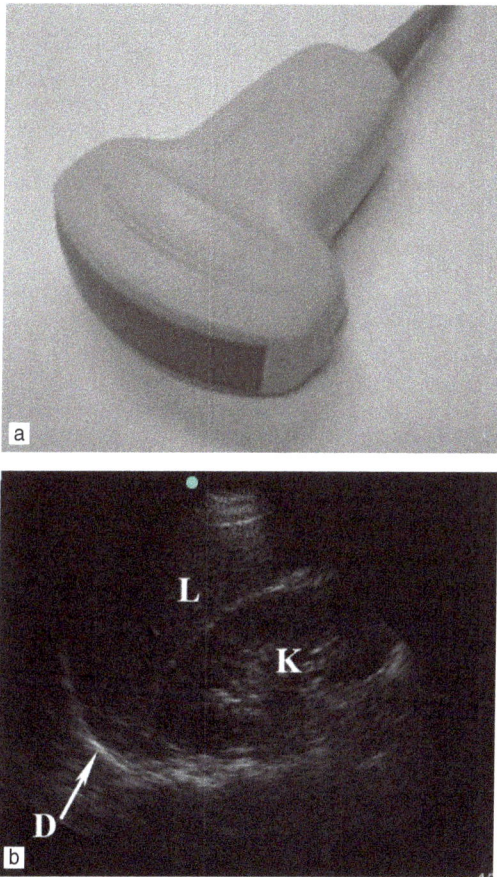

FIGURE 4-2 Curvilinear array probe (*a*). Right upper quadrant imaging using the curvilinear array probe (*b*). Note the sector shape produced by the probe. L: liver, K: kidney, D: diaphragm.

out of the beam, which results in a field of view that is wider than the probe's footprint. The image generated is sector shaped (Fig. 4-2*b*). These probes have frequencies ranging between 1 and 8 MHz, which allows for greater penetration, but less resolution. These probes are most often used in abdominal and pelvic applications. They are also useful in certain musculoskeletal evaluations or procedures when deeper anatomy needs to be imaged or in obese patients.

- Abdominal aorta
- Biliary/gallbladder/liver/pancreas
- Abdominal portion of FAST exam
- Kidney and bladder evaluation
- Transabdominal pelvic evaluation

ENDOCAVITARY PROBE

The endocavitary probe (Fig. 4-3a) also has a curved face, but a much higher frequency (8–13 MHz) than the curvilinear probe. This probe's elongated shape allows it to be inserted close to the anatomy being evaluated. The curved face creates a wide field of view of almost 180° and its high frequencies provide superior resolution (Fig. 4-3b). This probe is used most commonly for gynecological applications, but can also be used for intraoral evaluation of peritonsillar abscesses.

- Transvaginal ultrasound
- Intraoral (tonsillar) evaluation

PHASED ARRAY PROBE

Phased array probes (Fig. 4-4a) have crystals that are grouped closely together. The timing of the electrical pulses that are applied to the crystals varies and they are fired in an oscillating manner. The sound waves that are generated originate from a single point and fan outward, creating a sector-type image (Fig. 4-4b). This probe has a smaller and flatter footprint than the curvilinear one, which allows the user to maneuver more easily between the ribs and small spaces. These probes have frequencies between 2 and 8 MHz, but they usually operate at the

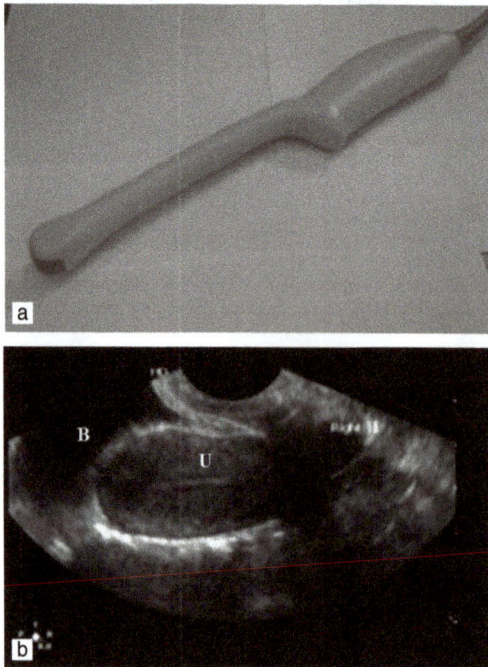

FIGURE 4-3 Endocavitary probe (a). Transvaginal ultrasound imaging using the endocavitary probe (b). This probe also produces a sector-shaped image, but a much wider field of view. U: uterus, B: bladder.

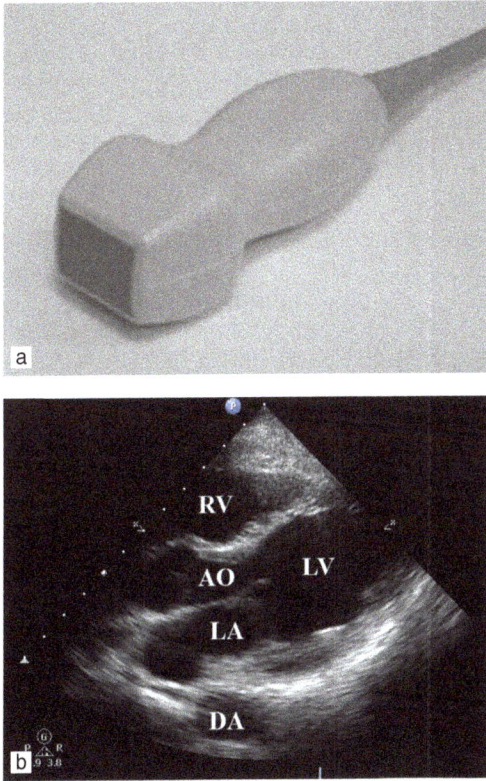

FIGURE 4-4 Phased array probe (*a*). Parasternal long-axis view using the phased array probe (*b*). Sound waves originate from a single point and fan outward, creating a sector-type image. RV: right ventricle, AO: aortic outflow, LV: left ventricle, LA: left atrium, DA: descending aorta.

higher end making them ideal for echocardiography. The phased array probe can also function at lower frequencies, which is useful for viewing the abdomen, pelvis, and for procedural guidance.

- Cardiac imaging
- Imaging between ribs in the flank or right upper quadrant
- May be used for transabdominal imaging if curvilinear probe not available

KNOBOLOGY

Although most ultrasound machines share some universal features, there is some variation in design between different manufacturers. It is important to become familiar with the particulars of the specific machine before scanning. The control panel of an ultrasound machine has various buttons and knobs that are used to adjust and record images.

ADJUSTING THE B-MODE IMAGE

B-mode, also known as basic, gray scale, or two-dimensional imaging, refers to the standard black and white image displayed on the ultrasound monitor.

Machine Presets   Most machines have settings that will adjust an image based on the anatomy being scanned. These presets are programmed to optimize images based on certain gain and power settings, focal zones, frame rates, and other settings. For instance, the echocardiography setting will automatically default to a higher frame rate in order to capture better cardiac imaging. The correct preset should be chosen before scanning is initiated.

Depth   The depth controls how much distance into the body the image displays in the far field. It is important to start out deep to not miss findings in the far field (Fig. 4-5a). Once the area of interest is identified and the far field has been surveyed, the depth can be decreased in order to focus in on the area of importance.

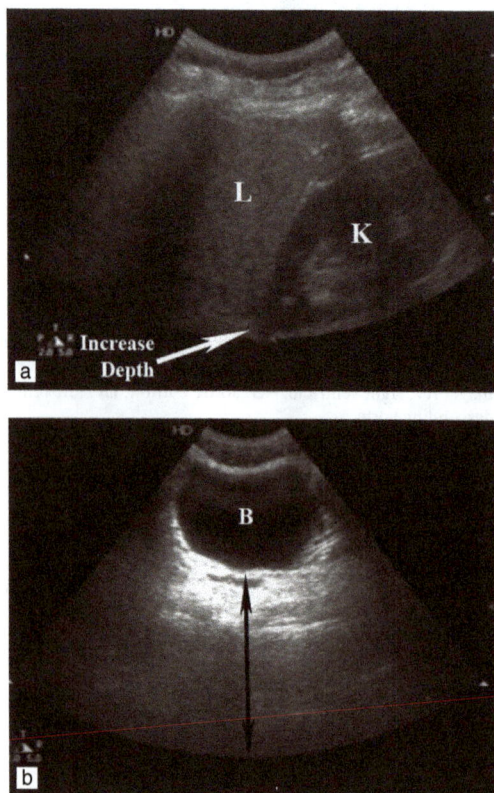

FIGURE 4-5 Right upper quadrant view illustrating too little depth (*a*). Note the liver (L) and kidney (K) appears shallow in this picture and are not fully imaged. Pelvic view (*b*) illustrating too much depth posterior to the bladder (B), and wasted space (black arrow).

When the depth is decreased, superficial structures will be magnified, which will improve resolution. Too much depth can be wasted space (Fig. 4-5b). Also, the larger the depth, the longer it takes for the machine to receive returning echoes, which can affect the quality and frame rate of the image display. Generally, depth should be adjusted to show the area of interest in the top two-thirds to three-quarters of the screen.

Gain   Gain adjusts how the machine "listens" for returning echoes. As the gain is increased, the strength of the returning echoes is amplified, which produces a brighter image. A decrease in gain will darken the image visualized on the monitor (Fig. 4-6a). Gain may be adjusted for the entire image (overall gain), or at depth, known as time-gain compensation (TGC). TGC may be set up as a column of sliding knobs, or may be adjusted with knobs for "near gain" and "far gain."

Appropriate gain is important for image quality, but too much gain can increase noise and wash out an image, making it appear too white on the screen (Fig. 4-6b). This error can obscure important findings, such as free fluid. This is a common mistake made by many novice sonographers, particularly behind a fluid-filled structure like the urinary bladder, where posterior acoustic enhancement brightens the image in the far field. Too little gain, particularly in an area in the middle of an image (such as when one of the TGC sliders is too far to the left) may be misinterpreted as an anechoic area of fluid. It is a good idea to check that the TGC sliders are in line prior to beginning the exam.

The gain on the machine should be set at a level that creates a clear image without appearing too bright or dark (see Fig. 4-2b). Many newer machines have an "image optimization" button that will automatically attempt to adjust gain appropriately throughout the image. It will help to darken the ambient lighting in the room to avoid using gain that is too high.

Zoom   The zoom function allows for the magnification of one area on the screen. The image appears larger, but the resolution of the magnified area does not change. Zoom generally works by selecting a square area, which can be sized and located on the screen by the user prior to zooming. This function is important when attempting to visualize a deep or small structure such as an intrauterine pregnancy or the common bile duct. The depth of an image should be optimized first before a sonographer zooms into a particular area.

Focus   The focus control optimizes the lateral resolution at a given depth. The best resolution of an object is found at the focal zone where the ultrasound beam is at its narrowest. Most monitors will display a small marking or arrow on the side of the screen indicating where the beam is focused. The focus is usually established for a specific application, but may need to be adjusted depending on what is being scanned. Focal zone is particularly important when trying to elicit shadowing from suspected gallstones.

Tissue Harmonics   When echoes are reflected off an object, they not only return at the fundamental frequency, but also at harmonic frequencies, which are at multiples of the fundamental frequency (2x, 4x, etc). These higher frequency waves experience less attenuation and less scatter and side-lobe artifact and may generate clearer images, particularly at the interface between fluid and tissue. Most machines will have a button called "tissue harmonic imaging" or THI, which will allow the transducer to use these harmonic frequencies. This imaging modality is used most commonly in cardiac applications.

Dynamic Range   Dynamic range refers to the range of echoes displayed and is expressed in decibels (dB). A high dynamic range is generally desirable as it will have a wider range of echo strength and will show more contrast, but the range may be reduced to minimize artifacts. Dynamic range is initially set based on the

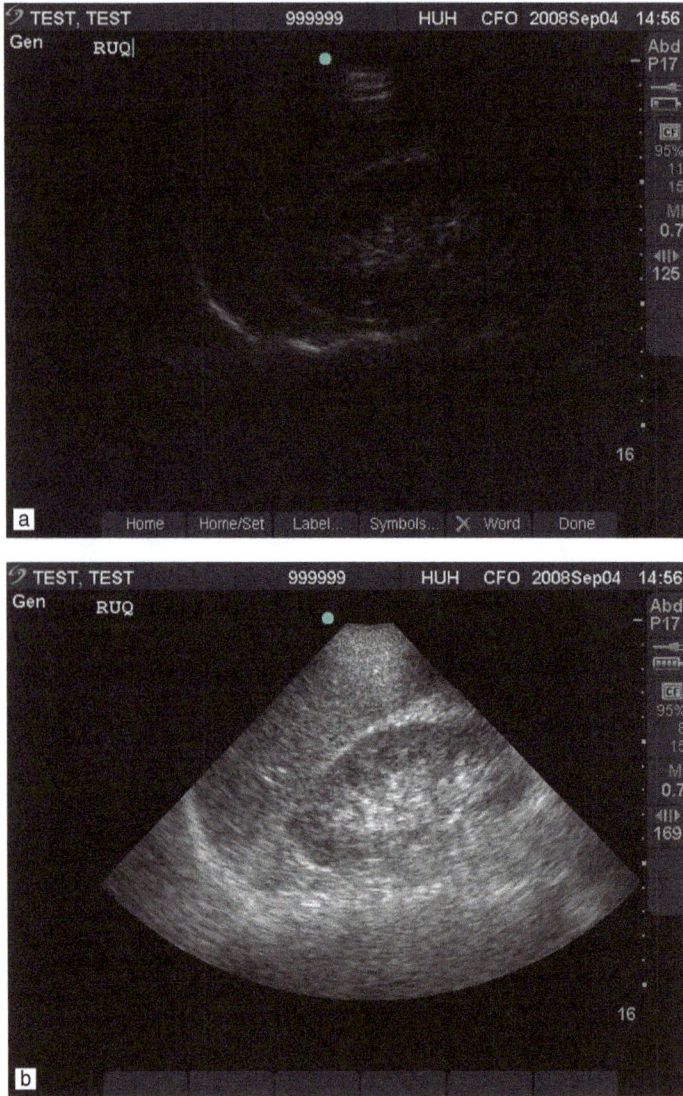

FIGURE 4-6 Right upper quadrant view demonstrating different gain levels. In (*a*) the image appears too dark and the gain needs to be increased. In (*b*) the image appears too bright and washed out which can obscure subtle findings such as free fluid. The overall gain needs to be decreased.

machine preset (ie, dynamic range for cardiac scanning is higher than abdominal scanning) but may be adjusted by the sonographer.

Frame Rate Dynamic or moving ultrasound is really just a series of still images displayed one after another to create motion. Frame rate refers to how many times per second a still image is displayed, measured in hertz (Hz) or frames per second. A high frame rate (30–40 Hz) is important for echocardiography, as the heart is moving quickly. A lower frame rate may allow for better individual images but may appear choppy. Frame rate is typically maximized for the depth and image aperture selected (ie, frame rate will increase as the field of view is decreased) but may be adjusted on the machine to a lower rate if desired.

OTHER MODES

M-Mode (Motion-Mode)   M-mode is used to visualize things that are physically moving. The motion occuring in a one-dimensional scan line is displayed on the vertical axis over time on the horizontal axis (Fig. 4-7). It is used in conjunction with B-mode scanning and should not be confused with Doppler imaging. The M-mode cursor (a single line) is placed over the moving object on the B-mode image, and the M-mode button is pressed. This mode is most commonly used in the evaluation of cardiac valves and fetal heart activity. It is also useful in measuring the respiratory variability of the inferior cava and in the evaluation of the lungs for pneumothorax.

Doppler   Doppler uses the frequency shift of sound waves to measure velocity, typically of blood (though tissue Doppler may measure myocardial motion). The most commonly used modes of Doppler are color-flow Doppler (CFD), power or angio Doppler, and spectral Doppler (pulsed [PW] and continuous wave [CW]).

Color Doppler displays the movement toward the probe as red and away from the probe as blue (Fig. 4-8). The use of color flow is helpful when attempting to identify a blood vessel and differentiate it from other surrounding structures.

Power (angio) Doppler measures flow within an object, but not direction. It also relies on a frequency shift to detect the presence of flow, but displays it in one color, usually orange, and therefore does not differentiate between flow toward or

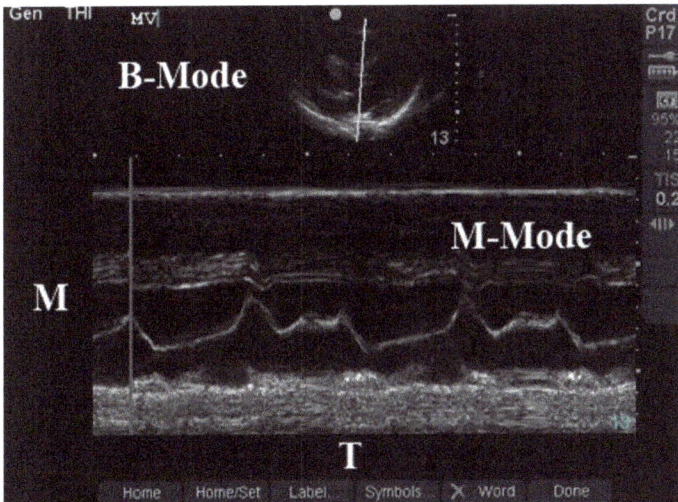

FIGURE 4-7 The use of M-mode in cardiac imaging. The upper image demonstrates a parasternal long-axis view of the heart seen in B-mode with the M-mode line placed across the mitral valve. The lower image depicts the motion (M) of the mitral valve on the Y-axis over time (T) on the X-axis.

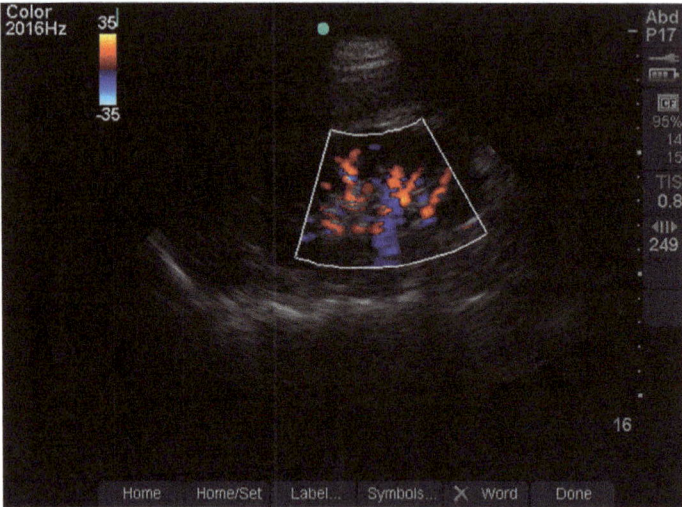

FIGURE 4-8 This image illustrates the use of color-flow Doppler in evaluating for renal blood flow. The red and blue colors represent flow toward and away from the probe, respectively.

away from the probe. It is more sensitive and less angle-dependent than color-flow Doppler at picking up low flow states, and therefore is useful for structures such as the testes. However, due to its sensitivity, small movements of the probe can create unwanted motion artifacts on the screen more commonly than other Doppler modes. Power Doppler is also useful in evaluating for urinary bladder jets in ruling out ureteral obstruction (Fig. 4-9).

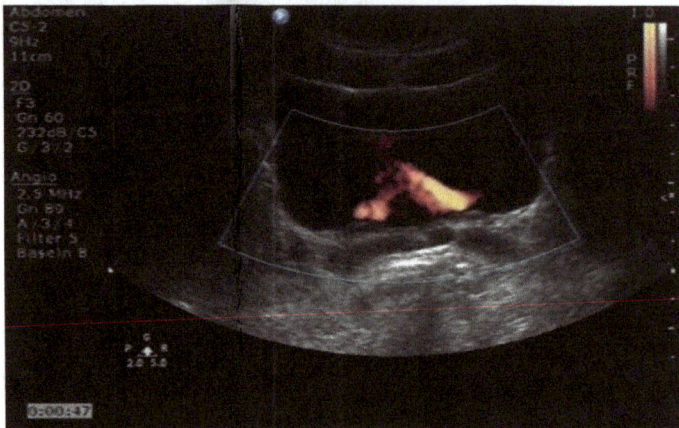

FIGURE 4-9 This image illustrates the use of power (angio) Doppler in evaluating for urinary jets within the bladder. Note the jets are present bilaterally, signifying no renal obstruction.

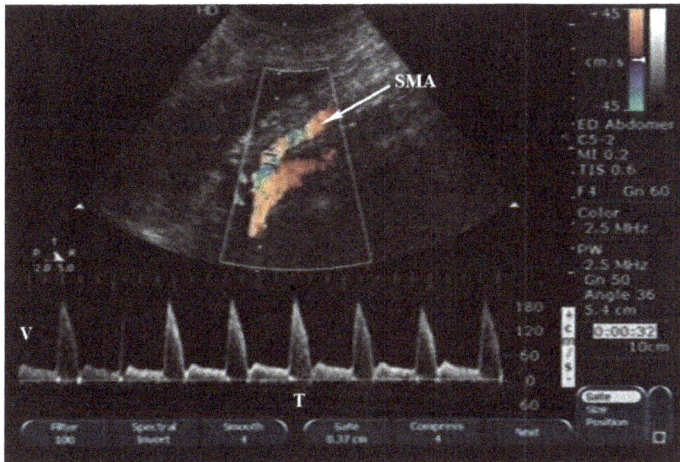

FIGURE 4-10 Pulsed-wave (PW) Doppler of the superior mesenteric artery (SMA). The image above shows the SMA with color flow. The PW Doppler calipers are placed over the blood flow within the lumen. The image below depicts the velocity (V) of blood flow on the Y-axis over time (T) on the X-axis.

Spectral Doppler displays velocity of flow on the X-axis against time on the Y-axis. Pulsed-wave Doppler (Fig. 4-10) allows the area of interest to be defined, but the maximum velocity is limited (the "Nyquist limit"). Continuous wave Doppler examines the maximum velocity along an entire scan line, and allows much higher velocity measurements, such as occurs in a stenotic valve (Fig. 4-11).

ADJUSTING THE DOPPLER IMAGE

Pulse Repetition Frequency (PRF) or Scale   Adjusting the PRF, sometimes labeled as the scale, adjusts the sensitivity of Doppler for flow velocity. A lower PRF will result in a lower scale, more sensitive for slower flows, but may cause more artifact (from "aliasing"). The scale will usually be displayed either on the side of the screen with corresponding colors for color and power Doppler, and along the Y-axis for spectral Doppler. On the lower end, the color Doppler scale may be as low as ~5 cm/s. Maximum scale for CW Doppler may go as high as 6 m/s.

Doppler Gain   Similar to the basic B-mode or two-dimensional image, gain may be adjusted for Doppler. Increasing Doppler gain will amplify returning signals, resulting in more color or a stronger spectral signal. As in B-mode imaging, too much gain will result in noise and artifact.

Baseline   Doppler can display flow either toward or away from the probe. Typically for color or spectral Doppler, the "zero" is in the center of the scale (or Y-axis). If you want to look only at the positive (or negative) flow, you can adjust the baseline up or down.

Wall Filter   Filter allows adjustment of the signal so that lower velocities up to a certain number will not be displayed, most applicable in color and power Doppler. A higher filter will reduce artifact but may limit visualization of lower flow.

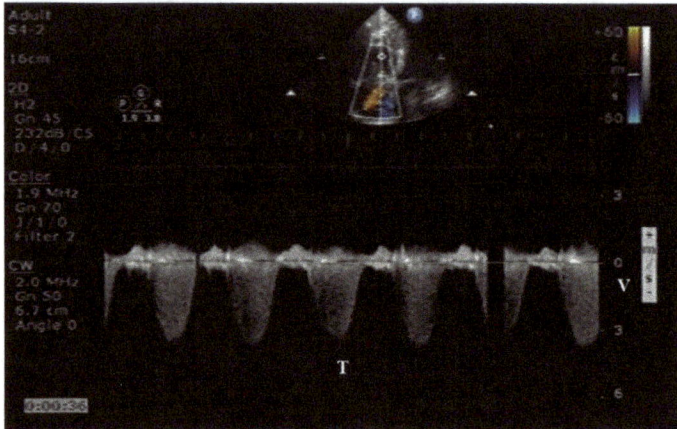

FIGURE 4-11 Continuous wave (CW) Doppler of the tricuspid valve (TV) in a patient with significant tricuspid regurgitation (TR). The image above shows an apical 4C view of the heart with the CW Doppler calipers placed over the TR flow. The image below depicts the velocity (V) of the TR on the Y-axis over time (T) on the X-axis. Note the wave produced by the Doppler tracing is depicted below the baseline, which represents blood flow away from the probe. CW Doppler is used in this situation due to its ability to pick up higher velocities, such as blood flow over turbulent valves.

MANIPULATING AND SAVING THE IMAGE

Freeze The freeze button is used to create a still image on the monitor. This control captures a single frame from a dynamic image. Most machines capture several seconds of still images, allowing selection of a previous image after pressing the freeze button. After freezing the scan, the sonographer can add text, make measurements or calculations, save or print the image.

Calculations Basic calculations, such as measurement, will be available on all images. Other calculations will be available based on the preset selected. For example, there are calculations specifically for fetal heart rate and gestational age in the obstetric setting. These calculations stress the importance of choosing the correct preset scanning mode.

Acquiring Images Images may be captured for archival or export. Still images may be saved by freezing the image and then hitting the appropriate button (acquire, save, store, etc). A moving image or "cineloop" is a dynamic clip, typically of several seconds, captured by acquiring the image without freezing it.

Most machines now store images digitally on an internal hard drive that can then be transferred to a more permanent storage location, either wirelessly or by connecting the machine to a storage device or ethernet cable. It is also possible to record much longer videos using an external videotape or DVD recorder if desired.

The industry standard for image storage is DICOM (Digital Imaging and Communications in Medicine), which may be an extra option on a machine. A picture archival communication system (PACS) uses DICOM and is the gold standard for image archival and review, although there are many ways to transfer, store, and print images.

OTHER EQUIPMENT

COUPLING MEDIA

Sound travels much better through liquid than air, and something to couple the face of the probe to the tissue is essential in obtaining an image. Most commonly gel is used, but standoff pads and water baths may also be used.

Gel is a water-based coupling medium that is more comfortable to the patient when warmed. It may be placed on the patient directly or on the probe first and should be used generously to avoid contact artifacts. Sterile gel should be used in contact with a mucous membrane or open wound, or in sterile procedures. Sterile gel is commonly available in packets (such as "Surgilube") or in sterile probe cover kits.

Superficial structures can be difficult to scan due to echoes that appear in the near field as a result of reverberation artifacts produced by the transducer. A standoff pad can be placed in between the probe and the skin, which places the structure of interest at the focal zone. This improves the lateral resolution and image quality. These are commercially available or the songrapher can create one using a gel pad or intravenous (IV) fluid bag.

A water bath can also be used in the scanning of superficial structures in place of gel. The patient's body part, usually the hand or foot, is placed inside a basin of water. The probe is then placed on top of the water surface and the area of interest is scanned from above. The water bath improves the resolution of the image and is also useful in avoiding direct contact of the probe with the skin surface, therefore improving patient comfort.

PROBE COVERS

Probe covers or sheaths protect probes from contamination and the patient from potential infection. Sterile probe covers are recommended for central line access, joint aspiration, and other procedures that have infection risks. Probe covers are also used for procedures that are not sterile, but involve exposure to mucous membranes, such as endovaginal or peritonsillar abscess evaluation. In these cases, a nonlatex condom should be used. Other nonsterile procedures that may benefit from probe covers include peripheral IV access and incision and drainage of an abscess. The use of a Tegaderm (or other cover such as a glove) can help protect the probe from contamination in these situations. Gel is required on both the inside and outside of any cover.

PROBE CLEANING

Probes and probe cords should be cleaned both before and after use. Any visible contamination can be removed by rinsing the probe using water and soap. Commercially available sprays are appropriate for basic disinfection. High-level disinfection (HLD) is a more thorough cleaning method that is often recommended for cleaning endocavitary probes after use, although the necessity of this level of cleaning when appropriate cleaning and probe covers are used is debated. HLD involves the use of a prolong soak in chemicals (eg, Cidex) requiring a designated area with ventilation/hoods.

PERIPHERAL INTRAVENOUS CATHETERS

Typical IV catheters for peripheral access are 1¼ in in length, and may infiltrate when used in deeper vessels identified by ultrasound. It is recommended that peripheral IVs be at least 1¾ in to over 2 in for ultrasound-guided peripheral access.

HAND TOWELS

Small cloth towels, kept with the machine, are helpful in cleaning gel off of patients, as well as probes and the machine.

Additional Reading

Goldberg RL, Smith SW, Mottley JG, Ferrara KW. Ultrasound. In: Bronzino JD, ed. *The Biomedical Engineering Handbook.* Florida, FL: CRC Press; 2006: chap. 65,1-23.

Hecht C, Wilkins J. Physics and image artifacts. In: Ma OJ, Mateer JR, Blaivas M, eds. *Emergency Ultrasound.* New York, NY: McGraw-Hill Companies, Inc; 2008:49-63.

Roberts PJA, Williams J. Imaging with ultrasound. In: Roberts PJA, Williams J, eds. *Farr's Physics for Medical Imag.* 2nd ed. London: W.B. Saunders Company; 2007.

Rose JS, Bair AE. Fundamentals of ultrasound. In: Cosby KS, Kendall JL, eds. *Practical Guide to Emergency Ultrasound.* Philadelphia, PA: Lippincott Williams & Wilkins; 2006:27-41.

Scruggs W, Fox C. Equipment. In: Ma OJ, Mateer JR, Blaivas M, eds. *Emergency Ultrasound.* New York, NY: McGraw-Hill Companies, Inc; 2008:15-47.

5 Ultrasound of the Aorta

Kristin Carmody and Christopher L. Moore

BACKGROUND AND INDICATIONS FOR EXAMINATION

Abdominal aortic aneurysm (AAA) has an adult incidence of 2%–4%, with approximately 10% of these cases occurring in people over the age of 65. The prevalence increases with risk factors for vascular disease, particularly smoking and hypertension. AAA has a male to female preponderance of 8:1 and may be present in as many as 10% of elderly male patients with at least one risk factor.

The rapid and accurate diagnosis of AAA at the bedside is important in decreasing the morbidity and mortality that may be associated with this disease entity. Bedside ultrasound has been shown to be a quick and reliable method to diagnose AAA in the critical care setting. Sensitivity and specificity of ultrasound are high when the aorta is visualized completely.

AAA rupture is among the top leading causes of death in the United States. When aneurysms rupture, they are highly lethal, with a mortality rate exceeding 50%. Ultrasound is not sensitive for rupture, as most ruptures occur into the retroperitoneum, which is a difficult area to visualize with ultrasound. In a stable patient, computed tomography (CT) still represents the best method for defining the extent of the aneurysm and the presence of leak or rupture. Although ultrasound does not detect rupture well, it has been shown to expedite care in patients who are hemodynamically unstable. In hemodynamically unstable symptomatic patients (abdominal pain, flank pain, back pain), the presence of an aneurysm is likely to mean leak or rupture and should prompt immediate preparation for operative intervention.

Ultrasound may also visualize aortic dissection. While ultrasound should not be used to rule out dissection (sensitivity is not good), specificity is high when a flap or false lumen is visualized. In particular, thoracic aneurysm and dissection are emergent, deadly diseases that may also be seen using bedside cardiac ultrasound, and may be a cause of pericardial effusion or tamponade. Contrast-enhanced CT, magnetic resonance imaging (MRI), and transesophageal echocardiography (TEE) remain the modalities of choice for thoracic aortic pathology.

Bedside ultrasound evaluation of the abdominal aorta should be performed in:

- The patient with undifferentiated hypotension, shock, or syncope
- The elderly patient with undifferentiated abdominal, flank, or back pain

PROBE SELECTION AND TECHNICAL CONSIDERATIONS

CURVILINEAR PROBE WITH A FREQUENCY OF 3.5–5.0 MHz

Lower frequencies, which provide better penetration, may be helpful in obese patients or when significant bowel gas is present.

TISSUE HARMONIC IMAGING

Tissue harmonics may help to sharpen the image and improve visualization of the aorta and associated deep vessels.

FOCAL ZONE

The focal zone should be adjusted and placed at the depth of the aorta. This improves the lateral resolution of the image.

COLOR-FLOW DOPPLER

Color-flow Doppler detects blood flow and therefore is helpful in identifying a blood vessel and distinguishing it from other artifacts that may be present in the abdomen. It is important to angle the probe in order to avoid having the beam perpendicular to the blood flow, which will erroneously appear on the screen as a lack of color. In addition, by decreasing the pulse repetition frequency (PRF, also known as scale) or increasing the color gain may help to detect color flow.

TIME-GAIN COMPENSATION

Time-gain compensation (TGC) can be adjusted in order to increase the far gain of the image. This produces an enhanced brighter signal returning from the far field and a resultant clearer image. Adjustment of this control may be useful in obese patients with difficult anatomy.

DEPTH

It is important to start with adequate depth, but it should be decreased appropriately once the landmarks are identified so that the structures of interest make up approximately three-fourths of the screen. An image that is either too deep or too shallow can be disorienting.

THORACIC AORTIC IMAGING

A cardiac probe, ideally a phased array with tissue harmonic imaging, should be used for all thoracic imaging.

NORMAL ULTRASOUND ANATOMY

THORACIC AORTA

The aorta originates at the left ventricular outflow tract (LVOT), distal to the aortic valve. The aortic root and descending thoracic aorta are usually best seen and measured with transthoracic echocardiography on a parasternal long-axis view of the heart. The descending aorta can be seen behind the heart on this view, which is illustrated in the echo chapter of this book. In some patients, the aortic arch can be seen using a suprasternal notch view. The sonographer can follow the carotid arteries down to their union with the brachiocephalic artery and the aortic arch. This view is challenging due to the presence of venous structures, as well as the lungs and trachea.

ABDOMINAL AORTA

The aorta enters the diaphragm through a hiatus at T12 to become the abdominal aorta. The vessel lies just anterior to the spine and follows its curvature anteriorly as it travels distally.

Landmarks   In a transverse view, the probe indicator should be pointed to the patient's right side. In this orientation, the vertebral body of the spine should be seen as a bright, curving hyperechoic structure that shadows distally. This is called the spine sign and serves as one of the landmarks for identifying the abdominal aorta. The normal aorta is circular in cross section and is seen anterior to the spine, on the right side of the screen (patient's left). The second important landmark is the inferior vena cava (IVC), which can also be visualized in this view, on the left side of the screen adjacent to the aorta, in a circular or teardrop conformation. The spine and IVC are thus the primary landmarks used to correctly identify the abdominal aorta, and should be routinely identified in order to avoid common pitfalls (Fig. 5-1).

Proximal Aorta   The first visible branch of the abdominal aorta is the celiac trunk. It exits anteriorly and branches into the splenic artery (coursing toward the right side of the screen), the common hepatic artery (coursing toward the left side of the screen), and the left gastric artery (not usually visualized on ultrasound). In a transverse orientation, the celiac and its two branches form the "seagull sign," with the splenic and common hepatic artery forming the wings (Fig. 5-2).

The next branch seen is the superior mesenteric artery (SMA), which branches anteriorly off the proximal aorta distal to the celiac trunk. In a transverse view, the SMA is seen as a circle with some surrounding hyperechoic fatty tissue with an appearance similar to a "mantle clock" (Fig. 5-3). The celiac trunk and SMA can also be seen in a longitudinal or sagittal view when the probe is rotated clockwise 90° with the indicator pointing cephalad (Fig. 5-4).

Also at this level, both the left renal and splenic vein can often be visualized. The left renal vein can be seen passing anterior to the aorta, between the aorta and the SMA to drain into the IVC. The splenic vein can be seen passing anterior to the SMA draining into the portal vein, which appears as a circular structure just anterior to the IVC (Fig. 5-5).

The renal arteries are more difficult to image, but can be seen at about the same level or slightly distal to the SMA. In a transverse view, they may be visualized exiting the aorta to the left or right of the screen. The right renal artery

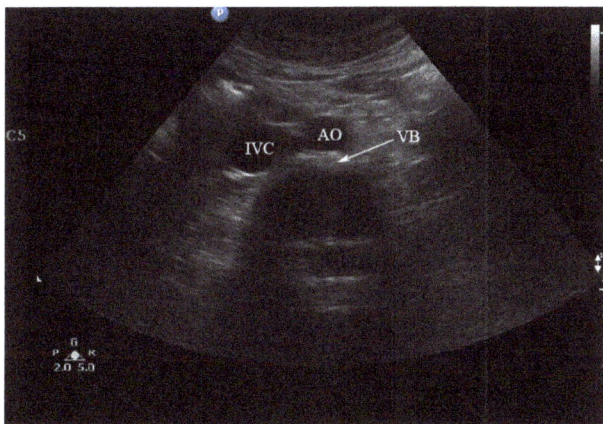

FIGURE 5-1   Transverse view of the aorta with landmarks. AO: aorta, IVC: inferior vena cava, VB: vertebral body.

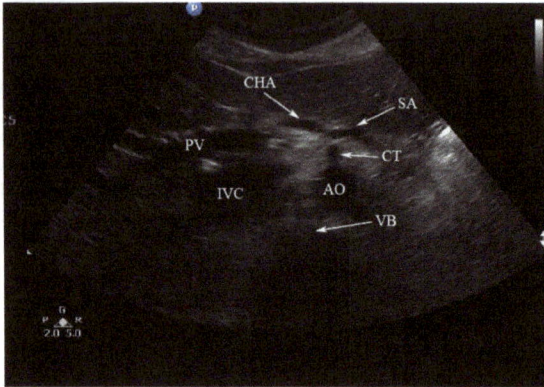

FIGURE 5-2 Proximal transverse aorta with celiac trunk and its branches (seagull sign). AO: aorta, IVC: inferior vena cava, PV: portal vein, CT: celiac trunk, SA: splenic artery, CHA: common hepatic artery , VB: vertebral body.

typically passes posterior to the IVC and may often be seen as a small circle that lies posterior to the IVC in a sagittal plane.

Mid-Aorta   Once the proximal aorta is appropriately imaged, the probe should be angled or moved more caudally until the above vessels disappear. At the level of the mid-aorta, usually only the spine, aorta, and IVC are visualized. Once again, the aorta should be imaged in both transverse and longitudinal orientations at this level.

Distal Aorta   The distal aorta bifurcates into the common iliac arteries at L4, approximately at the level of the umbilicus. The aorta is rarely visualized by placing the probe below this level. The iliacs will be visualized on the right side of the screen and the IVC will remain on the left, both still anterior to the vertebral bodies.

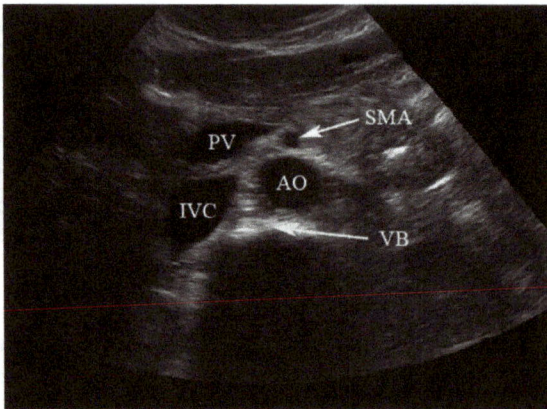

FIGURE 5-3 Proximal transverse view of aorta at the level of the superior mesenteric artery. AO: aorta, IVC: inferior vena cava, VB: vertebral body, SMA: superior mesenteric artery, PV: portal vein.

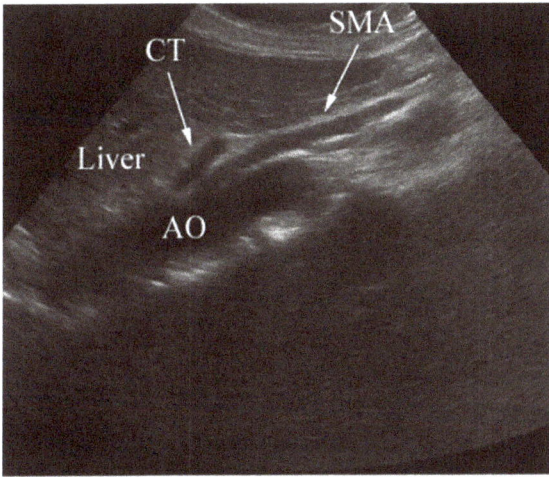

FIGURE 5-4 Proximal longitudinal (sagittal) view of aorta with branches. AO: aorta, SMA: superior mesenteric artery, CT: celiac trunk.

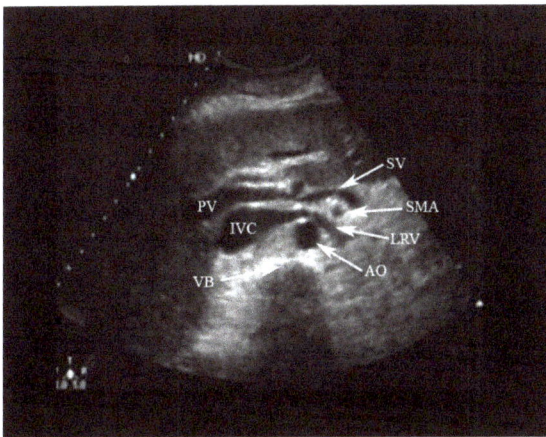

FIGURE 5-5 Transverse aorta at the level of the left renal and splenic veins. VB: vertebral body, IVC: inferior vena cava, AO: aorta, LRV: left renal vein, SMA: superior mesenteric artery, SV: splenic vein, PV: portal vein.

IMAGING TIPS AND PROTOCOL

TRANSVERSE VIEW

Imaging should begin with a proximal transverse view obtained by placing the probe on the patient's abdomen just below the xiphoid process, with the indicator pointing toward the patient's right (Fig. 5-6).

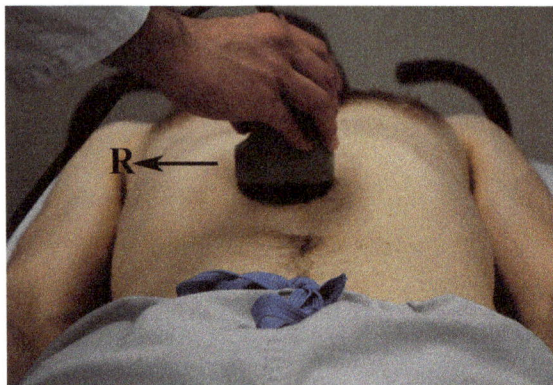

FIGURE 5-6 Position of probe on patient's abdomen just below the xiphoid process. The indicator is pointing toward the patient's right and the image obtained will be in a transverse view.

THE DIFFICULT PATIENT

Obesity typically presents the biggest challenge. Gentle, but persistent pressure with the probe, forcing bowel gas to the side, is probably the most important factor in obtaining an image. In some patients, the aorta may be best visualized from a coronal view through the right flank.

IDENTIFY LANDMARKS

Once below the xiphoid process, press firmly in order to displace any bowel gas that is obscuring adequate views. The probe should then be tilted in both cephalad and caudal directions until the landmarks (spine, IVC) come into view (see Fig. 5-1). If the spine and IVC are not easily visualized, the probe should be slid slowly in a caudal direction, pressing and rocking along the way, until an adequate image is obtained or the umbilicus is reached.

LONGITUDINAL (SAGITTAL) VIEW

Once the aorta and landmarks have been identified in a transverse plane, rotate the probe slowly into a sagittal (longitudinal) plane, keeping the aorta in view. This is accomplished by rotating the probe 90° in a clockwise fashion until the indicator is pointing toward the patient's head. It is important to correctly identify the aorta relative to the IVC in the transverse plane and keep it in view as the probe is rotated to assure that the IVC is not mistaken for the aorta in the long axis.

If the aorta is not well visualized anteriorly, patient positioning may help. If possible, the patient can turn on their left side into a decubitus position, which may help move bowel gas out of the way. It also may be possible to visualize the aorta in a coronal plane, with the probe placed in the right flank, similar to a FAST exam (Fig. 5-7).

THORACIC AORTA

Imaging of the thoracic aorta includes the parasternal long-axis view, detailed in the echo chapter of this book. The suprasternal notch view is challenging in many patients: a microconvex or phased array probe should be placed above the

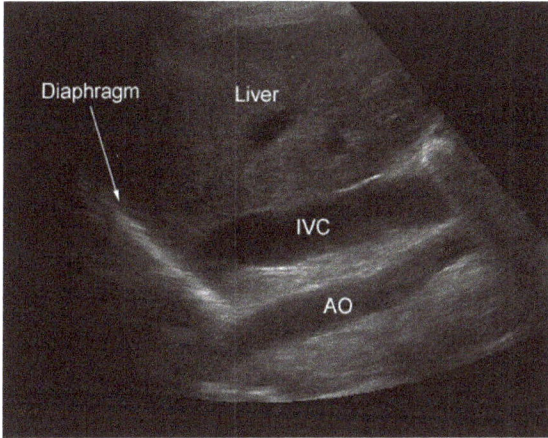

FIGURE 5-7 Coronal view of aorta and inferior vena cava. IVC: inferior vena cava, AO: aorta.

sternum with the probe indicator to the patient's right. The right common carotid artery should be followed down into the aortic arch, which should be examined for dilatation or dissection. One should be careful not to mistake the border between the superior vena cava and the aortic arch for dissection.

IMAGING PROTOCOL

Imaging of the abdominal aorta should ideally include complete visualization and measurement in two planes from the celiac axis down to the iliac bifurcation.

Measurements should be obtained in both the transverse and sagittal planes at the area of maximal diameter. The measurements should be obtained perpendicular to the axis of the aorta, extending from outside wall to outside wall, making sure that the entire aorta (not just the lumen) is adequately measured. Inclusion of the walls in the measurement ensures that intraluminal clots are identified and not mistaken as the border of the wall, which would result in an underestimation of the vessel size. If there is lower abdominal pain or suspicion of pathology, the iliac arteries should be visualized as well for evidence of aneurysm.

In some patients the exam may be limited, and in a small minority the abdominal aorta may not be visualized at all. In these cases, the exam should be documented as such and if clinical suspicion warrants, a CT scan should be obtained.

If indicated, visualization of the thoracic aorta should start with the parasternal long-axis view, with measurement of the aortic root and visualization of the descending thoracic aorta and pericardium. If available, a suprasternal notch view may visualize the arch. If transthoracic ultrasound does not show an aneurysm or dissection and one is suspected, more definitive imaging should be obtained such as TEE, MRI, or CT scan.

PATHOLOGIC ULTRASOUND FINDINGS

ABDOMINAL AORTIC ANEURYSM

An aneurysm is present if the aorta measures more than 3.0 cm, or is greater than 1.5 times the diameter of the proximal aorta. As described in the imaging protocol earlier, the measurement of an aneurysm should be taken in two planes (transverse and sagittal) at the point of maximal diameter, and should include the entire aorta (Fig. 5-8).

There are two basic types of aneurysms: fusiform and saccular. The vast majority of abdominal aneurysms are fusiform, and cause a portion of the aorta to dilate circumferentially. Fusiform aneurysms are atherosclerotic in nature and typically involve distal portions of the aorta. Saccular aneurysms are not as common, but should be kept in mind, as an isolated transverse view of the aorta may miss these types of aneurysms. This emphasizes the importance of visualizing the aorta in two planes.

The majority of aneurysms (>90%) involve the infrarenal aorta, although as many as 40% may involve the suprarenal aorta as well. Identification of the renal arteries allows classification into infra- or suprarenal aneurysm, which can have an impact on the surgical approach used. In some patients it may be difficult to visualize the renal arteries or proximal aorta, and therefore, CT scan is a more reliable way to classify aneurysm type and location. Isolated suprarenal aneurysms are unusual, but do occur, and thus, imaging of the abdominal aorta should always involve both the proximal and distal portions.

The abdominal aorta should be imaged down to the bifurcation, and if the iliacs are visible they should be measured as well. An iliac aneurysm is present if the diameter of either exceeds 1.5 cm.

Aortic aneurysms expand at a rate of approximately 0.3–0.4 cm/y, and this expansion accelerates as the aorta gets larger. Once the aortic diameter reaches 5.0 cm, the risk of rupture is about 5%/year, and increases with increasing diameter, prompting repair at this size if possible.

RUPTURED AAA

When an aneurysm ruptures, it is typically retroperitoneal. A leaking aneurysm may intermittently or slowly bleed into the retroperitoneum, or may rupture dramatically. Overall mortality exceeds 50% with rupture or leak, though it may be

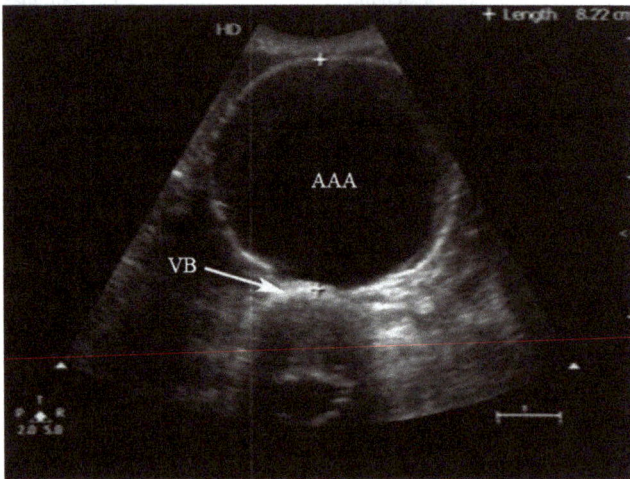

FIGURE 5-8 Transverse view of a fusiform abdominal aortic aneurysm. AAA: abdominal aortic aneurysm, VB: vertebral body.

improved with prompt recognition and operative intervention. Ultrasound is not reliable for detecting AAA rupture. When seen, visualization of the retroperitoneum may show heterogeneous clot around the kidney (more typically on the left) when bleeding is extensive. Occasionally aneurysms may rupture into the peritoneal cavity, with the ultrasound showing free intraperitoneal fluid, which is almost invariably fatal.

THORACIC AORTIC ANEURYSM

Thoracic aortic aneurysm is present if the diameter exceeds 4 cm. This diameter is measured at the aortic root or descending aorta visualized on the parasternal long-axis view, or at the arch using a suprasternal notch view (Fig. 5-9).

AORTIC DISSECTION

Aortic dissection may occur with or independently of an aneurysm. Dissections are not commonly seen on ultrasound, but when they are visualized they appear as a flap across the lumen that moves with aortic blood flow. Color-flow Doppler imaging may be used to differentiate the true from the false lumen. Ultrasound is not sensitive for dissection, but is specific if clearly visualized; however, the edge of a clot in an aneurysm may sometimes appear to be a dissection flap. The use of color-flow Doppler and the lack of movement of the flap help to distinguish clot from dissection (Figs. 5-10 and 5-11).

COMMON PITFALLS

PATIENT HABITUS AND BOWEL GAS

Obesity and bowel gas are the primary challenges a sonographer faces in attempting to visualize the abdominal aorta. Inadequate visualization can occur in up to 5% of patients due to these two factors. The impedance of obesity may be overcome by choosing the correct transducer and frequency settings (a curvilinear probe with lower frequency and better penetration) and by using tissue harmonics

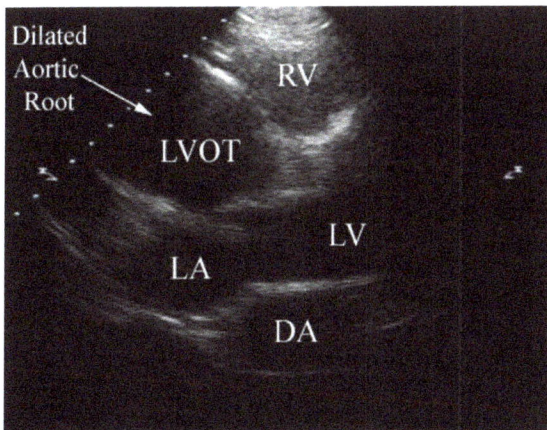

FIGURE 5-9 Parasternal long-axis cardiac view showing a thoracic aortic aneurysm. LVOT: left ventricular outflow tract, RV: right ventricle, LA: left atrium, LV: left ventricle, DA: descending aorta.

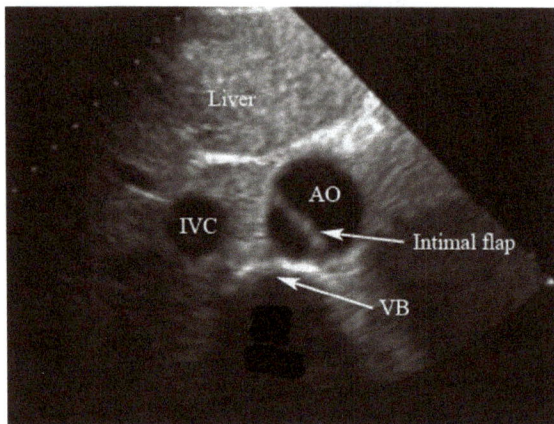

FIGURE 5-10 Transverse view of abdominal aortic dissection with flap. AO: aorta, IVC: inferior vena cava, VB: vertebral body.

to sharpen the image. Bowel gas can be pushed aside by applying firm pressure with the probe or by turning the patient into the left lateral decubitus position.

NOT PROPERLY IDENTIFYING THE AORTA

The aorta may be misidentified if landmarks are not clearly seen. These will be most clearly visualized in the transverse view, with adequate depth. The vertebral body and IVC should be visualized in the transverse plane, and depth adjusted so that the image takes up approximately three-fourths of the screen.

The IVC may be mistaken for the aorta. This may result in missing an aneurysm if the IVC is measured instead of the aorta. This can be avoided by visualizing the aorta relative to the IVC in a transverse view, and then rotating to a

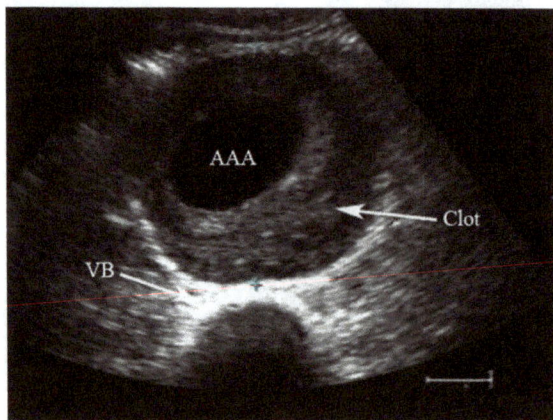

FIGURE 5-11 Transverse view of abdominal aortic aneurysm with large clot. AAA: abdominal aortic aneurysm, VB: vertebral body.

sagittal view, keeping the aorta in view. The IVC is more thin-walled than the aorta, is joined by the hepatic veins, and drains into the right atrium. The IVC does exhibit pulsations, and even though the wavy venous pulsations and respiratory variability of the IVC are different from the crisp arterial pulsations of the aorta, the presence of pulsations alone does not identify the aorta or rule out the IVC. In thinner patients, the IVC may be compressed by pressure with the probe.

INCORRECT MEASUREMENTS

The size of the aorta may be underestimated if both lumen and wall are not included. As mentioned earlier, the aorta should be measured from the outside wall to the opposite outside wall in a perpendicular fashion, including atherosclerosis or clot. This generous measurement increases sensitivity and makes missing AAA less likely. The size of the aorta may be overestimated if a measurement is taken in an oblique plane, not perpendicular to the axis of the vessel.

MISTAKING FLUID-FILLED STRUCTURES FOR AORTA

Other fluid-filled structures may be mistaken for a normal or aneurysmal aorta. These include the urinary bladder, the gallbladder, and cysts or pseudocysts of the kidney, liver or pancreas. This can be more of a problem if these fluid-filled structures are pathologic, large, painful, or abnormally placed. This pitfall can be avoided by using landmarks and by following a fluid-filled structure along its course. Color-flow Doppler can also help in this differentiation as the aorta will pick up color flow and these other fluid-filled structures will not.

OTHERS

Other potential pitfalls include mistaking the IVC or a hypoechoic aortic wall for aortic leak; mistaking aortic aneurysm with clot for dissection; and missing a suprarenal, iliac, or saccular aneurysm because of incomplete visualization of the aorta. These can be avoided by completely imaging the aorta and iliacs in two planes, and obtaining CT imaging if there is incomplete visualization and clinical suspicion.

INTEGRATION OF BEDSIDE AORTIC ULTRASOUND INTO CLINICAL CARE

Bedside ultrasound of the aorta should be an integrated part of the examination for patients who present with unexplained hypotension. It also should be used in the elderly and other patients with risk factors for AAA who present with abdominal, back, or flank pain. Ultrasound may be performed within minutes of arrival, in conjunction with other resuscitation measures. Ultrasound is very reliable in this situation for both ruling in and ruling out an aneurysm, allowing either expedient consultation and disposition or prompting a search for other causes of the symptoms.

When an aneurysm is identified on a bedside ultrasound in a patient who is asymptomatic or stable, definitive studies need to be performed to better delineate the extent of the aortic pathology, typically using contrast-enhanced CT scan. These patients should receive a confirmatory study, whether it be a CT scan, MRI, aortography, or TEE. If ultrasound shows an aneurysm in a symptomatic patient, particularly if signs of shock are apparent, definitive operative care should not be delayed for these other studies. An algorithm for both the stable and unstable patient summarizing the previously discussed clinical scenarios is shown in Fig. 5-12.

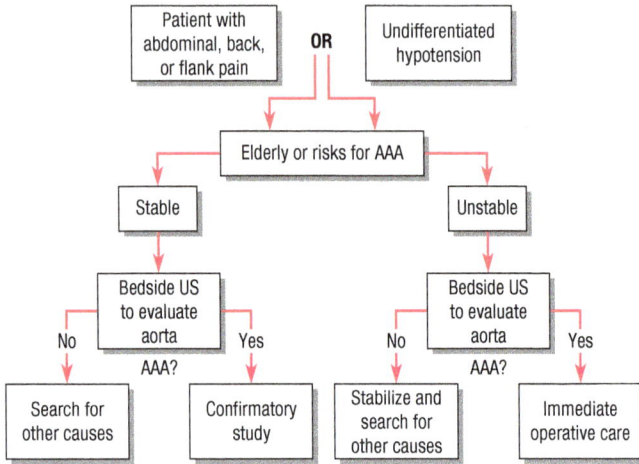

FIGURE 5-12 Algorithm for stable and unstable patients presenting with abdominal, back, or flank pain or those who present with undifferentiated hypotension.

Additional Reading

Costantino TG, Bruno EC, Handley N, et al. Accuracy of emergency medicine ultrasound in the evaluation of abdominal aortic aneurysm. *J Emerg Med.* 2005;29(4):455-460.

Fojtik J, Costantino TG, Dean AJ. The diagnosis of aortic dissection by emergency medicine. *J Emerg Med.* 2007;32(2):191-196.

Kuhn M, Bonnin RL, Davey MJ, et al. Emergency department ultrasound scanning for abdominal aortic aneurysm: accessible, accurate, and advantageous. *Ann of Emerg Med.* 2000;36(3):219-223.

Lederle FA, Johnson GR, Wilson SE, et al. Prevalence and associations of abdominal aortic aneurysm detected through screening. *Ann of Intern Med.* 1997;126(6):441-449.

Tayal V, Graf CD, Gibbs MA. Prospective study of accuracy and outcome of emergency ultrasound for abdominal aortic aneurysm over two years. *Acad Emerg.* 2003;10(8):867-887.

6 Echocardiography

Christopher L. Moore

BACKGROUND AND INDICATIONS FOR EXAMINATION

Ultrasound of the heart, or echocardiography (echo), is among the most challenging sonographic examinations to master. However, with goal-directed training clinicians can quickly and accurately answer some of the most critical questions using point-of-care echo:

- Is the heart pumping (and how well?)
- Is there significant fluid around the heart (pericardial effusion)?

Beyond these basic questions there is a wealth of information that echo can provide in critical care and emergency patients. The challenge is defining what can reliably be diagnosed based on the sonographer's experience. Understanding limitations and obtaining consultant-performed echo when available and appropriate is essential.

Echo should be used liberally in patients in whom a pericardial effusion is suspected. This includes patients presenting with chest pain, shortness of breath, tachycardia, hypotension, or syncope. Echo can expedite life-saving care in penetrating chest trauma. In a code or near-code situation, echo can rapidly identify some of the reversible causes of pulseless electrical activity (PEA). The finding of an enlarged heart on chest x-ray is an excellent indication for point-of-care echo, as this tends to be heart failure or pericardial effusion—both of which are readily diagnosed with echo but can be difficult to differentiate by physical exam and respond to very different treatments.

Echo may be easily integrated into algorithms for point-of-care sonography that include multiple goal-directed examinations, each designed to answer specific binary questions that can directly affect patient management. The extended focused assessment by sonography for trauma (FAST) exam includes goal-directed examinations of the peritoneum, pelvis, pleural cavities, as well as echo. Other indications where point-of-care echo should be incorporated into a diagnostic algorithm include unexplained hypotension (Chap. 25) and unexplained dyspnea (Chap. 26).

This section focuses on transthoracic echo (TTE). TTE is readily performed as a point-of-care examination at the bedside. While the anatomy and pathology remain the same, transesophageal echo (TEE) may provide superior images and diagnostic sensitivity, although it is more invasive, more technically challenging, and requires special equipment, sedation, and attention to airway management. Point-of-care TEE may be very helpful in a critically ill patient who is already endotracheally intubated.

NORMAL ULTRASOUND ANATOMY

The heart is best thought of as a cone, with a base and apex (Figs. 6-1 and 6-2*a* and *b*). The base, which contains the valves and atria, is positioned posteriorly and toward the right shoulder. The apex, where the ventricles come to a point, is directed obliquely and anteriorly toward the left hip. Thus, the "long axis" of the

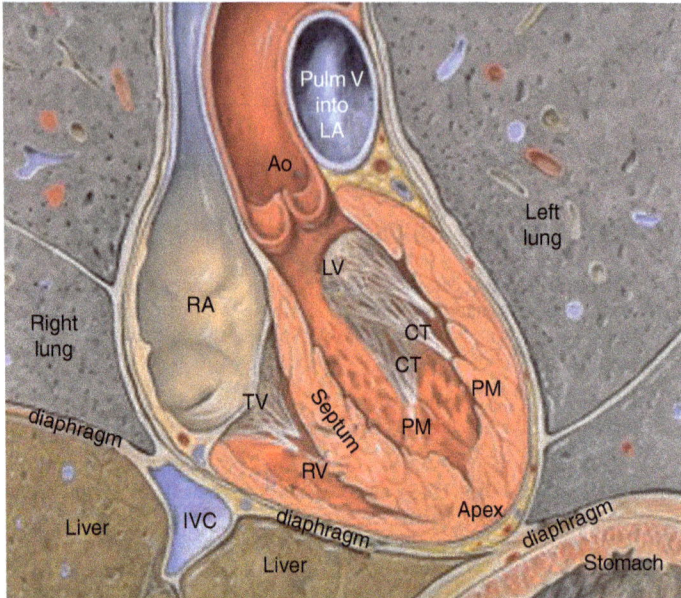

FIGURE 6-1 Cardiac anatomy, coronal plane. Inferior vena cava (IVC) courses through posterior to the liver to enter the right atrium (RA). Blood passes through the tricuspid valve (TV) to enter the right ventricle (RV). After leaving RV through the pulmonary valve (not shown) and coursing through the lungs, blood re-enters the heart via the pulmonary veins (pulm V.) draining into the left atrium (LA). Blood enters the LV through the mitral valve (not completely shown), which is tethered to the papillary muscles (PM) by the chordae tendinae (CT). Blood exits the LV through the aorta (Ao) to enter the systemic circulation. Apex is toward the left hip, while base includes the valves and atria. (*Patrick J. Lynch, medical illustrator; C. Carl Jaffe, MD, cardiologist.*)

heart is a line or plane directed from the right shoulder to the left hip. The "short axis" is perpendicular to the long axis, a line or a plane directed from the left shoulder to the right hip. Recalling geometry, when an ultrasound plane cuts through a cone along its axis a triangle results (long-axis view) (Fig. 6-3a), while when a plane cuts through a cone perpendicular to this axis it generates a circle (short-axis or "donut" view of the heart) (Fig. 6-3b).

Blood enters the heart from the inferior vena cava (IVC) as it drains into the right atrium, then passes through the tricuspid valve to enter the right ventricle (RV). The RV is more anterior (most frequently injured in stab or gunshot wounds), and can also be seen adjacent to the liver. The hepatic veins can be found in the liver and followed as they enter the IVC and ultimately the heart. The RV is a low-pressure, high-compliance chamber that can be thought of as wrapping around the conical and muscular left ventricle (LV) in a crescent shape.

Blood drains into the left atrium (LA) from the pulmonary veins (challenging to see on TTE). The LA is the most posterior structure of the heart and lies just anterior to the esophagus, providing a window for TEE. The mitral valve has an anterior and posterior leaflet and is attached to two papillary muscles via the chordae tendinae. The papillary muscles may be prominent on echo and should not be mistaken for clot.

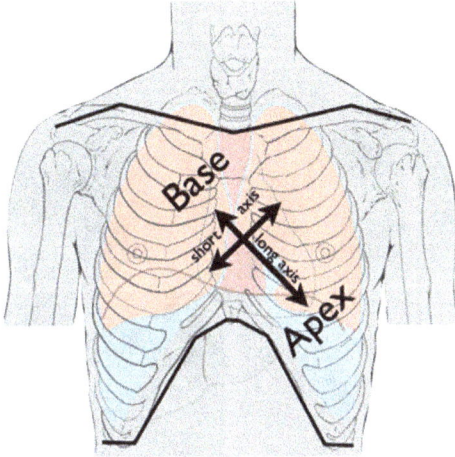

(a)

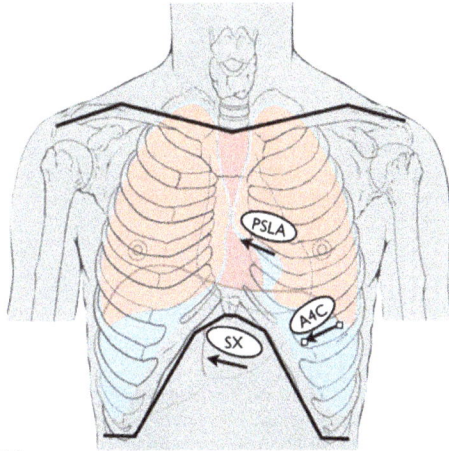

(b)

FIGURE 6-2 Probe positions on the chest. Arrows show indicator direction for a general EM/critical care orientation, with indicator corresponding to left of screen as it is viewed. (a) Long axis goes from base to apex (right shoulder to left hip). Short axis is perpendicular (left shoulder to right hip). (b) Parasternal long axis (PSLA) is shown in the third intercostal space. (rotate PSLA 180° to obtain cardiology PSLA view: "fourth and long"). Parasternal short axis (PSSA) is obtained by rotating probe 90° counterclockwise. Subxiphoid (SX) is shown using the liver as a window. Apical four chamber (A4C) at apex. (*Patrick J. Lynch, medical illustrator; C. Carl Jaffe, MD, cardiologist.*)

Blood leaves the LV through the three cusps of the aortic valve, which is located in the center of the heart, superior to the right atrium. The aortic root is best seen using a parasternal window. After arching out of view (unless a suprasternal window is available), the descending aorta may be seen posterior to the heart just anterior to the thoracic vertebral bodies on a parasternal view.

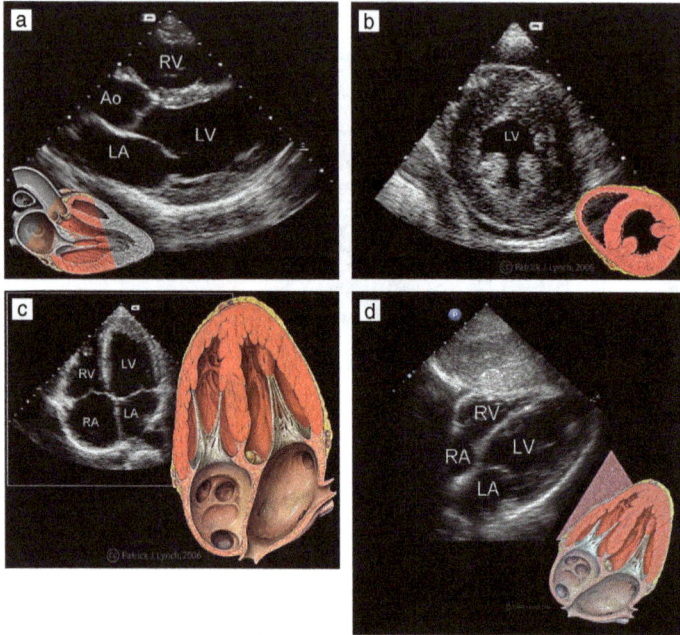

FIGURE 6-3 Basic cardiac windows. (*a*) Shows the parasternal long-axis (PSLA) window. (*b*) Shows the parasternal short-axis (PSSA) window, note papillary muscles. (*c*) Shows apical four-chamber view (A4C). (*d*) Shows a subxiphoid (SX) view. (*Patrick J. Lynch, medical illustrator; C. Carl Jaffe, MD, cardiologist.*)

PROBE SELECTION AND TECHNICAL CONSIDERATIONS

Perhaps more than any other exam, cardiac images may vary significantly depending on machine quality and probe selection/settings. While basic cardiac views (ie, looking for large effusion or cardiac motion in a FAST exam or code situation) may be accomplished with a curvilinear probe, much better images will generally be obtained using a phased-array probe. This is a small footprint probe, typically with a flat square face and a frequency from 2 to 5 MHz. The beam is electronically steered, and the image will often appear to generate from a point at the top of the screen. This narrow point of origination allows an image to be more easily obtained between ribs. Broadband imaging and the use of tissue harmonics will improve image quality.

It is important to use the cardiac setting as this will have a higher dynamic range (providing more contrast to see the endocardium) and appropriate persistence and frame rate (high-frame rate is important with a moving structure).

Due to longstanding imaging conventions, cardiologists use a probe orientation that is reversed from general abdominal and obstetrical scanning. This means that when a cardiac preset is chosen, the indicator will typically switch to the right side of the screen (rather than the correspondence with the left side of the screen as it is seen in general ultrasound). The indicator direction is often signified by a machine logo or dot on the screen. Gel can also be placed on the probe to determine the side of the indicator.

The different conventions in image orientation have caused confusion when providers performing point-of-care ultrasound do exams that incorporate echo with other imaging. Cardiologists and echo sonographers typically scan from the left side of the bed, using their left hand, while general ultrasound imaging is done from the right side of the bed. In addition to reversing the indicator/screen orientation, cardiologists also switch the indicator direction for most views (ie, directed to patient's left rather than patient's right). In practice, of the three primary windows that we emphasize in this text (parasternal, subxiphoid, and apical), only the parasternal long-axis (PSLA) view actually appears "reversed" on the screen when cardiologists perform it; that is, the apex of the heart in a cardiology PSLA is seen on the left side of the screen as it is viewed.

There are several potential solutions to this. When performing a point-of-care echo, the provider may adopt the complete cardiology convention, performing the exam from the left side of the bed with the left hand and the indicator reversed. Alternately, a general imaging orientation can be used, scanning from the right side of the bed. In order to develop consistent scanning patterns and hand–eye coordination for point-of-care ultrasound in general, it is the recommendation of this text that when possible ultrasound be performed consistently from the right side of the bed, using the right hand. Directing the indicator to the patient's right shoulder in a PSLA view will also provide an image orientation that is consistent with other point-of-care ultrasound orientation and echo and cause less confusion. However, if an image similar to that seen in cardiology texts is desired, the indicator may be directed to the patient's left hip in the PSLA view. This is the so-called "fourth and long" position: indicator is pointed to the 4 o'clock position for a long axis. The same structures will be imaged either way (see "current issues with emergency cardiac ultrasound probe and image conventions" in additional reading).

IMAGING TIPS AND PROTOCOL

There are three primary windows to the heart for TTE. These include the parasternal (long axis and short axis), apical four-chamber (A4C) view, and the subcostal (four-chamber and sagittal).

Probe positions on the body, with indicator directions, are shown in Figs. 6-2*a* and *b*, with resulting images in Fig. 6-3.

PARASTERNAL (LONG AXIS AND SHORT AXIS)

The PSLA view (EM/CC orientation) is obtained by placing the probe in the third or fourth intercostal space just to the left of the sternum, with the indicator directed to the right shoulder. The thumb should be placed on the indicator with the probe held similar to a pencil. Structures visualized should include the RV (anteriorly), the LA, mitral valve, LV cavity, LV outflow tract, and descending aorta (see Figs. 6-3*a* and 6-4). The parasternal view may be helped by having the patient turn on their left side, exhaling if possible. The PSLA is an excellent view for assessment of the LA, LV, and aortic outflow and is the most reliably obtainable window.

The parasternal short axis (PSSA) is obtained by rotating the transducer 90° counterclockwise so the indicator is toward the right hip (see Figs. 6-3*b* and 6-5). The plane of the ultrasound can then be tilted from apex to base through the four major levels of the PSSA: apex, LV papillary muscle level, mitral valve level (mitral valve has a "fishmouth" appearance in this view), and aortic valve level ("Mercedes" sign shows the three aortic cusps in the center of the heart). The PSSA is very good for determining overall LV systolic function.

APICAL FOUR CHAMBER

The A4C view is probably the most difficult of the three primary views to obtain consistently. However, when it is available and correctly obtained it provides excellent information about all four chambers and the tricuspid and mitral valves. This view is often helped significantly by getting the patient to roll on their left side, causing the heart to move against the chest wall. The probe should be placed just inferior and lateral to the nipple (under the breast in females), with the indicator directed toward the ceiling/patient's right side. The plane of the probe needs to be angled up into the chest between the ribs. When correctly obtained, the apex or point where the ventricles come together should be seen at the top of the screen, with the interventricular septum running vertically down the middle of the screen and the atria posteriorly (see Figs. 6-3*c* and 6-6). Commonly, the probe is placed too medially and results in a septum that runs along the screen at an angle. If possible, the probe should be moved laterally to obtain a true A4C view.

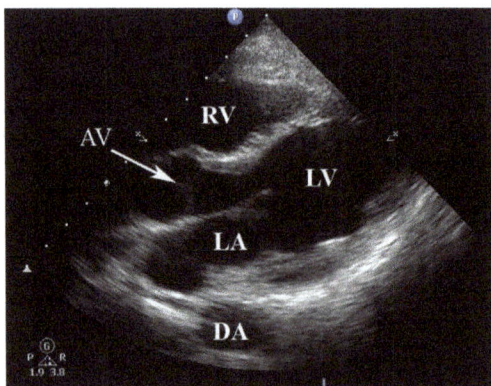

FIGURE 6-4 Normal parasternal long-axis (PSLA) view. RV: right ventricle, LV: left ventricle, LA: left atrium, AV: aortic valve, DA: descending aorta.

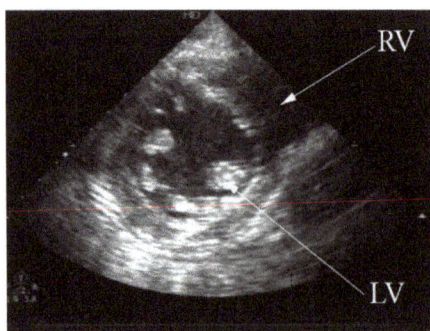

FIGURE 6-5 Normal parasternal short-axis (PSSA) view at the level of the papillary muscles. RV: right ventricle, LV: left ventricle.

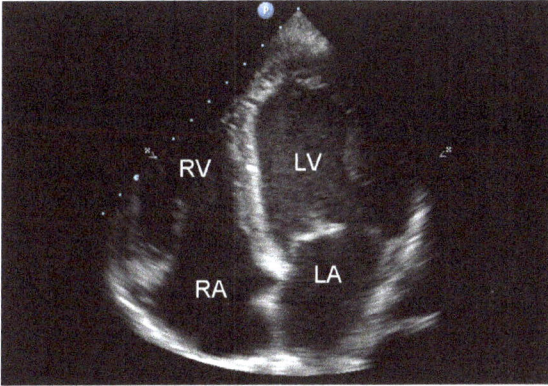

FIGURE 6-6 Normal apical four-chamber (A4C) view. RV: right ventricle, LV: left ventricle, RA: right atrium, LA: left atrium.

The A4C view is the preferred window for obtaining relative chamber size, and is excellent for assessing LV function.

SUBXIPHOID (FOUR CHAMBER)

The SX or subcostal view may be obtained by placing the hand over the probe with the thumb on the indicator directed toward the patient's right. The liver provides an excellent window into the heart and it may help to move the probe slightly to the right while angling up and into the left chest. The hepatic veins and IVC should be followed into the right atrium. The window will be improved by pressing the probe firmly down and up under the costal margin and by having the patient take a deep breath and hold it if they can. The subcostal four-chamber view includes the right atrium, tricuspid valve, RV (adjacent to liver), LA, mitral valve, and LV (see Figs. 6-3d and 6-7). The subcostal view is the preferred window for the detection of pericardial fluid as it images the most inferior part of the pericardium closest to the probe.

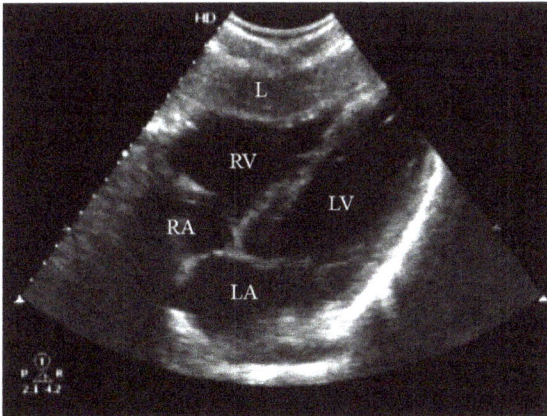

FIGURE 6-7 Normal subxiphoid (SX) view. RV: right ventricle, LV: left ventricle, LA: left atrium, RA: right atrium, L: liver.

A subcostal four chamber may be rotated to a subcostal sagittal view by turning the indicator toward the patient's head. The IVC should be seen along its course draining into the heart. This is the preferred way to visualize the IVC and assess fluid status (Chap. 8). Additionally, it shows the most inferior part of the pericardium very effectively.

When possible all three windows should be utilized to obtain a complete picture of the heart. However, some patients will have certain windows that are better than others, and sometimes a window that is not obtainable. For example, patients with chronic obstructive pulmonary disease (COPD) often have hyper-expanded lungs that push the heart down into the abdomen, providing an excellent SX window but limiting the parasternal view. Obesity or abdominal pain may cause the opposite situation. It is a rare patient who will not have any of the three windows available. In some patients, it may be a composite view such as the "low parasternal/high subxiphoid/medial apical window" that does not fit any one view exactly, but provides the necessary information.

Evaluation of the IVC for fluid status (covered in Chap. 8) is a valuable addition to the cardiac exam.

PATHOLOGIC ULTRASOUND FINDINGS

When performing a point-of-care echo, three primary questions should be answered:

- Is there a significant pericardial effusion?
- How well is the LV working?
- Are there signs of right-sided strain?

This can also be described as the "EEE" approach: effusion, ejection (LV function), and equality (RV<LV).

EFFUSION

A normal heart contains ~10 cc of serous fluid between the pericardium and endocardium, providing a lubricant as the heart beats. Malignancy, uremia, trauma, infection, and other causes may result in the buildup of fluid in the pericardial space (pericardial effusion). Pericardial effusion causes extrinsic compression of the heart that can prevent filling and leads to cardiovascular collapse (tamponade). The ability of the body to tolerate an effusion depends on how quickly it builds up—over time a malignant effusion can become massive while acute tamponade from a stab wound can result from a smaller amount of pericardial fluid.

Effusion typically collects in the inferior pericardium. Large effusions tend to be circumferential, although loculated/organized effusions are possible. Effusions should be seen as a black stripe between the ventricular wall and the pericardium (Fig. 6-8). Trivial effusions may appear as small pockets of black fluid that do not track fully around the pericardium. There are several different methods for grading effusion size, and there is some subjectivity to rating effusion size. Most commonly, the maximum pocket of fluid measured in diastole allows the following categorization:

- Small: <1 cm
- Moderate: 1–2 cm
- Large: >2 cm

At our institution (Yale-New Haven Hospital Emergency Department) effusions are graded as "no significant effusion" (includes trivial effusions), "small effusion" (<1 cm), or "moderate-to-large effusion" (>1 cm).

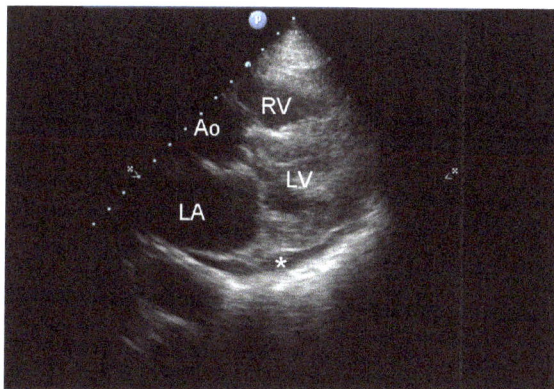

FIGURE 6-8 Small pericardial effusion (*) seen on a PSLA view. Note that the effusion is only visible posteriorly, not anteriorly.

Because effusions collect inferiorly, the SX view is the most sensitive and specific for effusion. In this view effusion will be seen as a black stripe between the pericardium (often adjacent to the liver) and the RV free wall. This can be either a SX four-chamber or a subcostal sagittal window. In a parasternal view, effusion should be seen as a black stripe posterior to the LV wall (inferior pericardium). Beware over-calling an effusion seen only anteriorly on the parasternal view (see Fig. 6-9 and pitfalls, below). In an A4C view effusion should be seen circumferentially.

Tamponade is a clinical diagnosis and occurs when there is hemodynamic col-lapse from the effusion. This results in extrinsic compression that restricts filling of the right heart. Beck's triad [hypotension, jugular venous distention (JVD), and "muffled" heart sounds] should be of only historical interest in diagnosing tamponade if point-of-care echo is available. Echo evidence of tamponade is

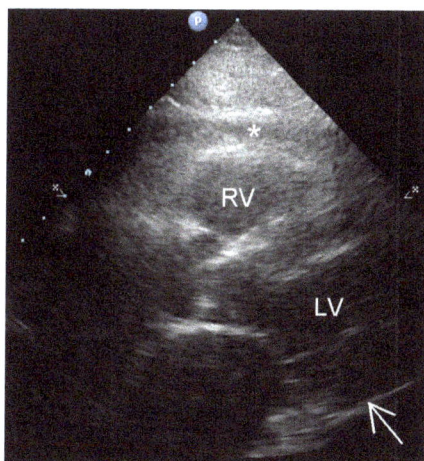

FIGURE 6-9 PSLA view with fat pad. While there is a hypoechoic (dark) space (*), it is not completely echo-free. There is no effusion seen between the left ventricle (LV) and posterior pericardium (arrow). When the image is moving, the anterior hypoechoic area nearly disappears in diastole.

present when there is right-sided diastolic collapse, seen as right ventricular or atrial inversion during diastole (Fig. 6-10). Be careful not to misinterpret ventricular or atrial systole for diastolic collapse. A full and non-collapsible IVC also indicates difficulty with venous return entering the heart (the ultrasound equivalent of JVD). Increased variation of mitral inflow velocity seen using pulsed-wave spectral Doppler is an advanced technique to diagnose tamponade (the ultrasound equivalent of pulsus paradoxus).

The first-line treatment for tamponade/impending tamponade is to raise preload by giving intravenous fluids. In cases where this does not relieve hemodynamic compromise, pericardiocentesis may be required emergently. Ultrasound guidance may be very helpful for pericardiocentesis. The needle approach may be either subcostal or parasternal, and may utilize dynamic or static ultrasound guidance. In either case, typically the largest collection of fluid that is closest to the skin surface is identified using ultrasound and this determines where and at what angle the needle should enter. If available, a pericardiocentesis "kit" that includes an appropriately stiff, well-sized catheter, and equipment for the Seldinger technique should be used.

EJECTION (LV FUNCTION)

Echocardiography has been used for decades to noninvasively assess ejection fraction (EF), a valuable measure of cardiac function. A normal EF is over 55%, and provides information on diagnosis, prognosis, and therapy. While many different measurement algorithms exist to determine EF using echo, in most cases visual estimate from an experienced observer is as good or better than the algorithms. With goal-directed training, the provider using point-of-care echo can become reasonably accurate at categorizing systolic function. We recommend grading function as "normal" (EF >50%), "mild-to-moderately depressed" (EF 30%–50%), or "severely depressed" (EF <30%). Occasionally the LV may actually be hyperdynamic, with almost complete cavity emptying. This should not be confused

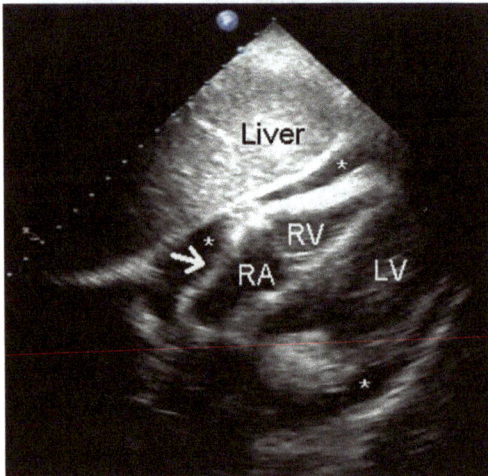

FIGURE 6-10 SX view, tamponade. The pericardial effusion can be seen circumferentially (*) with the arrow showing right atrium (RA) collapse ("scalloping").

with tachycardia (fast heart rate but normal EF). A hyperdynamic heart may occur in dehydration or sepsis and indicates the need for fluid resuscitation.

In order to accurately assess LV function, the heart should be visualized in as many of the three windows and planes as possible. Due to the possibility of focal wall-motion abnormalities, attempting to categorize function from a single view may be inaccurate.

In categorizing LV function, the sonographer should focus their attention on the LV endocardium. Tissue harmonic imaging is very helpful in identifying this border. A normal heart should contract with symmetric thickening of the myocardium. The PSSA at the papillary muscle level is often very good for looking at the "donut" view of the LV and assessing for circumferential contraction. In a PSLA or A4C a vigorously fluttering mitral valve indicates good function, while minimal mitral movement indicates poor function. The overall LV size will often indicate the presence of systolic dysfunction. An LV cavity measured in the PSLA perpendicular to the long axis with a maximum diameter of over 5.2 cm in diastole and/or 3.9 cm in systole indicates cardiac enlargement (Fig. 6-11).

It is not uncommon for a patient with congestive heart failure (CHF) to have normal systolic function. When the LV does not easily relax, filling is restricted and CHF due to diastolic dysfunction can result even with a normal ejection fraction. Doppler is generally required to investigate for diastolic dysfunction, including pulsed-wave interrogation of mitral inflow and tissue Doppler of the mitral annulus. A full discussion of this is outside the scope of this text.

While focal LV wall-motion abnormalities may be appreciated with increased experience and may be helpful in diagnosing ischemia if the wall motion was previously normal; they are also present with chronic scar. The interobserver variability on the determination of more subtle wall-motion abnormalities is usually high. Bundle branch blocks and other conduction abnormalities may also appear as focal wall-motion abnormalities.

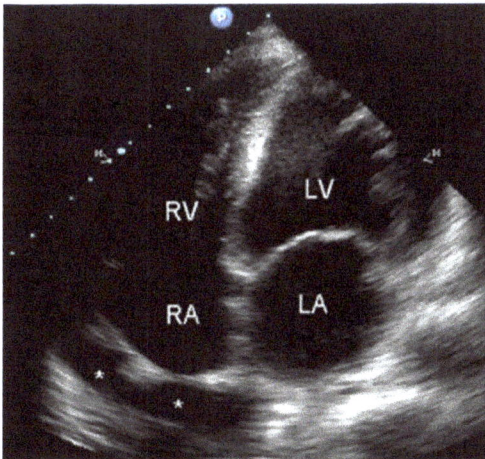

FIGURE 6-11 Dilated cardiomyopathy, A4C view. The moving images show poor left ventricle (LV) function. Note the centimeter marks on the side. Both the LV (>5.2 cm) and left atrium (LA, >4.0 cm) are dilated. Note the right pleural effusion (*) due to congestive heart failure. RV: right ventricle, RA: right atrium.

EQUALITY (RV STRAIN)

The presence of gross RV strain may provide valuable diagnostic and/or prognostic information in a patient with dyspnea, chest pain, or hypotension. In a normal heart, the ratio of RV:LV, measured across the tips of the valves in diastole, should be ~0.6. Increased pressure will cause the normally low pressure/high compliance RV to expand relative to the LV.

For simplicity and in order to maximize specificity (ie, true RV strain), we recommend calling RV strain as present if the RV:LV ratio is qualitatively assessed to be 1:1 or greater. If measured, this is ideally done in the A4C view across the tips of the tricuspid and mitral valves in diastole (Fig. 6-12).

Other signs of RV pressure overload include RV hypokinesis, a flattened or "D-shaped" septum, and paradoxical septal motion (ie, septum bows into LV in initial portion of diastole). McConnell's sign, which is defined as RV hypokinesis with apical "sparing", (ie, apex of the RV is the only portion moving well) has been found to be specific for acute RV strain from pulmonary embolism. A more advanced technique for measuring RV pressure involves measuring the peak velocity (V) of tricuspid regurgitation (typically present with RV pressure overload), using continuous wave spectral Doppler. The pressure gradient is calculated using the modified Bernoulli equation, $\Delta P = 4 \times V^2$. Tricuspid regurgitant velocity of 3 m/s (gradient over 36 mm Hg) or greater is elevated.

RV strain may be acute or chronic. Signs of chronic RV strain include RV hypertrophy (RV free wall >5 mm), and severely elevated RV pressures if they can be measured. Chronic RV strain frequently results from COPD, sleep apnea, or pulmonary hypertension. Acute RV strain in the patient with rapid onset of symptoms is concerning for pulmonary embolism.

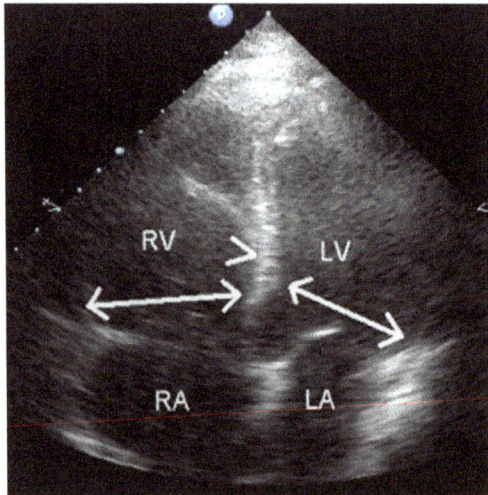

FIGURE 6-12 Right ventricle (RV) dilatation, A4C view. RV size in diastole is qualitatively and quantitatively bigger than left ventricle (LV), measured across and perpendicular to tips of valves. Note slight bowing of septum from RV into LV (arrowhead). RA: right atrium, LA: left atrium.

OTHER FINDINGS

Additional findings that are fairly straightforward include evaluating the size of the thoracic aortic root and descending thoracic aorta, atrial size, and presence of left ventricular hypertrophy (LVH).

The thoracic aortic root is best measured in the PSLA view just distal to the aortic valve. A normal aortic root is under 4.0 cm. While not sensitive, occasionally an aortic flap from dissection may be seen (Fig. 6-13). The presence of a pericardial effusion with chest pain should prompt the search for a proximal aortic dissection. The descending thoracic aorta may also be visualized and measured on the PSLA view. In some patients, the thoracic aortic arch may be visualized using a suprasternal notch view, obtained by placing a phased-array probe just above the sternum and angling down into the chest. The carotid arteries may be followed down to the aortic arch. Beware misinterpreting the adjacent superior vena cava as an aortic flap.

The LA is also easily visualized on the PSLA and A4C views. A diameter exceeding 4.0 cm indicates LA enlargement (see Fig. 6-11).

Echo is more sensitive and specific for LVH than electrocardiogram. LV septal thickness of 1.2 cm or more in diastole is a rough guide to the presence of LVH (Fig. 6-14). The presence of septal LVH, particularly in a young person presenting with syncope, should prompt the consideration of idiopathic hypertrophic subaortic stenosis (IHSS), a disease which may be fatal with exertion.

Occasionally, a cardiac mass may be seen in the atria or ventricles, often associated with valves. The differential includes thrombus, tumor (often myxoma), and vegetations in endocarditis. Consultant-performed echo should be obtained as soon as feasible. Beware of artifacts and the papillary muscles, which may be mistaken for cardiac masses.

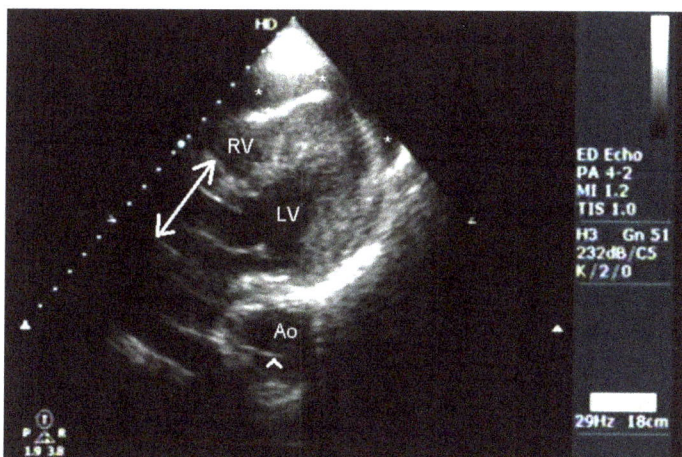

FIGURE 6-13 PSLA view, aortic dissection with pericardial effusion. The aortic root is dilated (arrow, >4.0 cm). A moderate to large pericardial effusion is seen (*). The descending aorta (Ao) is seen posteriorly, with a dissection flap seen (arrowhead). The flap is more apparent on the moving image. RV: right ventricle, LV: left ventricle.

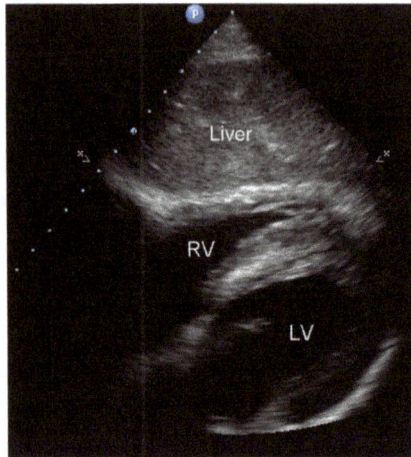

FIGURE 6-14 Left ventricular hypertrophy (LVH), SX view. Left ventricular (LV) septum, between right ventricle (RV) and left ventricle (LV), and LV posterior wall are both well over 1.2 cm (see centimeter marks on side).

Evaluation of the valves, cardiac output, and cardiac pressures may also be possible, but accurate diagnosis typically requires a thorough understanding and use of Doppler, which is outside the scope of this manual.

COMMON PITFALLS

MISTAKING A FAT PAD FOR PERICARDIAL EFFUSION

It is important not to mistake physiologic fluid or a pericardial/epicardial fat pad for effusion (see Fig. 6-9). As machines have improved, it is very common to see a trivial amount of fluid or a hypoechoic space around the heart due to fat. It is unlikely that this would be mistaken for a large effusion, and while a consultant-performed echo may be of help if there is a question in a stable patient, misdiagnosis may be much more problematic in an unstable patient. In particular, overcalling an effusion in an unstable trauma patient could lead to significant unnecessary intervention. It is extremely rare for a patient to have an effusion as a result of blunt trauma except in the case of cardiac rupture, which usually results in immediate death.

Fatty tissue will appear hypoechoic but will often have some echogenicity as opposed to a true effusion. Additionally, a fat pad or trivial effusion should nearly disappear as the heart expands in diastole. The most common place to see a pericardial or epicardial fat pad is in the anterior portion of the parasternal view. Because effusions collect posteriorly and inferiorly, if a hypoechoic space is only seen anteriorly on a PSLA view, the provider should be cautious about calling an effusion. When possible, a SX view should be obtained.

MISTAKING A PLEURAL EFFUSION FOR PERICARDIAL EFFUSION

Care should be taken not to mistake a pleural for a pericardial effusion (Fig. 6-15). This is of particular concern with a left pleural effusion, as a large fluid collection in the left pleural space may be seen adjacent to the LV. The descending aorta,

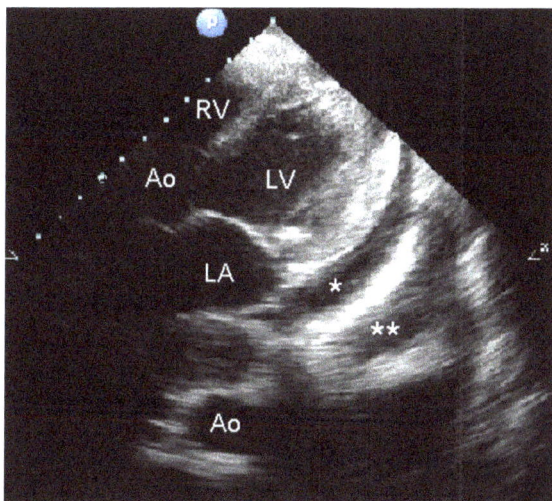

FIGURE 6-15 Pericardial and pleural effusion, PSLA view. Pericardial effusion (*) is separated from pleural effusion (**) by hyperechoic pericardium. Note descending aorta (Ao) in lower part of the screen. RV: right ventricle, LV: left ventricle, LA: left atrium.

seen best on the PSLA view, may help differentiate pleural from pericardial fluid. Pericardial fluid should interpose itself between the LV and descending aorta, while pleural fluid should track beside and behind the descending aorta. If a pleural effusion is suspected, a coronal view of the flank should be obtained to assess the pleural space (see Chap. 7).

MISTAKING ARTIFACTS FOR PATHOLOGY

Artifacts commonly encountered when performing echo include side lobe and mirror image. Side lobe artifact (see Chap. 2) may cause a hyperechoic area to appear inside one of the cavities. This is typically a shimmering area with indistinct borders and should not be mistaken for clot. Mirror image may cause cardiac or valvular motion to falsely appear behind a strong reflector, such as the pericardium.

INTEGRATION OF POINT-OF-CARE ECHO INTO CLINICAL CARE

Echo may be used as a standalone application or may be integrated into algorithms that incorporate chest imaging as part of a set of focused exams. In general, point-of-care echo should be used liberally whenever there is a possibility of significant pericardial effusion. Symptomatic presentations of chest pain, hypotension, dyspnea, or tachycardia, particularly with the presence of risk factors such as malignancy, are excellent indications for point-of-care echo. An echo may be invaluable in a code situation, and can be helpful in emergent cardiac procedures (pericardiocentesis and pacing).

The FAST exam is a longstanding example of an integrated exam that includes imaging of the peritoneum, pelvis, and thorax in addition to echo in the setting of trauma (Chap. 24). The use of echo in hypotension and dyspnea is discussed in Chaps. 25 and 26.

In the hands of trained users, echo is an incredibly valuable tool. However, it is important that users understand limitations and utilize consultant (cardiology)-performed echo when a comprehensive echo is indicated and available.

Additional Reading

Kaplan A, Mayo PH. Echocardiography performed by the pulmonary/critical care medicine physician. *Chest.* 2009 Feb;135(2):529-535.

Kimura BJ, Bocchicchio M, Willis CL, et al. Screening cardiac ultrasonographic examination in patients with suspected cardiac disease in the emergency department. *Am Heart J.* 2001 Aug;142(2):324-330.

Moore C. Current issues with emergency cardiac ultrasound probe and image conventions. *Acad Emerg Med.* 2008; 15(3): 278-284.

Plummer D, Brunette D, Asinger R, et al. Emergency department echocardiography improves outcome in penetrating cardiac injury. *Ann Emerg Med.* 1992;21(6): 709-712.

The Yale Atlas of Echocardiography. http://www.yale.edu/imaging/echo_atlas/contents/index.html. Accessed December 31, 2010.

7 Thoracic Ultrasound

Puncho Gurung and Peter Doelken

BACKGROUND AND INDICATIONS FOR EXAMINATION

Thoracic ultrasonography is useful for the evaluation of pleural, pulmonary, and chest wall pathologies. The major advantages of thoracic ultrasound include bedside availability, absence of radiation, and real-time guidance for therapeutic interventions. Traditionally, thoracic ultrasound was limited to exploration of pleural effusion, but with the availability of modern and smaller handheld units, the range of applications has broadened. Thoracic ultrasound is superior to standard chest radiography in the detection and characterization of pleural effusion, and it is indispensable for the guidance of pleural interventions at the bedside.

Thoracic ultrasound can quickly diagnose pneumothorax not only in the emergency department, but also in intensive care units and procedure suites where it is encountered as a complication of interventions such as central line placement or thoracentesis. In addition, bedside thoracic ultrasound is helpful in differentiating between consolidation, atelectasis, and pleural effusion, all of which may be visualized as an indeterminate opacity on a chest radiograph. It is also useful in the evaluation of pleural and chest wall pathology. The presence of pleural artifacts (B-lines or "lung rockets") indicates interstitial fluid and may help determine if there is pulmonary edema or acute respiratory distress syndrome (ARDS). In critical care units, thoracic ultrasound allows for earlier and more frequent assessments, and in many cases eliminates the transport risk associated with off-site CT scan.

Bedside thoracic ultrasound evaluation should be performed:

- In the patient with undifferentiated shortness of breath, hypoxemia, or chest pain
- In the patient with diminished breath sounds on lung exam
- To differentiate between effusion, infiltrate, and consolidation
- In the real-time guidance of thoracic procedures, such as thoracentesis

PROBE SELECTION AND TECHNICAL CONSIDERATIONS

LINEAR PROBE WITH A FREQUENCY OF 7.5–10 MHz

Higher-frequency transducers provide better resolution at the cost of depth. They are used for visualization of chest wall structures, which tend to be more superficial.

SECTOR SCANNING OR CONVEX-ARRAY PROBE WITH A FREQUENCY OF 3.5–5 MHz

Lower-frequency probes with smaller footprints should be used for the evaluation of pulmonary and pleural pathology. In particular a phased-array probe, which generates a sector image from a point using an electronically steered beam, may be ideal for getting a window between the ribs. These probes have an acceptable compromise between near-field resolution and depth of penetration.

TIME-MOTION MODE (M-MODE)

Time-motion mode (M-mode) displays motion as a one-dimensional line over time on the x-axis. It is useful for detecting lung sliding which is absent in the presence of a pneumothorax (the "seashore sign").

COLOR-FLOW DOPPLER

Color-flow Doppler imaging can be used to detect vascular flow within chest wall lesions and consolidated or atelectatic lung. Color Doppler helps to distinguish blood vessel flow from other structures that may be present in lung tissue. Power Doppler (angiography) has also been described as identifying pleural sliding (the "power slide" sign).

PROBE SETTINGS

An abdominal setting is often appropriate when imaging a simple pleural effusion. In the imaging of lung artifacts, a lower dynamic range/lower persistence, as is typically found in a cardiac setting (image appears more contrasted), will often display long rockets more effectively. Tissue harmonic imaging, when available, may also help. When using color flow or power Doppler, the scale or pulse repetition frequency (PRF) will need to be lowered in order to pick up flow without artifact, and gain may need to be increased.

NORMAL ULTRASOUND ANATOMY

RIBS AND RIB SHADOWING

The ribs are the first structures seen in thoracic ultrasound and help to serve as landmarks for other important structures. Similar to other bones, ribs block the ultrasound signal from getting through to more distal structures. They appear as semicircle hyperechoic structures anteriorly, and therefore appear at the top of the image on the monitor. Due to the inability of the beam to penetrate the ribs, a shadow is created behind the rib, which is seen as an anechoic area emanating from the rib surface posteriorly. The ribs and their shadows serve as landmarks in identifying the parietal and visceral pleura (Fig. 7-1).

CHEST WALL AND PLEURA

Higher-resolution probes of 7.5–10 MHz provide more detailed views of the various layers of the chest wall and pleura. Ultrasound examination of the pleura is affected by the presence of ribs and aerated lungs. Ribs absorb sound waves yielding a shadowing artifact, while air is a strong ultrasound reflector, making it impossible to directly visualize normally aerated lung. The normal pleura appears as an echogenic line between the chest wall and the aerated lung (see Fig. 7-1). In a longitudinal view, the succession of upper rib, pleural line, and lower rib outlines a characteristic pattern, the "bat sign." The visceral and parietal pleural layers cannot be distinguished from one another due to their thickness of only 0.2–0.4 mm. The entire costal pleura can be visualized using proper exam technique. The mediastinal and majority of the diaphragmatic pleura cannot be visualized due to the interposition of aerated lung. If there is a pleural effusion, or the interposed lung is not normally aerated, as in atelectasis or consolidation, examination of these areas is often possible. In addition, some parts of the heart or great vessels may be visible through the non-aerated lung or a pleural effusion. The diaphragm is visualized as an echogenic structure with respiratory movements.

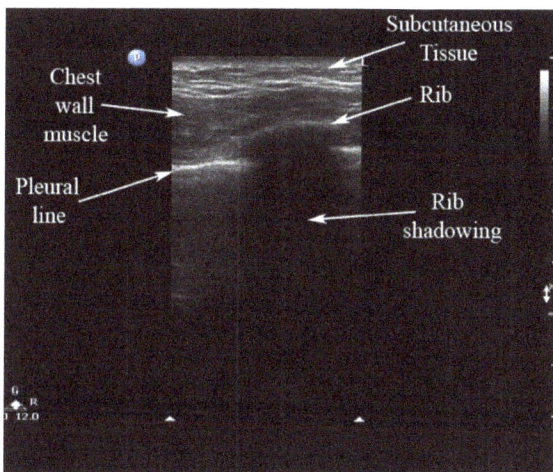

FIGURE 7-1 This figure illustrates common landmarks seen in thoracic ultrasound: ribs and rib shadowing with the pleural line in between. Anterior to the ribs, subcutaneous tissue and chest wall muscle are easily identified.

Lung sliding is the key finding in a lung without pneumothorax. While it may initially be subtle to novice observers, with practice it will be reliably seen as a "shimmering" movement at the pleural line. Lung sliding is a respirophasic movement of the lung and represents the visceral pleura moving against the parietal pleura, and is seen in both spontaneous breathing and mechanically ventilated patients.

LUNG ARTIFACTS

Because the lung is filled with air, it is not directly visualized unless there is consolidation. Instead, artifacts arising from the pleural interface are used. While artifacts often interfere with other imaging, they can be diagnostic in thoracic sonography.

There are two main types of lung artifacts that are commonly visualized: A-lines and "comet-tail" artifacts; both are types of reverberation artifacts (see Table 7-1). A-lines, also known as horizontal artifacts, are echogenic lines that appear between rib shadows that represent the repetition of the pleural line (Fig. 7-2). The presence of A-lines is considered normal, and should not be seen when B-lines or "lung rockets" are visualized.

Comet-tail artifacts are a type of reverberation artifact that occurs at a small air–fluid interface. They appear as vertical hyperechoic rays that arise at the pleural line. There are two major types of comet tail, often known as Z-lines and B-lines. Z-lines are tapering hyperechoic lines that do not reach the far side of the screen and are often seen in normal individuals. B-lines are comet-tail artifacts that arise from the pleural line, are well defined, spread to the edge of the screen without fading, erase A-lines, and move with lung sliding. A single B-line, or multiple B-lines in a dependent portion of the lung, is often found in normal subjects. Multiple B-lines, especially in the anterior/superior portion of the lung, are often

TABLE 7-1	LUNG ARTIFACTS IN THORACIC ULTRASOUND
Term	**Description**
Horizontal artifact (A-lines)	Horizontal echogenic line between rib shadows that represents the repetition of the pleural line. Seen in normal lung.
Comet-tail artifact (Z-lines)	Tapering vertical echogenic line that does not reach the edge of the screen. Often seen in normal patients.
Comet-tail artifact (B-lines)	Vertical echogenic reverberation artifact arising from the pleural line, spreads to the edge of the screen without fading, moves with the lung. Presence excludes pneumothorax. A single B-line or several in the dependent portion of the lung may be normal. Multiple B-lines ("lung rockets") are pathologic.

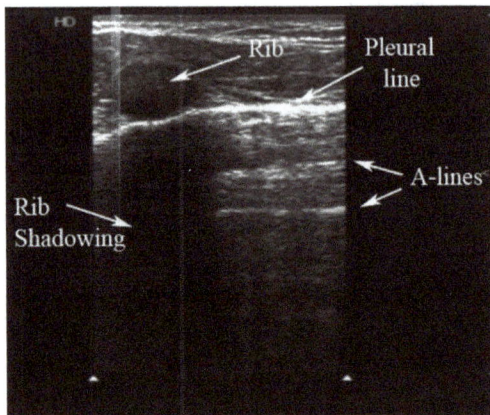

FIGURE 7-2 This figure illustrates a common normal artifact in lung imaging, A-lines or horizontal artifacts, which are echogenic lines that appear between rib shadows that represent the repetition of the pleural line.

termed "lung rockets," and are pathologic. The use of B-lines in diagnosis is discussed below (Fig. 7-3).

IMAGING TIPS AND PROTOCOL

Thoracic ultrasound is usually goal-directed. In emergency department patients, thoracic ultrasound is commonly used to diagnose a pneumothorax, pleural effusion, or in the real-time guidance of a thoracentesis. The critical care physician uses thoracic ultrasound for similar applications, but in addition it is often used to

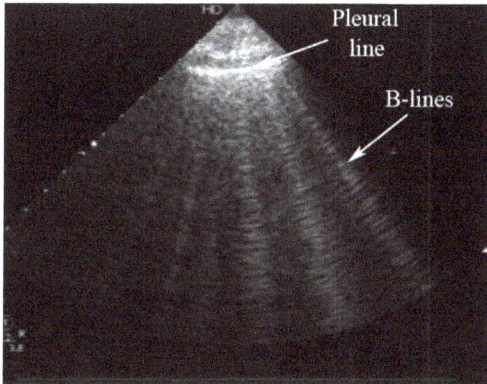

FIGURE 7-3 This figure illustrates B-lines or comet-tail artifacts, vertical, echogenic, ray-like, reverberation artifacts that have five main features, arise from the pleural line, are well-defined, spread to the edge of the screen without fading, erase A-lines, and move with lung sliding.

further characterize an opacity seen on chest radiograph or CT scan. The optimal positioning of the patient depends on such factors as what the physician is trying to image and if the patient is compliant and stable.

PATIENT AND PROBE POSITIONING

The anterior and posterior chest can be examined with the patient placed in a sitting position with both arms elevated. In the critically ill and in patients who are unable to sit upright, thoracic ultrasound may be performed in the supine or lateral position with one or more assistants helping to hold the patient.

By convention, the probe indicator is directed cranially and the corresponding mark on the screen can be seen in the upper left corner. Thus, the orientation of a typical thoracic ultrasound image is cephalad to the left and caudad to the right. The probe should be moved in longitudinal and then transverse directions to visualize the lung surface through the intercostal spaces, thereby avoiding the ribs. The parts of the lungs adjacent to the diaphragm may be examined from an abdominal window similar to a FAST examination of the right and left upper quadrants.

In the evaluation of a pneumothorax, the patient is best examined in the supine position where the most sensitive spot is in the evaluation of the lung apices. The probe should be placed in a sagittal orientation with the indicator pointing cephalad beginning at the second intercostal space midclavicular line (Fig. 7-4). The sliding of the parietal and visceral pleura should be evaluated in this view.

Optimally, pleural effusions are best identified using an abdominal view and a curvilinear probe, similar to the coronal right upper quadrant (RUQ) and left upper quadrant (LUQ) FAST positions. In these views, fluid can be identified superior to the bright hyperechoic diaphragm, appearing as an anechoic or hypoechoic area (Fig. 7-5). Pleural effusions can often be identified using the linear high-frequency probe in the same orientation as described earlier for pneumothorax. In this view, an anechoic or hypoechoic area representing the effusion may be seen between the pleural layers.

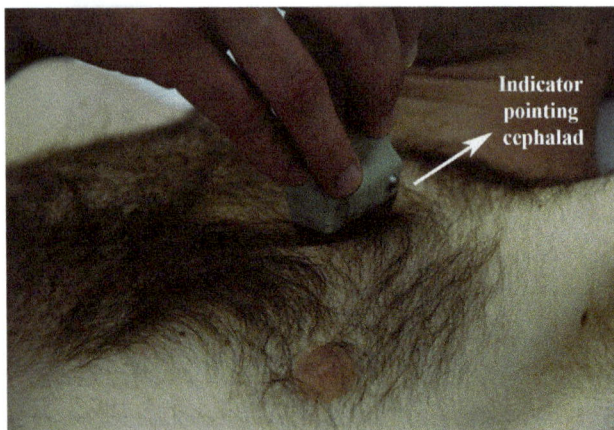

FIGURE 7-4 This figure illustrates correct probe positioning when evaluating for a pneumothorax. The probe indicator should be pointed cephalad, toward the patient's head, at approximately the second intercostal space midclavicular line.

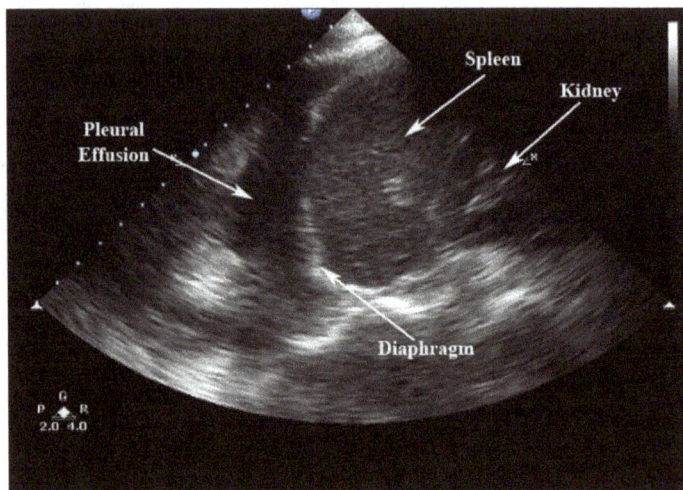

FIGURE 7-5 This image shows a moderately sized hypoechoic effusion, diaphragm, spleen, and kidney. This image was obtained with a curvilinear probe, in the coronal position, in the LUQ.

In order to further characterize an opacity seen on x-ray or CT, the patient and probe should be positioned at a point that best visualizes the ill-defined structure.

Ultrasound-guided thoracentesis is best performed with the patient in an upright position, leaning forward, with the probe placed posteriorly. In this position, lung is viewed through the patient's back in order to visualize the posterior lung and pleural effusion to be drained. Details of this procedure are described in Chap. 18.

IDENTIFY LANDMARKS

Once the probe is placed in a sagittal position on the patient's chest, the ribs and their corresponding shadows should be identified as landmarks. A rib will appear as a curved, slightly hyperechoic structure that blocks the ultrasound beam, therefore, producing an anechoic posterior shadow behind it (see Fig. 7-1). Ideally, an adequate thoracic image is obtained with the visualization of two ribs with their corresponding posterior shadows. The parietal and visceral pleura can be seen sliding between these two rib landmarks.

PATHOLOGIC SONOGRAPHIC FINDINGS

PLEURAL EFFUSION

Thoracic ultrasound can be used to confirm the presence or absence of pleural effusion suspected on the basis of physical findings or seen on a chest radiograph. Sonographic evaluation is superior to chest radiograph because it can differentiate pleural effusion from atelectasis and parenchymal lung disease, all of which may be seen as indeterminate opacifications on a radiograph. In addition, sonography differentiates between loculated pleural effusion and pleural thickening. It has been estimated that thoracic ultrasound can detect as little as 20 mL of pleural fluid, while an upright chest radiograph can require as much as 50–100 mL of fluid to be visible.

The diagnosis of pleural effusion can be made when an anechoic area of fluid is seen within the boundaries of parietal and visceral pleura with dynamic signs characteristic of pleural effusion (see Table 7-2). These signs include floating movement of atelectatic lung (floating lung or lung flapping), respirophasic changes in shape of the fluid collection, undulating movements of fibrinous stands, and a swirling motion of debris ("plankton sign") in the fluid collection. The boundaries of pleural effusion are defined by identification of adjacent organs, that is, diaphragm, lung, liver, spleen, kidney, heart/pericardium, spinal column, aorta, and inferior vena cava (see Fig. 7-5). The liver and spleen are seen in a subdiaphragmatic location. The adjacent lung in pleural effusion may be atelectatic, consolidated, or aerated. Aerated lung is visualized only indirectly by seeing artifacts such as A-lines or B-lines. In smaller effusions that cause less atelectasis, the aerated lung may move into the scanning field with inspiration

TABLE 7-2	**DYNAMIC SONOGRAPHIC SIGNS IN PLEURAL EFFUSION**
Term	Description
Floating lung	Floating movement of atelectatic lung within a pleural effusion. This is helpful to confirm the liquid nature of the suspected effusion.
Curtain sign	Movement of aerated lung into the field of view during inspiration, intermittently obscuring underlying effusion.
Sinusoid sign	Seen in M-mode when the visceral pleura moves toward parietal pleura during inspiration. Helps to distinguish liquid nature of anechoic shadow.
Plankton sign	Swirling motion of echogenic debris within pleural effusion.

creating the "curtain sign." In the presence of a pleural effusion, M-mode can be used to visualize the "sinusoid sign" which represents the movement of the visceral pleura toward the parietal pleura during inspiration (Fig. 7-6).

Thoracic ultrasound can also be used to estimate the volume of pleural effusion, reported as small, moderate, or large. Ultrasound has been found to be twice as accurate as lateral decubitus radiographs in predicting the volume of a pleural effusion.

Pleural effusions are further classified as anechoic, complex nonseptated, complex septated, or homogeneously echogenic based on their echogenicity (Figs. 7-7 and 7-8). An effusion is defined as anechoic if an echo-free space is present between the visceral and parietal pleura, complex nonseptated if echogenic material is seen within the anechoic effusion, complex septated when fibrin strands create a web of septa inside the pleural effusion, and homogeneously echogenic if the space between the parietal and visceral pleura is uniformly echogenic. The determination of echogenicity as hyperechoic, isoechoic, or hypoechoic is based on comparison with the echogenicity of the liver or spleen. The characterization of pleural effusion into these subclasses can help to distinguish between transudates and exudates. Transudates are anechoic, whereas an anechoic effusion can be transudative or exudative. Complex nonseptated, complex septated, and homogenously echogenic patterns are virtually always exudates. Sonographic findings of thickened pleura or associated parenchymal lesions are also indicative of exudates.

The echogenic swirling pattern is defined as numerous echogenic floating particles within a pleural effusion that swirl in response to respiratory movement or heart beat. Homogeneously echogenic effusions are seen in cases of hemorrhagic effusion and empyema, which may sometimes be confused with a solid lesion. Hemorrhagic effusions and empyemas will usually change shape with respiration or contain echogenic material swirling inside of them, unlike solid lesions.

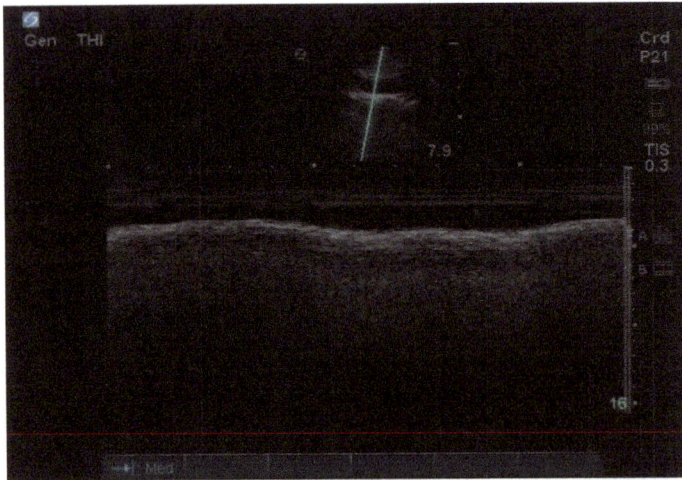

FIGURE 7-6 Composite 2D-mode image and M-mode image of a small pleural effusion. The 2D-mode image shows the cursor placement across the chest wall and an anechoic area between the chest wall and lung air artifact. The M-mode image demonstrates respirophasic movement of the lung toward the chest wall, called the "sinusoid sign," confirming the presence of pleural fluid.

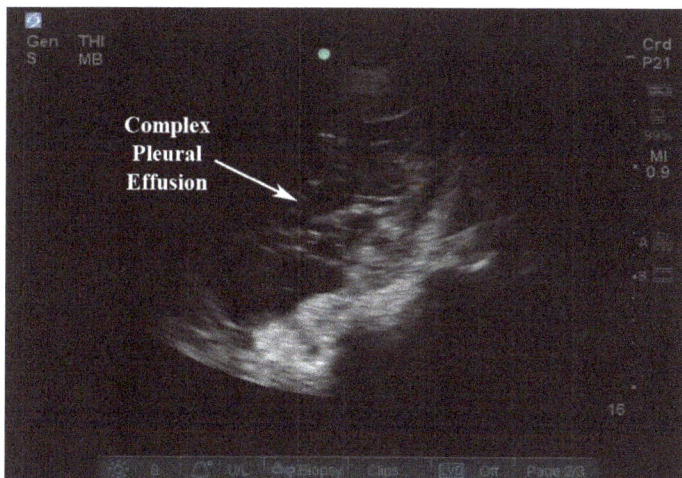

FIGURE 7-7 This image shows a complex nonseptated pleural effusion. These findings are due to malignant mesothelioma.

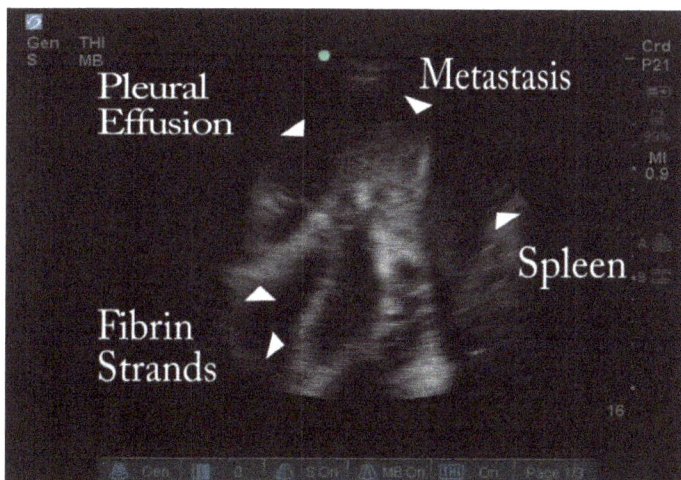

FIGURE 7-8 This image illustrates a complex septated pleural effusion with fibrin stranding and metastasis from a renal cell carcinoma on the thoracic surface of the diaphragm. The spleen is seen immediately below the metastatic lesion.

Rarely, cellular components may settle in the dependent parts of the pleural space in a pattern called the hematocrit sign.

In febrile critically ill patients, in the absence of malignancy, complex pleural effusion should lead to suspicion of complicated parapneumonic effusion or empyema. Empyemas are usually complex nonseptated (relatively hyperechoic), complex septated, or homogenously echogenic effusions. Thoracic ultrasound is superior to chest CT in visualizing stranding and septations in complex pleural effusion. These changes, which cannot be shown by CT, usually predict difficulty with tube drainage.

PNEUMOTHORAX

Thoracic ultrasound is now frequently used at the bedside to quickly exclude pneumothorax due to its higher sensitivity than supine chest x-ray and easy availability. Rapid identification of pneumothorax is urgent, particularly in trauma patients and those on mechanical ventilation. While supine chest x-ray is often used in the trauma bay for pneumothorax, the sensitivity of a supine chest x-ray has been reported to be as low as 40%, compared to ultrasound, which exceeds 80%. Supine chest x-ray may miss very large anterior pneumothoraces. CT scan is the gold standard for the diagnosis of pneumothorax and ultrasound may miss a small pneumothorax that is found on CT; however, the presence of anterior lung sliding essentially excludes significant lung collapse and may obviate the need for an immediate chest tube. In addition, sonographic evaluation of the chest, before and after invasive procedures that are associated with iatrogenic pneumothorax, provides immediate exclusion or confirmation of a collapsed lung. Evaluation for the presence of a collapsed lung relies on the recognition of the dynamic signs of a pneumothorax on ultrasound (see Table 7-3) and accurate interpretation of sonographic artifacts generated by the lung.

The key sonographic finding in pneumothorax is the absence of lung sliding. In a pneumothorax, the presence of air between the parietal and visceral pleura prevents visualization of lung air artifact, and therefore no lung sliding is seen. The presence of lung sliding reliably excludes a large pneumothorax. In addition, the evaluation of lung sliding over the anterior, lateral, and posterior chest helps in quantifying the size of the pneumothorax. Air will first move to the most superior part of the hemithorax unless limited by significant adhesion. Therefore, in small pneumothoraces, with the patient supine, lung sliding would only be absent in the anterior portion of the chest. Therefore, in the supine trauma patient, the apices should be examined first by placing the probe in a sagittal position, midclavicular line at approximately the second intercostal space (see Fig. 7-4). In larger pneumothoraces, lung sliding will be absent in much more lateral and even posterior locations.

TABLE 7-3	**DYNAMIC SONOGRAPHIC SIGNS IN PNEUMOTHORAX**
Term	Description
Lung sliding	Respirophasic movement at the pleural line caused by inspiratory excursion of lung. Its presence excludes pneumothorax at the area under the probe.
Seashore sign	Lung sliding in M-mode is depicted by wave-like pattern located above the pleural line and a sand-like pattern below it. With a pneumothorax, this sign is replaced by the "stratosphere sign" showing only the motionless layer of the chest wall.
Lung point sign	Indicates the area in which the lung intermittently comes in contact with the chest wall during inspiration with a slight increase in lung volume. It is 100% specific for pneumothorax.

Lung sliding is not a specific sign and may be absent in conditions other than pneumothorax. Other conditions that cause an absence of lung sliding include pleural symphysis, (adherence of the parietal layers, often following pleurodesis), pleural fibrosis, loss of lung compliance as in atelectasis, blebs in chronic obstructive pulmonary disorder (COPD), and lung contusion. In this subset of patients with absent lung sliding, the specificity of the sonographic exam for pneumothorax can be further improved by additional evaluation for A-lines (see Fig. 7-2). The presence of A-lines in patients with absent lung sliding increases the specificity of the sonographic exam for pneumothorax to 94%. When present, B-lines that move with the lung rule out pneumothorax with a negative predictive value of 100% (see Fig. 7-3).

Lung sliding can also be evaluated by M-mode sonography. In the time-motion mode, a clear distinction between a wave-like pattern located above the pleural line and a sand-like pattern below it can be made. This is referred to as the "seashore sign" (Fig. 7-9). It depicts the granular pattern from respirophasic movement of lung underlying the horizontal motionless layers of the chest wall. In a pneumothorax, this sign is replaced by the "stratosphere sign," which shows only the motionless layers of chest wall as the air prevents visualization of the movement of the underlying lung (Fig. 7-10).

The lung point sign is the most specific sonographic sign for pneumothorax. The lung point sign occurs when the lung intermittently comes into contact with the chest wall during inspiration and represents the edge of the pneumothorax. It will be seen in real time when absent lung sliding at the pleural line is briefly replaced by sliding during inspiration. Visualization of multiple rib spaces may be required to find the lung point. When present, it is 100% specificity for a pneumothorax. The lung point sign can also be used to estimate and mark the size of pneumothorax, and may be helpful for serial monitoring of pneumothorax progression or resolution.

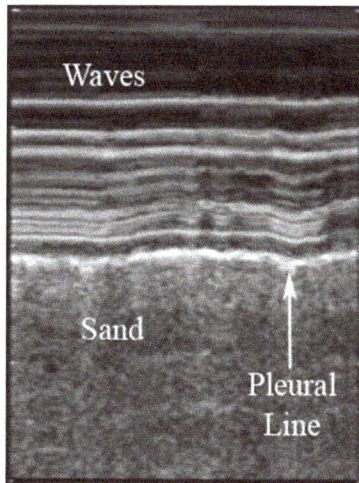

FIGURE 7-9 This M-mode image depicts the "seashore sign" where a clear distinction between a wave-like pattern located above the pleural line and a sand-like pattern below it can be made. The granular area below the pleural interface is caused by lung sliding.

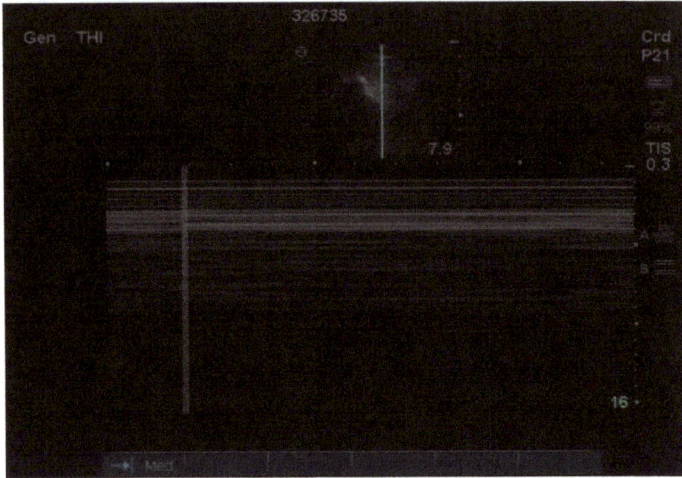

FIGURE 7-10 This M-mode image illustrates the "stratosphere sign." The granular area is not seen signifying absence of lung sliding (see Fig. 7-9 for comparison).

PLEURAL-BASED LESIONS

Thoracic ultrasound is ideally suited for further characterization of pleural lesions localized by chest CT or conventional radiography. Chest CT is more sensitive for the initial detection of pleural thickening and in the identification of focal masses involving the pleura and chest wall. Pleural thickening is seen as a peel of tissue accompanying pleurisy or empyema. Benign pleural thickening does not infiltrate the chest wall and ribs, and is demarcated against aerated lungs. Tumor infiltration may present as diffuse, irregular, nodular parietal, or visceral pleural thickening. Thoracic ultrasound has better sensitivity and specificity in assessing chest wall involvement compared to chest CT.

Metastatic nodules are echogenic and well demarcated from the surrounding tissue or pleural fluid (see Fig. 7-8). Pleural carcinomatosis is difficult to detect by sonography due to the small size of the tumor seeding. In addition, carcinomatosis of the visceral pleura is more difficult to detect because of reflection artifacts that arise from the lung surface. In a patient with known primary malignancy, the combined findings of pleural effusion and nodules, or sheet-like thickening, are highly suggestive of metastatic disease. Mesotheliomas are usually visualized as diffuse irregular thickening of the pleura with localized nodules and are frequently associated with large pleural effusions (see Fig. 7-7).

CONSOLIDATION

Thoracic ultrasound is frequently used to differentiate between alveolar consolidation, atelectasis, and pleural effusion. In the evaluation of the critically ill patient, thoracic sonography has a sensitivity of 90% and a specificity of 98% for detecting alveolar consolidation; however, it requires a comprehensive survey of the pleura to reach a sensitivity this high. Alveolar consolidation is seen as a tissue-like pattern visible at the chest wall devoid of centrifugal inspiratory dynamics. While it may appear sonographically similar to liver or spleen, it will be superior to the diaphragm. The air bronchogram is a typical ultrasound sign of consolidation. This is usually visualized as air-filled bronchi producing hyperechoic punctiform or linear elements. The superficial boundary of consolidation is at the level of the pleural line or at the boundary of a pleural effusion, if present. The deep boundary is usually irregular in the case of aerated lung or regular in the case of whole lobe involvement. Absence of the "sinusoid sign" (described earlier under Pleural Effusion) in M-mode differentiates alveolar consolidation from potentially associated pleural effusion. Normal lung sliding can also be impaired with consolidation.

ATELECTASIS

Thoracic sonography can also be used for bedside evaluation of atelectasis. Complete atelectasis usually results in absent lung sliding and visualization of a tissue-like pattern. This tissue-like pattern is better visualized if the atelectatic lung is in contact with the chest wall or if there is a pleural effusion present in between the chest wall and the atelectatic lung which improves transmission of the ultrasound waves. Usually, the atelectatic lung abuts the posterior chest wall in dependent atelectasis.

Lung pulse is the recording of pulsations that are synchronized with heart activity at the pleural line. It is seen in the early stages of atelectasis when the non-ventilated lung is still inflated prior to collapse. It is explained by the presence of a parenchymatous cushion transmitting cardiac vibrations through the motionless non-ventilated lung. This pattern can be observed in M-mode as well. Lung pulse is sensitive and specific for the diagnosis of ensuing radiographic atelectasis of the left lung following selective intubation of the right lung. Lung pulse is seen before any visible changes in conventional radiographs. When the lungs are ventilated, physiological lung sliding becomes dominant and obliterates this heart signal.

ALVEOLAR-INTERSTITIAL SYNDROME

A single comet tail (B-lines) in the anterior lung, or multiple comet tails confined laterally to the tenth or eleventh intercostal spaces, can be seen in up to one-third of healthy volunteers. Alveolar interstitial syndrome (AIS) is a radiologic diagnosis that may be seen on chest x-ray, CT, or ultrasound, and encompasses any process which may cause interstitial involvement and impaired alveolocapillary exchange. AIS includes acute conditions such as pulmonary edema, interstitial pneumonia, or ARDS, and chronic conditions such as pulmonary fibrosis. Using ultrasound, AIS is defined as the presence of more than two B-lines in a given lung region and is often termed "lung rockets" (see Fig. 7-3). These multiple comet-tail artifacts that fan out from the pleural line to the edge of the screen are related to small subpleural water-rich structures surrounded by air.

B-lines that are 7 mm apart correspond to thickened interlobular septa (corresponding to interstitial fluid—the ultrasound equivalent of "Kerley B-lines"), while B-lines that are 3 mm apart or less correspond to ground-glass areas indicating alveolar edema. It has been shown that ultrasound may be helpful in the spectrum of re-aerating lungs, which may vary from complete alveolar consolidation, to alveolar fluid (B-lines 3 mm or less apart), to interstitial fluid (B-lines ~7 mm apart), to normal, and this may be helpful in assessing positive end-expiratory pressure-induced alveolar recruitment in ventilated patients.

COMMON PITFALLS

PATIENT HABITUS AND EDEMA

Obesity and edema can degrade image quality and make it difficult to discern ultrasound interfaces. The sonographer may sometimes find it necessary to use a lower-frequency curvilinear probe, which will provide better penetrance in order to visualize thoracic structures in more obese patients.

IMAGE ARTIFACTS

Image artifacts are common in thoracic ultrasonography. Rib shadowing and lung air reflections are present to some degree in every image (see Fig. 7-1). Rib shadows should not be misinterpreted as anechoic fluid. Artifacts related to the beam itself, such as reverberation, mirroring, marginal, and scatter artifacts, may confuse the operator. Translational artifacts that occur when the patient is breathing at a high respiratory rate may make it difficult to discern dynamic pleural movement. Subcutaneous emphysema can cause reflection artifacts that make ultrasound examination difficult. Artifacts are typically visible in a single plane of scanning and attenuate or disappear when the probe angle is changed. Therefore, if a potential pathologic finding is questioned, gentle fanning of the probe from side to side can sometimes help the sonographer distinguish artifacts from real findings. Artifacts tend to disappear with slight adjustment of the probe and plane, while pathological findings will usually exist in more than one view.

HEPATORENAL AND SPLENORENAL RECESS

The curvilinear line between the liver and kidney (hepatorenal recess) or spleen and kidney (splenorenal recess) can be seen as a bright hyperechoic structure on ultrasound. In both of these views, the sonographer should be careful to not mistake these recesses for diaphragm (Fig. 7-11).

INADEQUATE COUPLING MEDIUM

Inadequate use of coupling medium, such as gel, can result in excess artifacts. The sonographer should always make sure to use adequate gel when scanning.

FALSE POSITIVES

The sonographer should be particularly aware of the fact that absent lung sliding may not indicate a pneumothorax. While a lung point sign is much more specific,

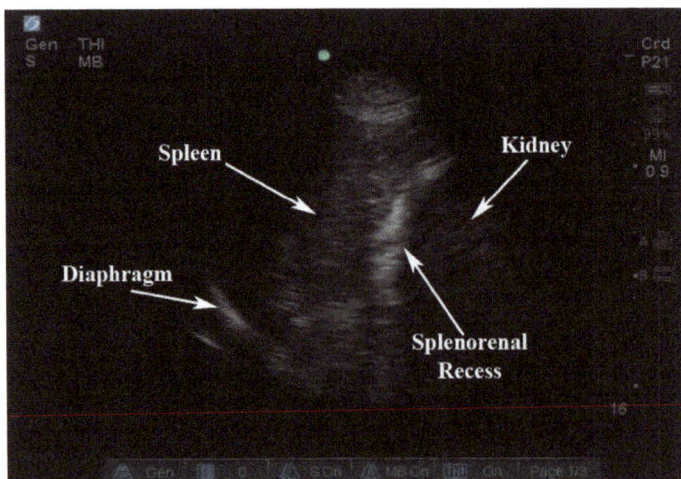

FIGURE 7-11 This image depicts the splenorenal recess as a bright curvilinear structure. The splenorenal recess is located between the upper pole of left kidney and spleen and may be confused with the diaphragm. The hepatorenal recess in the RUQ can have a similar echogenic appearance.

another study (chest x-ray or CT) should be performed prior to thoracostomy, except in extreme circumstances.

INTEGRATION OF THORACIC ULTRASOUND INTO CLINICAL CARE

Recent technological advances have led to the wider availability of affordable, portable ultrasound machines in emergency rooms, procedure suites, and critical care units. Thoracic ultrasound should be considered an extension of the physical examination. Sonographic examination of the pleural space can be easily learned by clinicians for the diagnosis and characterization of pleural effusions, pneumothorax, consolidations, atelectasis, pleural-based lesions, and in AIS.

The presence of lung rockets is closely correlated with serum B-type natriuretic peptide level in congestive heart failure (CHF). In patients presenting acutely, ultrasound may help to differentiate between two of the most common causes of dyspnea: COPD (A-lines, no B-lines) and CHF (lung rockets, no A-lines). Ultrasound has been used to demonstrate the development of high altitude pulmonary edema using portable ultrasound at Everest Base Camp. Initial reports have shown some promise in using ultrasound to identify acute chest syndrome in sickle cell anemia patients. As described earlier, ultrasound may be used in place of or in addition to the chest radiograph to help assess progress in ARDS, pneumonia, and adequacy of mechanical ventilation.

Ultrasonography of the pleural space should be used to provide guidance for invasive procedures such as thoracentesis and pleural biopsy.

Ultrasound should be integrated into the extended FAST exam to assess for pneumothorax in trauma, and may be used following any procedure that carries a risk of iatrogenic pneumothorax.

In summary, thoracic ultrasound should be considered in any patient presenting with undifferentiated shortness of breath, hypoxemia or chest pain, in the patient who has diminished breath sounds on physical examination, and in the real-time guidance of all thoracic procedures.

Additional Reading

Beckh S, Bolcskei PL, Lessnau KD. Real-time chest ultrasonography: a comprehensive review for the pulmonologist. *Chest.* 2002;122(5):1759-1773.

Blaivas M, Lyon M, Duggal S. A prospective comparison of supine chest radiography and bedside ultrasound for the diagnosis of traumatic pneumothorax. *Acad Emerg Med.* 2005;12(9):844-849.

Lichtenstein DA. Pleural effusion and introduction to lung ultrasound. In: Lichtenstein *General Ultrasound in the Critically Ill.* Berlin: Springer-Verlag; 2005: 96-104.

Lichtenstein D, Meziere G, Biderman P, et al. The comet-tail artifact: an ultrasound sign of alveolar-interstitial syndrome. *Am J Respir Crit Care Med.* 1997;156: 1640-1646.

Mayo P, Doelken P. Pleural ultrasonography. *Clin Chest Med.* 2006;27:215-227.

Ultrasound of the Inferior Vena Cava

Martin L. Mayse

BACKGROUND AND INDICATIONS FOR EXAMINATION

Ultrasound evaluation of the inferior vena cava (IVC) provides rapid, noninvasive assessment of a patient's hemodynamic status at the bedside. The size of the IVC and its respiratory variability has been shown to correlate with right atrial pressure (RAP) and intravascular volume. These observations are valuable in estimating RAP, detecting changes in intravascular volume, and monitoring a patient's response to volume resuscitation.

Structurally, the IVC is a thin-walled, highly compliant vessel. Its size and dynamics vary with respiration and changes in intravascular volume. The development of negative intrathoracic pressure during inspiration increases the venous blood return from the extrathoracic veins into the right heart. This leads to an increase in the blood flow through the IVC and a subsequent decrease in its blood volume, resulting in a reduction in intraluminal pressure. These changes decrease the diameter of the IVC during inspiration relative to expiration. These observations are reversed with positive pressure ventilation in which IVC diameter increases during inspiration.

In patients with a low RAP and/or intravascular volume, the IVC size is relatively decreased and its respiratory variability is increased. If RAP is very low, the IVC can collapse completely during spontaneous inspiration. In patients with high RAP and/or intravascular volume, the IVC size is increased and its respiratory variability is decreased. The IVC is very compliant, but its capacity to distend is not unlimited and is restricted by connective tissue in its walls and surrounding structures.

Traditionally, central venous pressure (CVP) and volume status in the acute care setting have been measured by placing a central line. Central lines are invasive, time consuming to insert, and may cause significant complications. Bedside ultrasound has been shown to provide a good estimation of CVP in place of more invasive methods. The clinician can perform serial IVC measurements on an ill patient in order to guide their decision in providing more intravenous fluids or to administer more aggressive medication therapy.

Bedside ultrasound evaluation of the IVC should be performed in:

- The patient who requires an estimation of intravascular volume status, who does not have a central line, or is at a facility that does not have the ability to measure CVP
- Any patient undergoing fluid resuscitation in order to monitor their response and need for additional fluids or medications

PROBE SELECTION AND TECHNICAL CONSIDERATIONS

CURVILINEAR OR PHASED-ARRAY PROBE

To visualize the IVC, a phased-array (frequency of 2.0–4.0 MHz) or curvilinear probe (frequency of 3.5–5.0 MHz) should be used. These relatively low-frequency probes provide better penetration and visualization of deep structures.

DEPTH

Depth of field should be adjusted to allow complete visualization of the IVC and its entrance into the right atrium. The depth needed will mostly depend on the habitus of the patient. Obese patients will naturally have deeper vessels and therefore require an increased depth setting.

TIME GAIN COMPENSATION

Time-gain compensation or far gain should be adjusted in order to account for loss of signal that can occur in the far field, and to provide a relatively uniform intensity across the entire depth of the image.

COLOR-FLOW DOPPLER

Color-flow Doppler is used to detect the presence, magnitude, and direction of blood flow. It is useful in differentiating blood vessels from other structures and artifacts in the abdomen.

M-MODE

M-mode ultrasound detects the motion of structures located along a single axis as they move toward or away from the transducer over time. This method is particularly useful in displaying changes in the IVC that occur during respiration and is the preferred method for quantifying IVC size and its respiratory variability.

NORMAL ULTRASOUND ANATOMY

The IVC is the largest vein in the body. It drains blood from the lower extremities, abdominal wall, and the visceral structures of the abdomen and pelvis and returns it to the right heart.

The IVC is formed by the union of the common iliac veins at the level of the fifth lumbar vertebrae. It ascends cranially through the abdomen along the right side of the aorta. It passes anterior and to the left of the right kidney where it is joined by the renal veins at the level of the second lumbar vertebrae. It continues its ascent along the left border of the descending part of the duodenum before it passes behind the intestine and enters a groove on the posterior-inferior surface of the liver between the right and caudate lobes (Fig. 8-1). It then passes

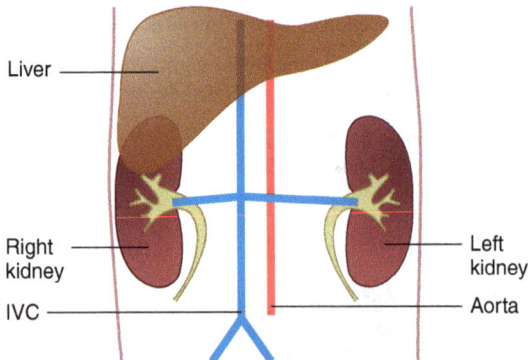

FIGURE 8-1 Anatomic relationships of the IVC to the aorta, kidneys, and liver.

posterior to the portal vein and is joined by the hepatic veins prior to passing through the diaphragm at the eighth thoracic vertebrae. Its course ultimately ends at the right atrium of the heart into which it drains blood from the lower body.

The IVC can be visualized in a transverse (short-axis) or in a sagittal (long-axis) orientation while scanning the abdomen. Imaging is performed with the patient in a supine position using the liver as an acoustic window. It is recommended to begin with a transverse view, with the probe indicator to the patient's right side just below the xiphoid process. In this orientation, the vertebral body of the spine is seen as a bright hyperechoic structure with posterior shadowing. The aorta is seen in cross section just anterior to the spine as an anechoic blood-filled circular structure. The IVC is seen adjacent to the aorta on the patient's right side as an anechoic circular or teardrop structure (see Chap. 5). The image on the screen will depict the IVC on the left side and the aorta on the right. As the IVC is followed toward the heart, the left, middle, and right hepatic veins will be seen to enter the IVC just before it enters the right atrium.

Care should be taken not to confuse the IVC and aorta. The IVC will be thinner-walled, more compressible, and will often have a teardrop shape as opposed to a circular conformation in a transverse view. The IVC will show respiratory variation and may pick up pulsations from the adjacent aorta so "pulsatility" seen on two-dimensional imaging should not be used to differentiate the two. Color-flow Doppler may be used to confirm characteristic arterial flow in the aorta.

After completing the transverse view, a sagittal (longitudinal) view is obtained by rotating the probe 90° clockwise so the indicator is toward the patient's head. This is also called a subcostal long view and will display the IVC in its long axis, with the left side of the screen toward the head and the right side toward the feet (Fig. 8-2). This image will depict the IVC coursing along the posterior border of the liver, crossing the diaphragm, and draining into the right atrium. It is often recommended that the sonographer obtain a subxiphoid cardiac view first and then rotate the probe 90° into the subcostal long orientation in order to obtain an adequate image.

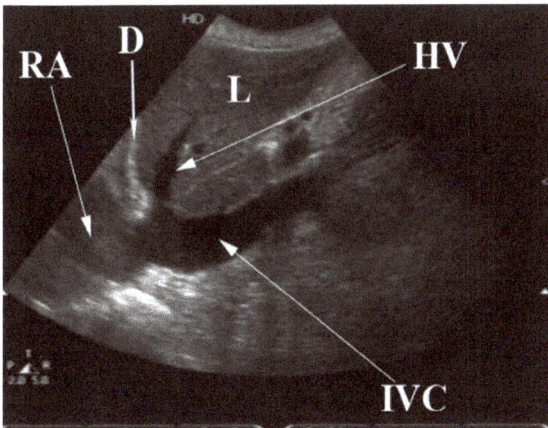

FIGURE 8-2 Sagittal (subcostal long) view of the inferior vena cava (IVC) draining into the right atrium (RA). The probe indicator is pointed toward the patient's head over the inferior portion of the liver (L). The left side of the screen is toward the patient's head and the right toward the feet. Note the hepatic vein (HV) draining into the proximal IVC just distal to the diaphragm (D).

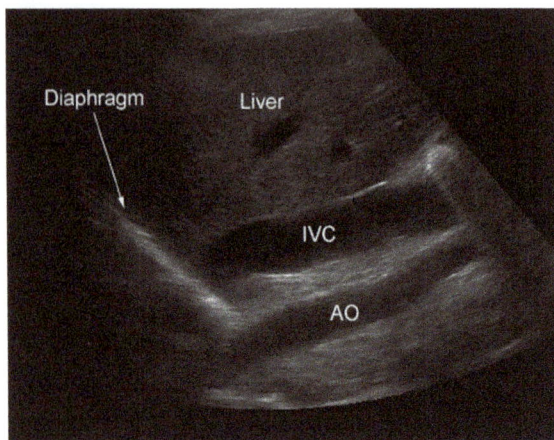

FIGURE 8-3 Coronal (longitudinal) view of the IVC and aorta (AO) traveling parallel to one another across the posterior border of the liver toward the diaphragm. The probe is pointing toward the patient's head and placed in the anterior to midaxillary line over the lower right intercostal spaces. The IVC lies anterior to the aorta in this orientation.

The IVC can also be visualized in its long axis in a coronal orientation similar to a FAST exam. The probe is oriented toward the patient's head in the anterior to midaxillary line on the patient's right side in between the lower intercostal spaces. Figure 8-3 depicts the IVC traveling parallel and anterior to the aorta along the posterior border of the liver as they both cross the diaphragm.

If the above two views are difficult to obtain, the patient can be asked to turn to their left side in a lateral decubitus position. The IVC is then visualized through the liver in a subcostal location, as described earlier, or by placing the probe on the patient's right flank.

IMAGING TIPS AND PROTOCOL

A transverse view of the IVC may be helpful to identify the landmarks as described earlier; however, the IVC diameter and collapsibility should be estimated and measured in the sagittal plane. Care should be taken to visualize the long axis of the IVC at its widest diameter, and not on the side of the vessel. Measurements of IVC diameter should be taken approximately 2 cm caudal to where the IVC passes through the diaphragm and enters the right atrium.

The IVC can also be measured with the patient in the left lateral decubitus position. Imaging of the IVC is adequate in this position, but variations in the hydrostatic pressure can cause estimates of the IVC diameter to differ significantly from those obtained with the patient in a supine position.

Measurements of the IVC and its respiratory variability correlating to CVP have been well described in the literature. A quick estimate of a patient's fluid status is extremely helpful in this setting, especially when CVP measurements are not available. The "collapsibility index" (CI) or "caval index" represents the change in IVC diameter that occurs during respiration relative to the maximum IVC diameter and is defined as:

$$\frac{D_{IVC-\max} - D_{IVC-\min}}{D_{IVC-\max}}$$

- $D_{IVC-\max}$: The maximum anteroposterior diameter of the IVC that occurs during respiration
- $D_{IVC-\min}$: The minimum anteroposterior diameter of the IVC that occurs during respiration

The $D_{IVC-\max}$ is measured during expiration in spontaneously breathing patients and during inspiration in patients receiving positive pressure ventilation. The $D_{IVC-\min}$ is the opposite and is measured during inspiration in spontaneously breathing patients and during expiration in patients receiving positive pressure ventilation.

Once an adequate image of the IVC is obtained, it should ideally be measured 2–3 cm caudal to the IVC-hepatic vein junction or 2 cm distal from its entrance into the right atrium. At this location, the anterior and posterior walls of the IVC are well delineated and parallel. The diameter of the vessel should be measured from wall to wall perpendicular to its long axis and collapse during inspiration should be determined.

M-mode, which detects motion over time, may be used to identify changes that occur during respiration. Measurements can be done with the IVC either in its short or long axis. The M-mode line should be placed perpendicular to the long axis ~2 cm below the atrial junction. Ensuring a perpendicular cut by the M-mode can be done by angling the probe or using directional M-mode if available. Figure 8-4*a* and *b* shows the IVC with respiratory variations in its diameter. The image can be frozen and the diameter of the vessel can be measured at its widest and thinnest parts in order to determine the amount of collapse during inspiration.

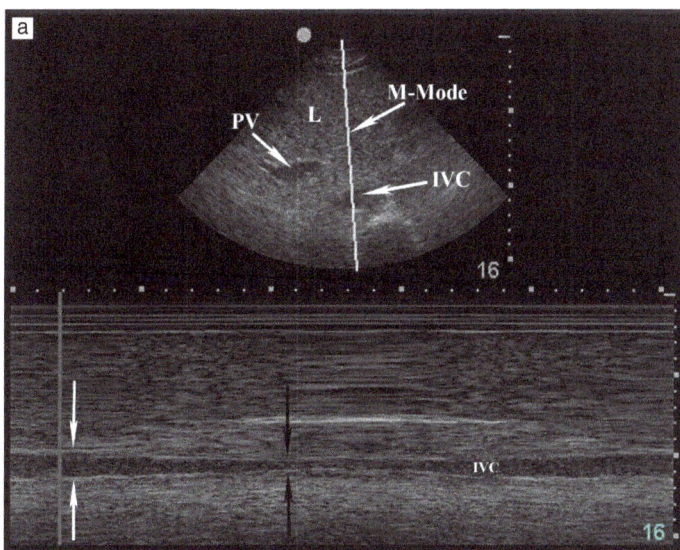

FIGURE 8-4(*a*) Transverse view of the inferior vena cava (IVC) using M-mode imaging during inspiration and expiration of a spontaneously breathing patient. Note the M-mode axis line is through the lumen of the IVC. The white arrows point out the maximum IVC diameter ($D_{IVC-\max}$) and the black arrows the minimum IVC diameter ($D_{IVC-\min}$). PV: portal vein, L: liver.

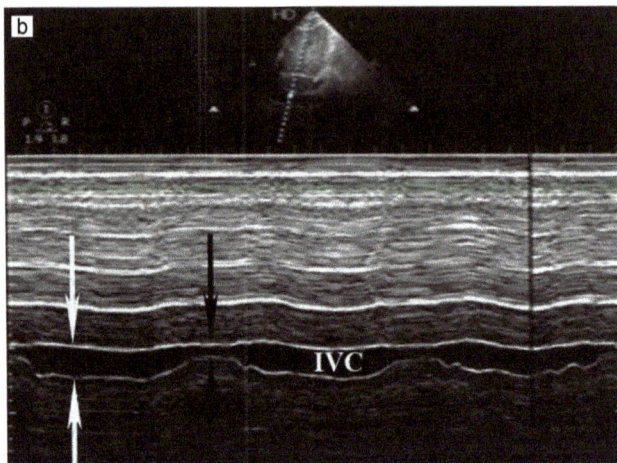

FIGURE 8-4(*b*) Longitudinal view of the inferior vena cava (IVC) using M-mode imaging during inspiration and expiration of a spontaneously breathing patient. The white arrows point out the maximum IVC diameter (DIV_{C-max}) and the black arrows the minimum IVC diameter (DIV_{C-min}).

PATHOLOGIC ULTRASOUND FINDINGS

FLAT IVC AND/OR COLLAPSE >50% ON INSPIRATION

A normal IVC has a diameter anywhere between 1 and 2 cm and collapses by approximately 50% with inspiration. This corresponds to a normal CVP (10 mm Hg) and fluid status. An IVC diameter <1.5 cm and/or an inspiratory collapse >50%, indicates a low CVP (<5–8 mm Hg) and volume depletion. Using the CI equation discussed earlier, an index >50% corresponds to a low CVP.

Typical causes for a decreased CVP include:

- Hypovolemia most often due to dehydration or blood loss
- Distributive shock due to septic, anaphylactic, or neurogenic causes

These findings guide the physician in their resuscitation efforts. For instance, patients who have a low CVP due to hypovolemia will either need more intravenous fluids or blood products. The patient who has a low CVP due to shock may need to be started on vasopressors or inotropes. The sonographic findings of a flat or largely collapsible IVC need to be combined with the patient's clinical situation in order to determine the best course of treatment. This becomes crucial in patients who may require careful fluid management, such as in those with a history of congestive heart failure (CHF) or end-stage real disease (ESRD). This is also helpful in the elderly patient who could easily be pushed into cardiac failure when given too much fluid over a short period of time. In this situation, repetitive sonographic measurements of the IVC can guide the clinician on how much fluid is needed by monitoring the changes in their intravascular volume status.

PLETHORIC IVC AND/OR COLLAPSE <50% ON INSPIRATION

If the IVC has a diameter greater than 2.5 cm and shows minimal collapse on inspiration, the IVC is considered plethoric and the CVP high (>15 mm Hg). A collapsibility index of less than 20% is specific for a high CVP.

Typical causes for an elevated CVP include:

- Hypervolemia most often due to CHF, ESRD, or liver failure, but can be due to iatrogenic fluid resuscitation
- Tension pneumothorax
- Cardiac tamponade
- Pleural effusion

The sonographic signs of an elevated CVP along with the clinical presentation of the patient help the physician in making treatment decisions. For instance, patients who have an elevated CVP due to hypervolemia may need nitrates, diuretics, or dialysis. If the patient's condition is a result of clinician-administered intravenous fluids, resuscitative efforts can be stopped and the patient reevaluated. The finding of an elevated CVP may aid in making the diagnosis of a tension pneumothorax or cardiac tamponade. Repeated sonographic measurements of the IVC can monitor changes in the patient's intravascular volume status.

COMMON PITFALLS

PATIENT HABITUS AND BOWEL GAS

Obese patients and bowel gas are common obstacles when attempting to visualize the IVC. If the IVC cannot be found in a subcostal long orientation, a coronal right upper quadrant view or left lateral decubitus view can be attempted. The sonographer should apply firm pressure with the probe while scanning, which helps to push bowel gas out of the way.

MISTAKING THE AORTA FOR THE IVC

The IVC and the aorta run parallel to one another and often have a similar diameter, thus making it possible to mistake one for the other. It is important to remember the anatomical relationship of these great vessels and to identify the IVC to the right of the aorta on a transverse view. Once the IVC is found in its short axis, the sonographer should keep it in view while turning the probe 90° into the longitudinal orientation.

The IVC is more compressible and has thinner walls than the aorta. The venous pulsations of the IVC are usually less distinct than the arterial pulsations of the aorta, but this characteristic should not be fully relied on to differentiate the two.

INCORRECT MEASUREMENTS

The size of the IVC may be under- or overestimated if it is not measured at the correct location or along the proper axis. The IVC should be measured from one wall to the opposite wall in a perpendicular fashion, taking note of the axis of the vessel. The size of the vessel may be calculated erroneously if the measurement is taken in an oblique plane. Also, the vessel should be measured at its maximal and minimal locations to ensure accurate determination of its respiratory variability.

MISTAKING FLUID-FILLED STRUCTURES FOR THE IVC

Other fluid-filled structures may be mistaken for the IVC. These include the urinary bladder, the gallbladder, kidney, liver, pancreatic cysts, and pseudocysts, which also appear as anechoic structures within the abdomen. This pitfall can be avoided by using landmarks and by following a fluid-filled structure along its course. Color-flow Doppler can also help in this differentiation, as it will detect blood flow in the IVC unlike these other fluid-filled structures.

IVC DIAMETER NOT RELIABLE

There are certain clinical situations in which the IVC diameter may not correlate well with a patient's intravascular volume status. These situations include right-sided heart failure, severe tricuspid insufficiency, and positive pressure ventilation.

INTEGRATION OF BEDSIDE ULTRASOUND OF THE IVC INTO CLINICAL CARE

Sonographic measurement of the IVC diameter is a useful noninvasive method in evaluating a patient's intravascular volume. The IVC diameter and its respiratory variability combined with the patient's clinical scenario can guide a clinician's treatment decisions and resuscitation efforts. While some studies have questioned a reliable quantitative correlation between IVC measures and preload, the qualitative assessment of volume status and response to therapy is useful in many situations.

IVC assessment can determine the presence of hypovolemia and monitor the response to fluid therapy. Bedside ultrasound of the IVC can easily be integrated into the FAST exam protocol. It should be routinely used as part of the sonographic evaluation of patients who present with unexplained hypotension to help identify a cause and course of treatment. IVC assessment is helpful in unexplained dyspnea, specifically in determining the presence of fluid overload and CHF.

Additional Reading

Brennan JM, Blair JE, Goonewardena S, et al. Reappraisal of the use of the inferior vena cava for estimating right atrial pressure. *J Am Soc Echocardiogr.* 2007;20:857-861.

Cheriex EC, Leunissen ML, Janssen HA, et al. Echography of the inferior vena cava is a simple and reliable tool for estimation of 'dry weight' in haemodialysis patients. *Nephrol Dial Transplantation.* 1989;4:563-568.

Feissel M, Michard F, Faller JP, et al. The respiratory variation in inferior vena cava diameter as a guide to fluid therapy. *Int Care Med.* 2004;30:1834-1837.

Perera P, Mailhot T, Riley D, Mandavia D. The RUSH exam: rapid ultrasound in shock in the evaluation of the clinically ill. *Emerg Med Clin North Am.* 2010; 28:29-56.

Yanagawa Y, Nishi K, Sakamoto T, et al. Early diagnosis of hypovolemic shock by sonographic measurement of inferior vena cava in trauma patients. *J Trauma.* 2005;58:825-829.

9 Ultrasound Evaluation of Peritoneal Fluid

Jonathan S. Thierman

BACKGROUND AND INDICATIONS FOR EXAMINATION

Bedside ultrasound is an optimal first-line imaging modality for the evaluation of peritoneal free fluid. The "focused assessment with sonography in trauma" (FAST) examination is one of the common applications used in evaluating the patient for free peritoneal fluid from hemorrhage. Ultrasound has been shown to be sensitive and specific for significant hemoperitoneum. Ultrasound has long been accepted as a life-saving tool in the hypotensive trauma patient, but its benefits have expanded beyond this. Bedside ultrasound is now readily used to search for free fluid in the non-traumatic patient and in other disease processes. It can be used to evaluate for free peritoneal fluid in patients with end-stage liver disease, renal disease, or congestive heart failure.

In addition, the evaluation for peritoneal fluid is invaluable in other patients who may present with abdominal or flank pain. For example, intraperitoneal free fluid in a pregnant patient with abdominal or pelvic pain usually indicates a ruptured ectopic pregnancy that will require operative intervention. The rapid diagnosis of free fluid at the bedside can expedite patient care and definitive treatment.

Bedside ultrasound evaluation for peritoneal free fluid should be performed in:

- The acute trauma patient with blunt or penetrating torso injuries
- The pregnant or pediatric trauma patient
- The subacute trauma patient with a delayed presentation who complains of worsening abdominal pain
- The elderly patient with undifferentiated abdominal or flank pain
- The pregnant patient with abdominal or pelvic pain
- The patient with undifferentiated shock or dyspnea

PROBE SELECTION AND TECHNICAL CONSIDERATIONS

- The abdomen and pelvis are best imaged using a wide footprint curvilinear probe with an operating frequency between 3.5 and 5.0 MHz. Lower frequencies may help with more obese patients while higher frequencies can be used in thin or pediatric patients.
- The phased-array or microconvex transducer in the 2.0–5.0 MHz range can also be used to evaluate the abdomen and pelvis for free fluid. The small footprint allows imaging between the ribs, which is particularly helpful in young thin patients.

TOTAL GAIN AND TIME-GAIN COMPENSATION

The total gain can be increased to brighten the signal returning from the structure of interest and improve the image on the machine monitor. Often times, the near field has adequate gain, and therefore does not need to be adjusted. In order to compensate for signal loss in the obese patient, time-gain compensation (TGC, far gain) may be increased to enhance the attenuated signal reflecting from deeper tissues in the patient. Decreasing the far gain is often required to adjust for the posterior acoustic enhancement artifact that appears behind the bladder in the pelvic window. The TGC controls should be equalized prior to beginning an exam in order to avoid a false-positive "stripe" that can result when the TGC is set too low.

DEPTH

The sonographer should start with a depth of 15 cm or more and scan through the entire far field before focusing in on the more superficial structures of interest. This ensures that abnormal findings are not missed in the deeper fields, and helps to orient the sonographer. Once the deeper areas are interrogated, the depth can be decreased resulting in the structure of interest using approximately three-fourths of the screen.

NORMAL ULTRASOUND ANATOMY

There are three views of the peritoneal cavity that should be evaluated when searching for free fluid. These are the perihepatic [right upper quadrant (RUQ), hepatorenal, "Morison's pouch"], perisplenic [left upper quadrant (LUQ), splenorenal], and suprapubic views. While Morison's pouch is the most sensitive single view for significant free fluid, acquiring multiple views increases overall sensitivity. Evaluation of the paracolic gutters was initially advocated in some descriptions of the FAST exam, but have not been found to improve sensitivity.

PERIHEPATIC (RUQ, HEPATORENAL, "MORISON'S POUCH") VIEW

The perihepatic view examines the RUQ and is typically the first abdominal view obtained, as it is the most sensitive for free peritoneal fluid and the most reliably imaged. This view visualizes Morison's pouch, the potential space between the liver and the right kidney, which is an extension of the right paracolic gutter. This view should also include evaluation of the right hemithorax above the diaphragm for pleural effusion or hemothorax.

The main imaging plane for the RUQ is the right coronal view. The transducer is placed on the right flank with the probe indicator pointing toward the patient's head. It should be positioned in the midaxillary line over the eighth to eleventh intercostal rib spaces (Fig. 9-1). The resulting image is a coronal plane with the left side of the screen toward the head, the feet toward the right, more superficial structures at the top of the screen, and deeper structures at the bottom (Fig. 9-2). The exam should focus on the potential space between the liver and kidney (Morison's pouch). Tilting the probe superiorly should allow visualization of the right hemithorax above the diaphragm. An adequate examination is obtained when the liver, including the inferior liver tip, is visualized in the same plane as the inferior pole of the right kidney. Interrogation of the inferior liver tip is important, as this is the most dependent region, and may contain a subtle collection of free fluid.

A normal Morison's pouch will be visualized as a lack of anechoic or hypoechoic fluid in between the liver and right kidney interface. A normal right hemithorax will be visualized as a mirror image artifact in which the liver appears to be on both sides of the diaphragm (see Fig. 9-2). This artifact is normal and assures the sonographer that there is no free fluid in the pleural space. Free fluid above the diaphragm will appear as an anechoic (black) or hypoechoic space and represents a hemothorax or pleural effusion depending on the clinical scenario.

It is sometimes difficult for the sonographer to fully interrogate the RUQ due to rib shadowing. In this situation, the probe should be angled in between the ribs. This right intercostal oblique view is obtained by orienting the probe in the

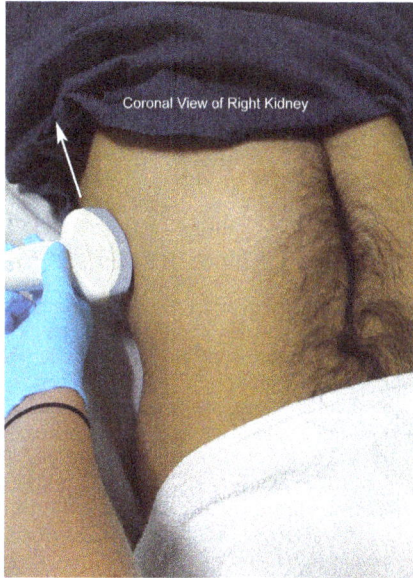

FIGURE 9-1 The proper positioning of patient and probe for RUQ imaging. Notice the probe is in a coronal orientation with the indicator pointing toward the patient's head (arrow) in the mid-to-anterior axillary line.

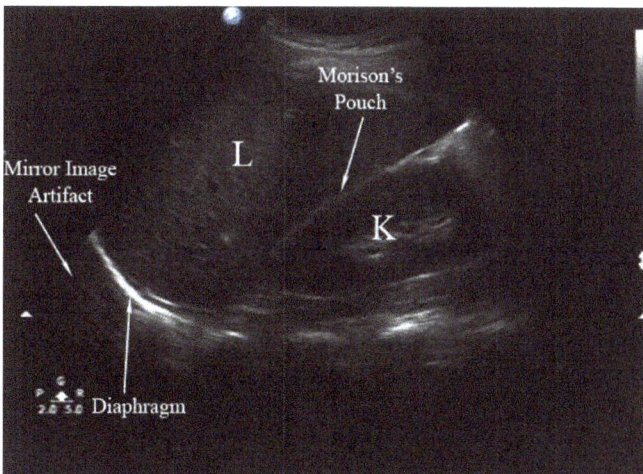

FIGURE 9-2 A normal coronal view of the RUQ with landmarks. The left side of the image is toward the patient's head. The bright white hyperechoic diaphragm can be seen with a mirror image artifact of the liver above it, which signifies a normal pleural space without fluid. A normal Morison's pouch is seen between the liver and kidney. The patient's feet would be directed toward the right side of the screen. Note the inferior tip of the liver and kidney are both imaged on the right where fluid often collects first. K: kidney, L: liver.

midaxillary line between the lower rib spaces angling slightly toward the patient's posterior body surface. The transducer can be subtly rotated both anteriorly and posteriorly to optimize the image and reduce artifacts from rib shadowing. A smaller footprint or phased-array probe may also help in this situation.

PERISPLENIC (LUQ, SPLENORENAL) VIEW

The LUQ view is used to assess for left pleural effusion, and for free fluid in the subphrenic and splenorenal recesses, which communicate with the left paracolic gutter. The probe can then be tilted superiorly to image the diaphragm and lower chest. This view is typically more difficult than the RUQ view to obtain for a few reasons. The kidney is anatomically more superior and posterior on the left, and the spleen does not provide as large of a sonographic window as the liver. This more posterior position can add additional rib shadows on the left that obscure the anatomy. In addition, the operator stands on the patient's right side and must lean over the patient in order to place the transducer in the LUQ. "Knuckles on the bed" is a phrase often used to describe the LUQ view as it emphasizes the need to reach all the way around the patient posteriorly in order to obtain an adequate window.

As on the right, start with a coronal view. The probe should be placed on the left flank in the posterior axillary line over the seventh to ninth intercostal spaces with the indicator pointing toward the patient's head. Once again, the positioning will need to be more superior and posterior than the RUQ and the sonographer will typically have their hand against the bed to obtain the best view. If the patient is cooperative, inspiration may help the view. The patient may have to be placed in the lateral decubitus position, if tolerated, in order to optimize the image (Fig. 9-3). If rib shadows are obscuring important anatomy, an intercostal oblique view

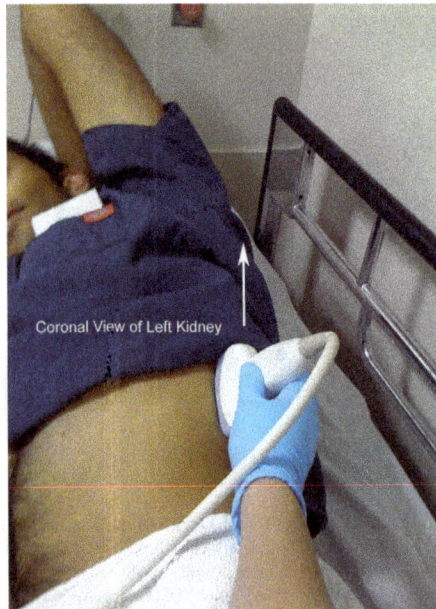

Coronal View of Left Kidney

FIGURE 9-3 The proper positioning of patient and probe for LUQ imaging. The patient is in a lateral decubitus position with the probe in a coronal orientation with the indicator pointing toward the patient's head (arrow) in the posterior axillary line.

should be attempted by rotating the transducer slightly and directing it posteriorly. Sometimes a more anterior view through the rib cage can visualize the structures needed.

The orientation is similar to the RUQ view, with the left side of the screen toward the patient's head and the right side of the screen toward the patient's feet. An adequate LUQ view should visualize the spleen, left kidney, and the subphrenic space (Fig. 9-4). As opposed to the right side, free fluid will often collect in the subphrenic space first before collecting in the splenorenal recess. Therefore, adequate imaging should always include good views of the interface between the spleen and diaphragm. As with the perihepatic view, the operator should make sure to visualize the inferior tip of the spleen lying adjacent to the inferior pole of the left kidney in order to be complete. The inferior thorax can be visualized by angling the probe superiorly, and having the patient take a breath in if they are able to.

A normal subphrenic space and splenorenal recess will be visualized as a lack of anechoic or hypoechoic fluid in between the spleen and both the diaphragm and left kidney. A normal left hemithorax will be visualized as a mirror image artifact above the diaphragm that gives the illusion of spleen appearing on both sides (see Fig. 9-4). This artifact assures the sonographer that there is no free fluid in the pleural space.

SUPRAPUBIC (PELVIC) VIEW

The suprapubic view is the most dependent potential space for free fluid to collect. The posterior cul-de-sac or pouch of Douglas, also called the rectouterine space, is the dependent continuation of the peritoneal cavity between the rectum

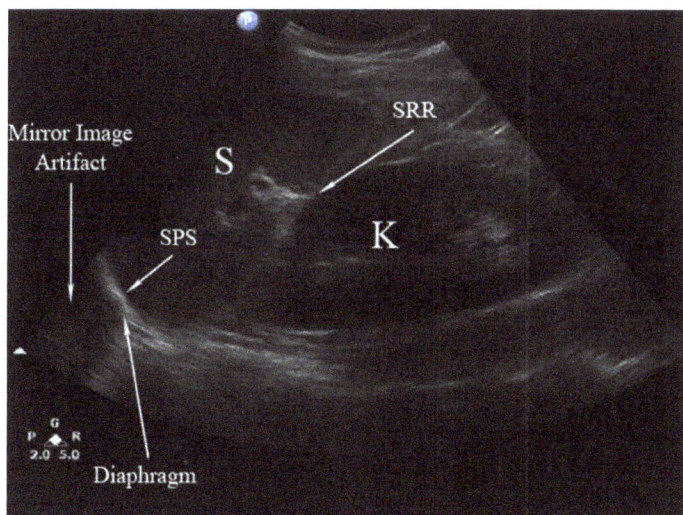

FIGURE 9-4 A normal coronal view of the LUQ with landmarks. The bright white hyperechoic diaphragm can be seen with a mirror image artifact of the spleen above it, which signifies a normal pleural space without fluid. A normal subphrenic space (SPS) is visualized between the spleen and diaphragm. A normal splenorenal recess (SRR) is visualized between the spleen and left kidney. Note the inferior tip of the spleen and kidney are both imaged on the right. K: kidney, L: liver.

and the back wall of the uterus in the female patient. In a male patient, the most dependent area is a similar space posterior to the bladder and anterior to the rectum, known as the rectovesicular space.

The suprapubic view is easier to obtain when the bladder is full because it provides a large sonographic window and views should be obtained prior to Foley catheter placement if possible. The suprapubic view looks for free fluid in the pelvis. While fluid in blunt trauma is assumed to be blood, it may also be urine or ascites. In young women, a small amount of physiologic fluid may be a result of the normal menstrual cycle.

The suprapubic view is obtained by positioning the transducer on the lower abdomen just above the pubic symphysis. In the sagittal view, the transducer should be oriented longitudinally with the indicator pointing toward the patient's head and angled inferiorly. When full, the bladder is easily found due to the large sonographic window it provides and because there are no ribs or other bony structures obstructing the view. In a female patient, the uterus can be seen superiorly and posteriorly relative to the bladder (Fig. 9-5). There may be bowel gas, which can scatter the ultrasound signal, but usually, sliding and/or angling the probe more inferiorly will reduce this impediment. The imaging plane should be swept through the entire volume of the bladder in the left-to-right directions while the operator looks for a black anechoic stripe behind the bladder or uterus.

After the entire area is surveyed in the longitudinal orientation, the transducer is then rotated 90° counterclockwise so that the probe indicator is oriented toward the patient's right (Fig. 9-6). The bladder and the area behind it are then scanned by angling the probe from superior to inferior. A normal transverse suprapubic view demonstrates the bladder as a trapezoidal or oval-shaped anechoic structure (Fig. 9-7).

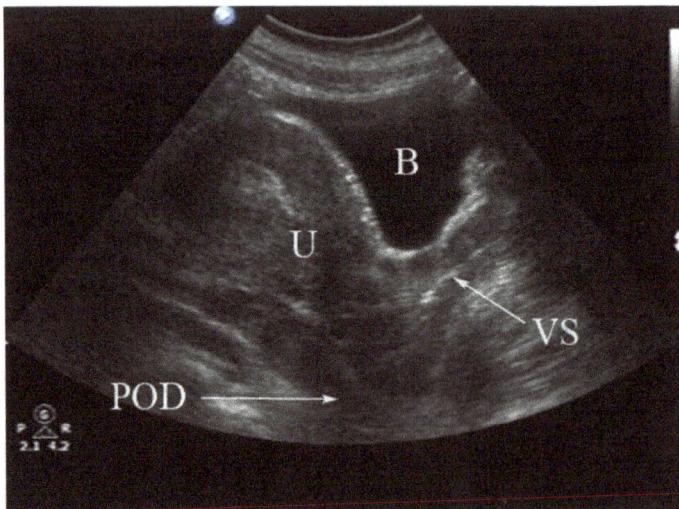

FIGURE 9-5 A normal sagittal suprapubic view with the probe oriented toward the patient's head. The patient's head is to the left of the screen, the feet to the right, the anterior surface is at the top of the screen, and posterior surface is at the bottom. The bladder (B) is seen anteriorly and inferiorly to the uterus (U) in this orientation. The arrow points to the pouch of Douglas (POD), the most dependent area where free fluid will collect first. Notice that there is no black anechoic area behind the posterior wall of the uterus, which would signify possible free fluid. VS: vaginal stripe.

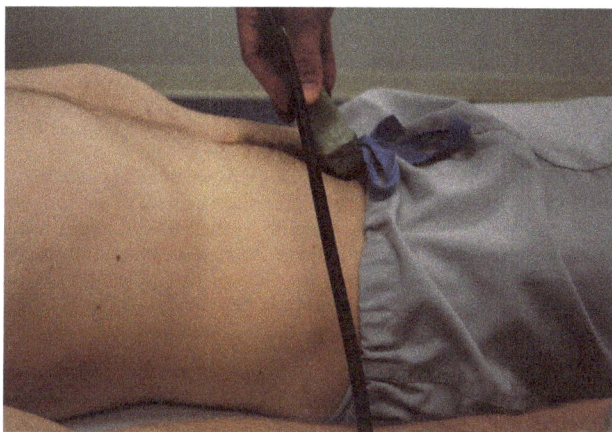

FIGURE 9-6 Proper positioning of the patient and probe to obtain a transverse view of the bladder. The probe is placed above the pubic symphysis in a transverse orientation with the indicator pointing toward the patient's right side. Notice the probe is angled inferiorly looking down into the pelvis.

The uterus and cervix can often be seen as circular homogenous tissue posterior to the bladder. Similarly, the prostate can be visualized inferiorly in the male patient. Fluid will be seen behind the bladder and may wrap around it if there is a large enough amount present. Large amounts of fluid in the pelvis may actually look like the bladder, particularly if the bladder is decompressed. The probe must be angled inferiorly enough to image the entire bladder.

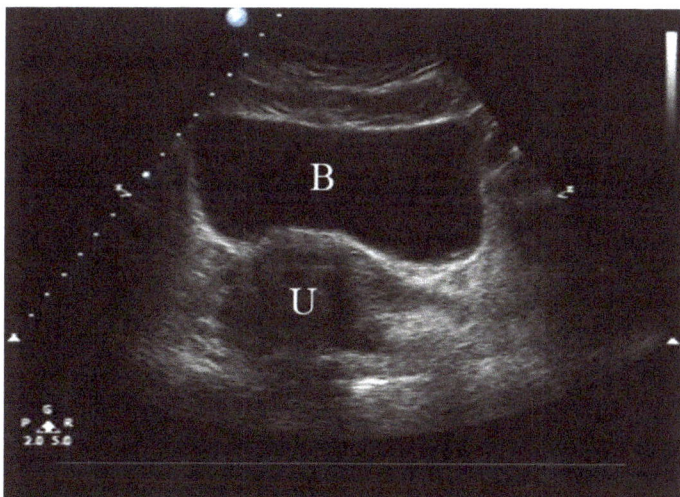

FIGURE 9-7 A normal transverse suprapubic view with the probe oriented toward the patient's right side. The bladder (B) is seen anterior to the uterus (U) in this orientation. Notice that there are no black anechoic areas surrounding the organs, which would signify possible free fluid.

IMAGING TIPS AND PROTOCOL

THE DIFFICULT PATIENT

Patients will not always have the easiest anatomy to visualize, especially the LUQ view which typically is the most challenging. The most common impediment the sonographer faces is obesity. Lowering the probe frequency or applying more pressure may improve visualization. If the patient is compliant, they can be asked to roll into a lateral decubitus position, which helps to bring the organs out from under the ribs. A Trendelenburg position can also help, as this will cause fluid to accumulate in the upper quadrants and increase the sensitivity for free fluid. The image can also be improved by asking the patient to take a deep breath in, which can help to slide the organs down from beneath the ribs and limit shadowing obscuring important anatomy.

IMAGING PROTOCOL

Proper transducer selection, adequate application of ultrasound coupling gel, and imaging a patient with a full bladder are essential for obtaining adequate image quality. The probe indicator should point toward the patient's right side or superiorly toward the patient's head to maintain the convention for the resulting images.

Multiple views of the abdominal examination will increase sensitivity for free fluid. This means that the sonographer should attempt to obtain all of the views discussed above if possible.

In the trauma patient there may be subtle signs of free fluid present, unlike the patient with ascites who may have a more dramatic presentation. Therefore, it is imperative that the sonographer image the spaces where potential fluid collects first. This means full visualization of the RUQ and LUQ, including the inferior tips of both the liver and spleen. In addition, in the LUQ view, a thorough image of the subphrenic area between the spleen and diaphragm needs to be obtained. The suprapubic view should be imaged in both the sagittal and transverse orientations, although the sagittal view often provides more information, particularly in the female pelvis. In females of childbearing age, the uterus should be visualized in two planes for evidence of pregnancy, which may occur prior to a human chorionic gonadotrophin test.

The inferior thoracic cavity should be investigated as part of the RUQ and LUQ for pleural effusion or hemothorax.

In some patients, the exam may be limited despite attempts to improve the image, and in a small minority the appropriate images may not be visualized at all. Even with excellent views, abdominal sonography is not completely sensitive for free fluid or intrabdominal injury, and a CT scan should be obtained with an inadequate or negative FAST if there is significant suspicion for intrabdominal injury.

PATHOLOGIC ULTRASOUND FINDINGS

FREE FLUID IN THE ABDOMEN, PELVIS, OR CHEST

Free fluid will appear as a black, anechoic signal. The sensitivity of ultrasound for free fluid varies with the amount of fluid present. While as little as 100 mL of fluid can be detected in some cases when multiple views are obtained, the examination is most sensitive when there is 500 cc or more.

In the RUQ, free fluid will typically appear in Morison's pouch as a black stripe between the liver and right kidney (Fig. 9-8). The fluid should track around and between the organs, creating acute angles at the edges. Rounded angles may

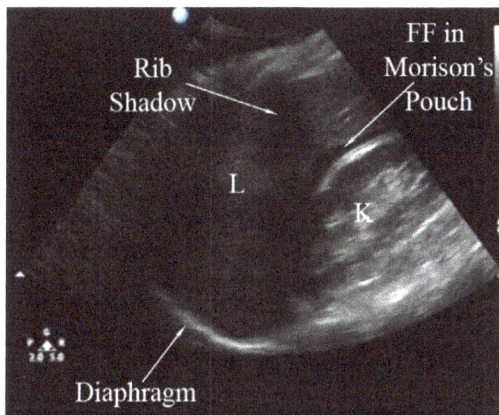

FIGURE 9-8 A RUQ coronal view of a young man with a splenic laceration from a motor vehicle accident showing free fluid (FF) in Morison's pouch between the liver (L) and right kidney (K). Notice the rib shadow in the middle of the image obscuring part of the liver and pouch. The sonographer must be aware of this potential interference and attempt to optimize the image around the rib shadows or free fluid could be missed.

indicate a contained fluid collection such as a cyst or the gallbladder. The fluid should be followed to make sure it is not a vessel (such as the hepatic veins draining into the inferior vena cava [IVC]). If the fluid is subtle, it may only appear around the inferior tip of the liver. In patients with chronic ascites, fluid may also be seen in Morison's pouch, but a larger amount will typically be seen beyond the tip of the liver as well as between the liver and diaphragm (Fig. 9-9). In addition, the liver will often appear shrunken and more heterogeneous.

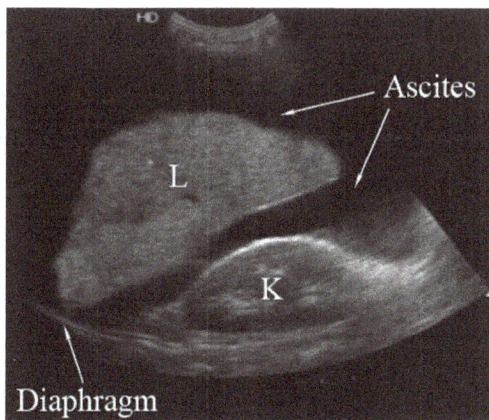

FIGURE 9-9 RUQ coronal view in an elderly woman with ascites due to liver cirrhosis. This view demonstrates fluid, seen as dark black anechoic areas, surrounding the whole liver (L). Notice the difference in fluid distribution compared to the trauma patient in Fig. 9-8. In addition, the liver appears shrunken, heterogeneous with irregular surfaces, another clue that this free fluid is due to ascites. K: kidney.

In the LUQ free intraperitoneal fluid will collect in the subphrenic space between the diaphragm and spleen, in the splenorenal recess between the spleen and left kidney, or in the left paracolic gutter (Fig. 9-10). A black stripe or pocket in any of these locations indicates fluid. Once again it is important to visualize the inferior tips of both the left kidney and spleen.

In the suprapubic view, free fluid will appear as a black anechoic collection outside the bladder. In a patient with a large amount of pelvic free fluid, the collection may actually be mistaken for a distended bladder. The pelvic walls can surround a fluid collection and resemble the bladder. It is essential to properly identify the bladder and its walls, and to follow any fluid to see if it is contained within the bladder walls or tracks into the pelvis (Fig. 9-11). The probe must be angled inferiorly enough over the symphysis pubis and into the true pelvis to find the bladder. In a female patient, the most sensitive area for finding fluid is in the rectouterine space or pouch of Douglas, the most dependent area in the pelvis (Fig. 9-12). Larger amounts of fluid may track into the anterior cul-de-sac or the utero-vesicular space between the uterus and bladder (see Fig. 9-11). The female pelvis should be evaluated for sonographic signs of pregnancy, particularly if a CT is being considered. In the male, the most dependent area where fluid collects first is in the rectovesicular space, between the bladder and rectum (Fig. 9-13).

ULTRASOUND OF THE PLEURAL SPACES

The inferior thorax should be imaged as part of the coronal view of the right or left upper quadrant. A black anechoic area in the costophrenic space represents fluid (Fig. 9-14). The presence of a mirror image artifact (appears that the liver or spleen is superior to the diaphragm) essentially rules out a pleural effusion. Ultrasound is more sensitive for thoracic fluid than chest radiograph, and may detect 50 cc or less. Free fluid in the pleural space in a trauma victim on the right or left most often represents a hemothorax. In a non-trauma patient (or a trauma patient with chronic disease), pleural fluid might be an effusion from congestive heart failure, renal failure, malignancy, or various pulmonary causes.

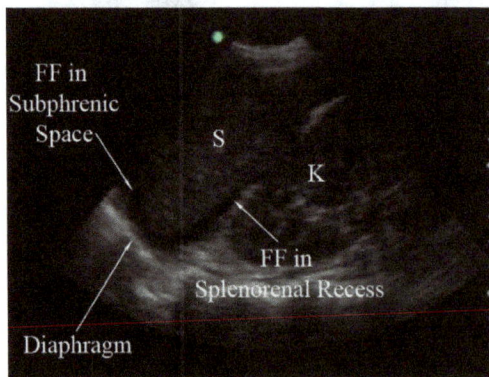

FIGURE 9-10 LUQ coronal view in a man with cirrhosis and ascites illustrating free fluid (FF) in both the subphrenic space between the spleen (S) and diaphragm and in the splenorenal recess between the spleen and left kidney (K). In a trauma, free fluid in the LUQ will often be more subtle than this.

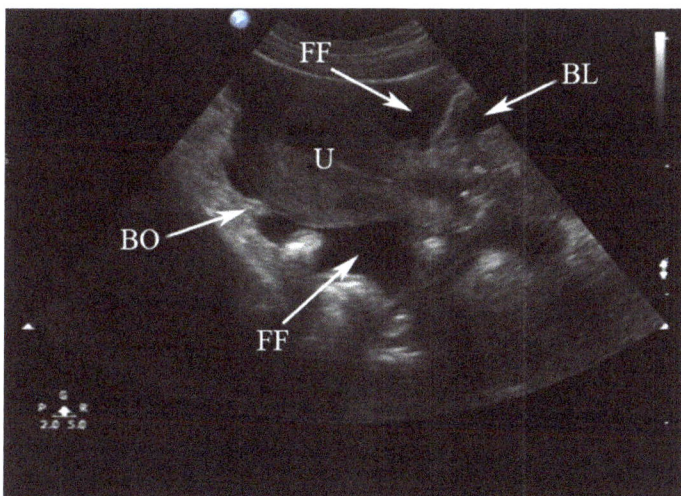

FIGURE 9-11 Sagittal suprapubic view in a woman with a ruptured cyst. Note the extensive amount of free fluid (FF) that appears in both the anterior and posterior cul-de-sacs. The free fluid in the utero-vesicular space is adjacent to the bladder (BL), which lies anterior to the uterus (U). Note the bladder has thick walls with well-contained anechoic urine inside of it as opposed to the poorly defined free-flowing pelvic fluid surrounding it. Free fluid can also be identified by the presence of loops of bowel floating inside of it (BO). It is important for the sonographer to not mistake free fluid that appears anteriorly as the bladder.

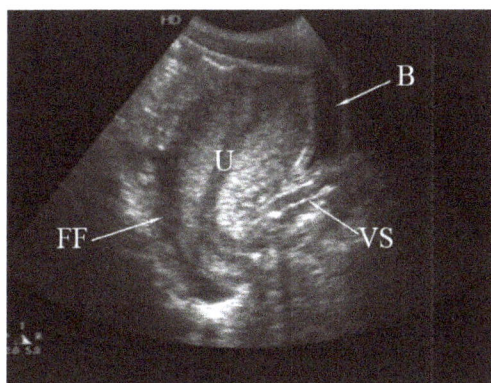

FIGURE 9-12 Sagittal suprapubic view in a woman with a ruptured ectopic pregnancy. The probe is oriented toward the patient's head, which is to the left of the screen, the feet are to the right, the anterior surface is on top, and posterior surface on the bottom. The uterus (U) with vaginal stripe (VS) is seen superior and posterior to the bladder (B) and free fluid (FF) is visualized as an anechoic area behind the uterine wall in the pouch of Douglas.

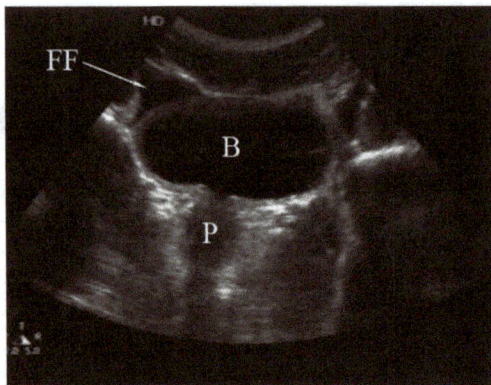

FIGURE 9-13 Transverse suprapubic view in a male patient suffering a gunshot wound to the abdomen. The probe is oriented toward the patient's right side where free fluid (FF) can be seen collecting around the bladder (B). Note the prostate (P) located posterior and inferior to the bladder.

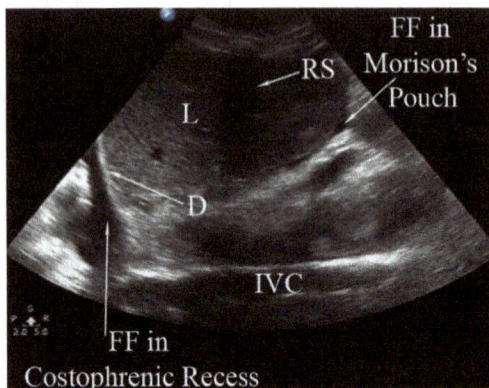

FIGURE 9-14 RUQ coronal view in a patient with end-stage renal disease illustrating free intraperitoneal fluid in Morison's pouch and also a right-sided pleural effusion. Note on the left side of the image the bright white hyperechoic diaphragm (D) with a black anechoic area above it representing fluid in the costophrenic space. The inferior vena cava (IVC) can be seen at the bottom of the screen crossing over the diaphragm to drain into the right atrium. L: liver, RS: rib shadow.

OTHER PATHOLOGICAL FINDINGS

Occasionally, when looking for free peritoneal fluid, the clinician may directly detect injury in a solid organ such as the spleen or liver. Acute solid organ lacerations may appear as fragmented areas of varying echogenicity, but may be difficult to detect during ultarsound. The laceration may cause a subcapsular hemorrhage, which appears as a crescent-shaped hypoechoic stripe surrounding the organ. Fluid from a kidney injury or aortic aneurysm leak may also collect in the retroperitoneal space, where it will be seen as an anechoic or hypoechoic collection surrounding the kidney but not tracking into the peritoneal cavity. These injuries are difficult to diagnose using ultrasound; therefore, when a solid organ injury or retroperitoneal fluid is suspected, a CT examination will be more sensitive.

COMMON PITFALLS

INADEQUATE VIEWS

In all three peritoneal views, subtle findings can be missed if the sonographer is not scanning through the entire area where free fluid may collect. A small amount of fluid may collect in the most dependent inferior regions and this may be the only abnormal ultrasound finding on the exam. The transducer should be adjusted on the patient as much as possible to optimize the view and the patient repositioned to increase the sensitivity of the exam.

The sonographer must also remember to position the probe more superiorly and posteriorly in order to adequately visualize the LUQ. Once again, the operator must often lean over the patient while standing on the patient's right side in order to reach the LUQ with the transducer. The imaging of the LUQ can sometimes be improved by having the patient roll into the right lateral decubitus position, but this is not always realistic in a sick patient.

The operator may position the transducer too superiorly and the bladder is either missed entirely or obscured by bowel gas. If the bladder is not readily identified, the operator should first attempt to reposition the probe more inferiorly. Another helpful hint is to perform the suprapubic view before a Foley catheter is placed because a full bladder greatly enhances the ease of imaging. There are studies that have shown that free fluid in the pelvis will often be missed without a full bladder. If a Foley catheter has been placed, the suprapubic view may be enhanced by infusing 200 mL of normal saline in order to temporarily fill the patient's bladder.

PATIENT HABITUS AND BOWEL GAS

Obesity and bowel gas are common challenges a sonographer faces in attempting a thorough exam. Inadequate visualization of important interfaces can occur in a good number of patients due to these two factors. Visualization may be enhanced in obese patients by choosing the correct transducer and frequency settings (a curvilinear probe with lower frequency and better penetration). Bowel gas can be pushed aside by applying firm pressure with the probe or by turning the patient into the lateral decubitus position.

MISINTERPRETING THE FINDINGS OF FREE FLUID

As discussed earlier, patients with ascites will have a significant amount of free intraperitoneal free fluid on their abdominal exam. In a trauma situation, it is important to understand these findings within the context of the patient's presentation. The finding of free fluid due to ascites is often more dramatic than what is found in a trauma situation. Free fluid from ascites will often track over the liver, delineating the liver edge (which is often shrunken or nodular with ascites from cirrhosis) as seen in Fig. 9-9, while acute intraperitoneal fluid is typically found just between the kidney and liver as seen in Fig. 9-8. The amount of free fluid due to ascites is often very large and would be incompatible with life if it were truly due to a trauma. It is important for the sonographer to use these findings in combination with the patient's pertinent past medical history. If necessary, a diagnostic peritoneal tap can help distinguish ascites from blood, as can Hounsfield units on CT scan.

Female patients of menstruating age may have a small amount of physiologic free fluid in the pelvis. As a general rule, when free fluid extends more than 50% along the uterine wall in the posterior cul-de-sac or any fluid anterior to the uterus (in the utero-vesicular space) is considered abnormal.

MISTAKING FLUID-FILLED STRUCTURES FOR FREE FLUID

The operator may sometimes mistake a stomach full of food, fluid, or gas for free fluid in the LUQ or for abnormal splenic architecture (Fig. 9-15). The clinician can avoid confusing the stomach contents for free fluid by ensuring that the imaging plane is not too far anterior or medial so that the stomach does not obscure important left-sided structures. The operator should be aware of the appearance and position of the stomach. It is typically found somewhat deep to the spleen but anterior and medial to the kidney. Fluid seen in the stomach will be encased by the stomach walls and rugae may be seen; fluid in the stomach also will not track into crevices around the spleen.

Fluid-filled cysts can also be interpreted as free fluid if they are not imaged thoroughly. These cysts can appear in the kidneys, liver, or spleen and can sometimes obscure the interface between two organs where the examiner is actually searching for free fluid. This pitfall can be avoided by carefully scanning through the whole area in full and noticing that these cysts will be more regular-appearing, have definitive borders, and are self-contained, unlike the appearance of free fluid. The appearance of cysts and examples are discussed more fully in Chap. 10. The gallbladder is another fluid-filled contained structure that may occasionally be found between the kidney and liver and should not be mistaken for free fluid. Again, following the borders of the fluid and understanding biliary anatomy (Chap. 11) can help avoid this pitfall.

The IVC courses along the posterior border of the liver before emptying into the right atrium of the heart. As this vessel is filled with blood, its lumen will appear black and anechoic, similar to free-fluid findings in Morison's pouch. Any fluid collection should be followed to see where it leads to—the hepatic veins will drain into the IVC, which will then drain into the right atrium. If there is any

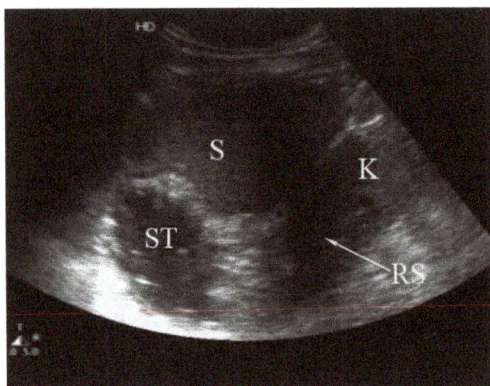

FIGURE 9-15 LUQ coronal view illustrating the fluid-filled stomach (ST) overlying the superior and posterior surface of the spleen (S). Notice the splenic architecture looks distorted due to this finding. The sonographer can improve this image by moving the probe more posterior and superior. K: left kidney, RS: rib shadow.

question, color-flow Doppler may show blood flow in the IVC that would not be present with free fluid (see Fig. 9-14).

The seminal vesicles in a male patient, located lateral and posterior to the bladder, can appear hypoechoic or anechoic and should not be mistaken for free fluid. The sonographer can avoid this by carefully fanning through the bladder and noticing that these structures are contained and regular unlike the appearance of free fluid.

RIB SHADOWS

Rib shadows can obscure important anatomy in both the perihepatic and perisplenic views. There are a few maneuvers that the sonographer can attempt in order to move the important organs out from beneath the ribs. Using a microconvex or phased-array probe may help to image between the ribs. The intercostal oblique view, discussed earlier, may provide a window between the ribs. Avoidance of the ribs can also be achieved by moving the probe a little inferiorly and simultaneously rotating the probe in the anterior/superior directions to capture the correct imaging plane. The success of this maneuver will vary greatly on the patient size and body habitus. Finally, asking the patient to take a deep breath in and out can help slide the organs out from beneath the rib cage.

PERINEPHRIC FAT

Depending on the habitus of the patient, there may be a significant amount of hypoechoic perinephric fat surrounding the kidneys, which should not be mistaken for free fluid. Perinephric fat is contained within the renal capsule and surrounds the architecture of the organ, unlike free fluid due to trauma or ascites. It also contains echoes and does not have the typical anechoic black appearance of free fluid.

GAIN

Certain artifacts can obscure free fluid in the FAST exam. Too much total gain or far gain (TGC) can actually "wash out" important parts of the image. This can be especially apparent in views through the bladder where the posterior enhancement (a bright white area behind the fluid-filled bladder) can obscure small amounts of anechoic free fluid that may have settled around this organ. This can be avoided by decreasing the far gain or TGC.

AVOIDING FALSE POSITIVES

As noted above, there are several situations where it may appear that there is free fluid when it does not exist. The abdominal portion of the FAST exam should be very specific in experienced hands, and reasonably sensitive for significant free fluid. However, the novice sonographer should be very sure that fluid is truly present before making clinical decisions based on the FAST exam.

INTEGRATION OF BEDSIDE ABDOMINAL ULTRASOUND INTO CLINICAL CARE

Bedside ultrasound evaluation for free fluid should be incorporated into the evaluation of both the traumatic and non-traumatic patient. Ultrasound is rapid, noninvasive, and sensitive for detecting significant fluid in the thoracoabdominal cavity. The equipment is relatively inexpensive and the exam requires no preparation, making it relatively easy to perform at the bedside of the trauma or critical care patient. Ultrasound does not expose the patient to contrast medium or ionizing radiation like CT scan imaging and can prevent the unstable patient from being transported out of the department.

A new finding of free fluid by ultrasound in a trauma patient is assumed to be hemorrhage until proven otherwise, and usually indicates significant injury. However, CT scan remains a more sensitive modality for many significant traumatic injuries and is more specific at defining the exact injury when it is present. In a stable patient with either a positive FAST or a negative fast and a significant suspicion of thoracoabdominal injury, a CT examination should still typically be performed.

In the non-traumatic situation, bedside ultrasound in the evaluation for free fluid can help secure the diagnosis and expedite treatment in certain patients. A pregnant patient with abdominal pain and/or hypotension and free peritoneal fluid most likely has a ruptured ectopic pregnancy that will require operative intervention. A patient with a history of liver or renal disease who complains of abdominal pain or fever may be diagnosed with new ascites and peritonitis. A quick search for free fluid in any of these patients may save time, resources and improve patient treatment and survival. An ultrasound evaluation looking for free fluid should be incorporated into the algorithm of any patient presenting with undifferentiated abdominal pain or hypotension.

Additional Reading

Hosek W, McCarthy M. Trauma ultrasound and the 2005 Cochrane Review. *Ann Emerg Med.* 2007;50(5):619-621.

Jehle D, Stiller G, Wagner D. Sensitivity in detecting free intraperitoneal fluid with the pelvic views of the FAST exam. *Am J Emerg Med.* 2003;21(6):476-478.

McGahan JP, Richards JR. Blunt abdominal trauma: the role of emergent sonography and a review of the literature. *AJR Am J Roentgenol.* 1999;172:897-903.

Melniker L, Leibner E, McKenney M, Lopez P, Briggs W, Mancuso C. Randomized controlled clinical trial of point-of-care, limited ultrasonography for trauma in the emergency department: the first sonography outcomes assessment program trial. *Ann Emerg Med.* 2006;48:227-234.

Stengel D, Bauwens K, Schouli J, et al. Emergency ultrasound-based algorithms for diagnosing blunt abdominal trauma. *Coch Rev.* 2005;18(2):1-19.

10 Renal and Urinary System Ultrasound

James Q. Hwang and Cori McClure Poffenberger

BACKGROUND AND INDICATIONS FOR EXAMINATION

The urinary system is very amenable to imaging with ultrasound. The liver and spleen provide windows through which the kidneys can be visualized. The bladder is located directly behind the pubic symphysis and is readily seen from the suprapubic approach, particularly when full. Ultrasound of the kidneys and bladder can play a vital role in the effective management of patients in the emergent and critical care setting. Focused renal and urinary ultrasound can determine the presence of hydronephrosis, directly visualize stones, and measure bladder volume. Ultrasound easily identifies renal cysts, and may identify masses or clots in the kidneys or bladder. Ultrasound may guide urinary procedures such as ensuring correct Foley catheter placement, and suprapubic bladder aspiration.

Focused renal ultrasound should be incorporated into the examination of any patient with undifferentiated flank or abdominal pain. Ureteral stones can be difficult to visualize because they are retroperitoneal, but the presence of hydronephrosis on the side of the pain is very specific for ureterolithiasis as the cause of the patient's symptoms. Patients with abdominal, back, or flank pain may also have more serious diagnoses such as abdominal aortic aneurysm or dissection, cholecystitis, ovarian torsion, ruptured ectopic pregnancy, and others. Bedside ultrasound may be helpful in diagnosing other causes of pain although other imaging modalities such as consultant-performed ultrasound or CT may be required if the diagnosis remains uncertain.

Bedside ultrasound evaluation of the urinary system should be performed in patients presenting with the following:

- Acute renal failure
- Abdominal pain or flank pain suspicious for renal colic
- Back, abdominal, or pelvic pain of uncertain cause
- Urinary retention
- Palpable abdominal or flank mass
- Renal trauma
- Gross hematuria

PROBE SELECTION AND TECHNICAL CONSIDERATIONS

CURVILINEAR PROBE WITH A FREQUENCY OF 3.0–5.0 MHz

When imaging the kidneys and bladder, the curvilinear probe with a frequency of 3.0–5.0 MHz should be utilized. Alternatively, a phased-array probe with a frequency of 2.0–4.0 MHz can be used to visualize the kidneys through the intercostal spaces. Lower frequencies, which improve penetration, can provide better visualization in obese patients.

TISSUE HARMONIC IMAGING

Another ultrasound machine setting that can be of particular use in renal imaging is tissue harmonics. Renal stones, which are often made up of calcium, block the penetration of the ultrasound beam and produce an acoustic shadow. Tissue harmonics enhance acoustic shadowing and may improve the identification of nephrolithiasis.

DEPTH

The sonographer should start with adequate depth in order to not miss abnormalities in the far field. This is important for findings such as free fluid around the bladder, which is easily missed if subtle. Once the far field is fully interrogated, the depth can be decreased in order to make sure the kidneys or bladder are taking up most of the screen.

GAIN AND TIME-GAIN COMPENSATION

The overall gain can be adjusted in order to brighten the image if needed. In patients with difficult anatomy or obesity, the far field is often what is difficult to visualize. In these patients, the far gain or time-gain compensation can be turned up to improve the deeper parts of the image. However, with a full bladder the sound travels so easily that the brightness in the far field can "wash out" the image and cover up pathological findings, especially free fluid. This is known as posterior acoustic enhancement and reducing the far-field gain may help minimize this issue.

FOCAL ZONE

To optimize the image, the focal zone (area of maximal lateral resolution) should be positioned at the depth of the kidney or bladder.

COLOR-FLOW AND POWER DOPPLER

Color-flow Doppler may help distinguish renal vasculature from hydronephrosis, both of which can appear as anechoic areas in the renal hilum. Vessels should show color flow while hydronephrosis does not. Power Doppler, which shows the presence of flow only without regard to velocity and direction, is good at picking up low-flow states. Doppler can help to evaluate the presence of urinary bladder jets in ruling out obstruction, which is discussed later in this chapter. Doppler placed over kidney stones may display a "twinkling" artifact that can help identify stones.

NORMAL ULTRASOUND ANATOMY

KIDNEYS

The kidneys lie within the retroperitoneum, in a space that also includes the adrenal glands, proximal collecting system, and perinephric fat. Typically, the left kidney is positioned more superiorly and posteriorly than the right kidney, while the right kidney is often slightly larger in size. A difference in size up to 2 cm between the kidneys may be normal. The kidneys generally lie between T12 and L4 or between the eighth and eleventh ribs. Their average size is 9–13 cm in length, 4–6 cm in width, and 2.5–3.5 cm in depth (Fig. 10-1). The right kidney is surrounded by the liver anteriorly, the diaphragm superiorly, and the psoas and quadratus lumborum muscles posteriorly. The left kidney is surrounded by the spleen, large and small bowel, and stomach anteriorly, the diaphragm superiorly, and the psoas and quadratus lumborum muscles posteriorly.

Each kidney is surrounded by three outer layers: closest to the kidney lies the true fibrous capsule, next is a layer of perirenal fat, and finally, Gerota fascia,

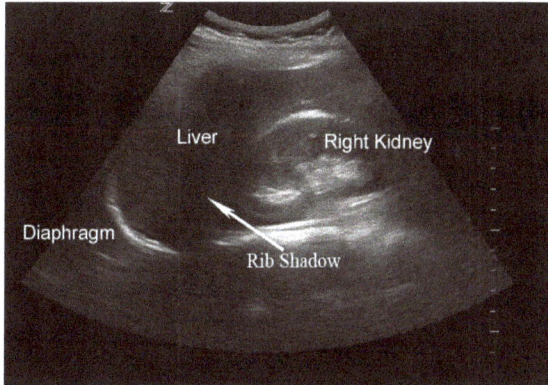

FIGURE 10-1 A longitudinal view of a normal right kidney. This image was obtained with the probe in a coronal position, pointed toward the patient's head, in the mid-to-anterior axillary line. Also visualized are the liver and right hemidiaphragm. Within the architecture of the liver is a black anechoic stripe representing a rib shadow. Rib shadows can obscure important findings, and therefore, the sonographer must attempt to scan around them. This can be achieved by asking the patient to take a deep breath in and out, which will move the liver and kidneys out from beneath the ribs. In addition, the probe can be moved down a rib space, it can be angled more obliquely in between the ribs, or a probe with a smaller footprint may be used.

which also encloses the adrenal glands. The true fibrous capsule is quite echogenic, is easily visualized on ultrasound, and outlines the kidney. The kidney itself can be further subdivided into the renal parenchyma and the renal sinus. The renal parenchyma is considered the body of the kidney and consists of the renal cortex and the renal medulla. The cortex and medulla are divided by an imaginary line running along the outside of the medullary pyramids. The cortex contains the filtration apparatus of the nephrons and appears more hypoechoic and less echogenic than either the liver or spleen. The medullary pyramids have their base toward the cortex while the papillae drain into the renal fornices. The fornices, in turn, empty into the calyces, which then merge to form the renal pelvis. As the urine-producing segment of the kidney, the renal medulla typically appears less echogenic than the renal cortex. The renal sinus is the central portion of the kidney and consists of the calyces, vasculature, lymphatics, and peripelvic fat. Due to the peripelvic fat, the renal sinus usually appears echogenic or bright. In general, there are 8–18 minor calyces that coalesce to form 2–3 major calyces. The major calyces empty into the renal pelvis and proximal ureter. The renal hilum can be defined as the entrance to the renal sinus and is occupied by the renal artery, renal vein, and the proximal ureter. The renal vasculature consists of the main renal artery, which branches into interlobar arteries, followed by arcuate arteries, and finally interlobular arteries. The arcuate arteries course along the base of the medullary pyramids and can be important sonographic landmarks. The renal veins run parallel to the course of the arteries.

URETERS

The ureters drain the renal pelvis and are retroperitoneal structures that run along the anterior and medial surface of the psoas muscle. In the pelvis, they course anterior to the iliac vessels and enter the bladder at a postero-inferior angle. They are approximately 6 mm in diameter and can be difficult to image through their entire course as they often become obscured by bowel gas. Typically, the ureters are not well visualized unless they are markedly dilated. The three most common places for ureteral obstruction due to kidney stones are: (1) where the renal pelvis begins to drain into the ureter (the ureteropelvic junction or UPJ), (2) as the ureter crosses the pelvic brim, and (3) where the ureter enters the bladder (the uretero-vesicular junction or UVJ).

Ureteral jets are intermittent streams of urine expressed into the bladder by the normal peristalsis of the ureters. While they may be seen with B-mode or gray-scale imaging, power or color-flow Doppler can more easily visualize these jets. When using Doppler, the pulse repetition frequency, also known as scale, needs to be decreased in order to detect these lower-flow velocities. Ureteral jets are seen as bursts of color entering from the base of the bladder and flowing toward its center. These jets occur at regular intervals, approximately every 15–20 seconds in a well-hydrated patient, and typically last under a second (Fig. 10-2). When scanning for ureteral jets, it is important to scan slowly through the bladder, focus-ing over the trigone, looking for these intermittent pulsatile contractions. If ure-teral jets are not visualized, this can suggest the presence of obstruction, particu-larly if a unilateral jet is seen on the unaffected side. Conversely, documenting the presence of bilateral ureteral jets suggests the lack of significant obstruction.

BLADDER

The bladder is a triangular structure located within the pelvis, directly behind the pubic symphysis. The apex or vertex of the bladder is located anteriorly and is connected to the umbilicus by the median umbilical ligament, which is the rem-nant of the urachus. The bladder can be further divided into the fundus, body, trigone, and neck. The fundus or base of the bladder faces posteriorly toward the rectum, along the back of which run the seminal vesicles and terminal portions of the vas deferens. The neck of the bladder leads to the urethra. The ureters enter the

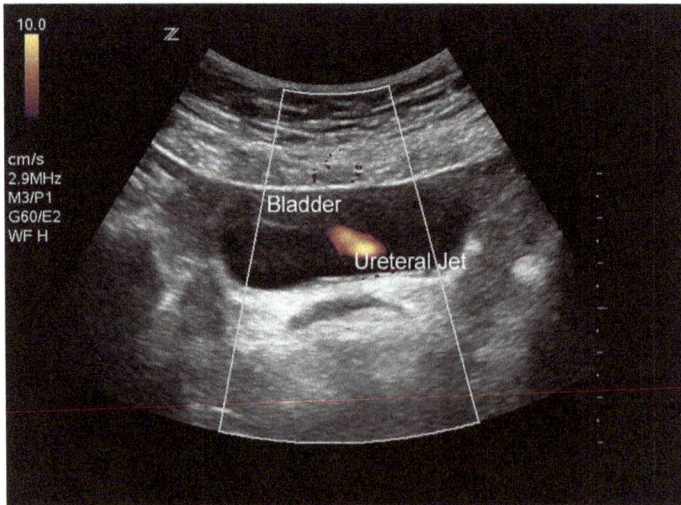

FIGURE 10-2 Transverse view through the trigone of the urinary bladder illustrating a left ureteral jet using power Doppler. The left ureteral jet is seen entering from the base of the bladder and flowing toward the center.

bladder at a postero-inferior angle. In most people, the bladder is a thin-walled, anechoic, urine-filled structure with a wall that is 3–6 mm thick (see Fig. 10-2). In males, the prostate is located posterior and inferior to the bladder and in females the cervix occupies this posterior position. The prostate normally measures less than 5 cm in its maximum dimension. A diffusely enlarged prostate may be consistent with benign prostatic hypertrophy, while an asymmetric or irregular deformity of the prostate may be more suggestive of possible malignancy. Ultrasound does not reliably differentiate between hypertrophy and carcinoma; therefore, any concerning abnormalities should be referred for further management.

IMAGING TIPS AND PROTOCOL

KIDNEYS

In a patient with suspected pathology, the sonographer should begin with the unaffected side, in order to have a baseline image to compare the potentially abnormal kidney to. The patient should be placed in a supine or lateral decubitus position to help bring the kidneys out from beneath the ribs. The kidneys should be viewed primarily in a coronal plane, although other planes may be helpful. The right kidney is more easily visualized due to the large acoustic window provided by the liver. In order to obtain a coronal view, the probe should be placed in the mid-to-anterior axillary line between the eighth and eleventh rib spaces with the transducer pointing toward the patient's head (Fig. 10-3a). The left kidney is

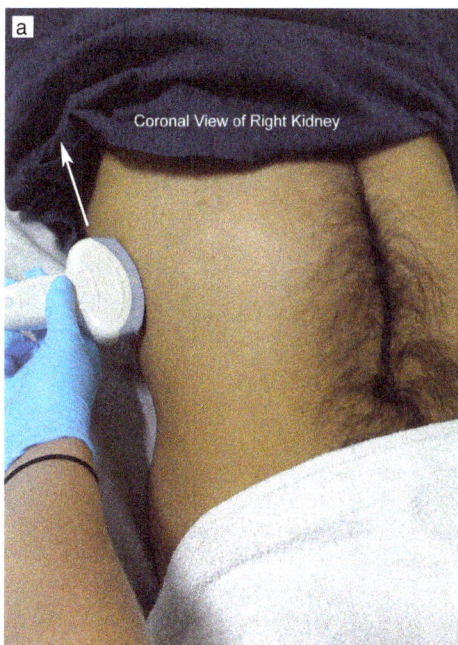

Coronal View of Right Kidney

FIGURE 10-3(a) The proper positioning of patient and probe for right kidney imaging. Notice the probe is in a coronal orientation with the indicator pointing toward the patient's head (arrow) in the mid-to-anterior axillary line.

more difficult to visualize due to its slightly more posterior and superior location. The probe position on this side should be adjusted accordingly and placed in the posterior axillary line between the sixth and ninth rib spaces (Fig. 10-3b). Oftentimes, the lateral decubitus position or the use of a phased-array probe to image between the ribs is required to adequately image the left kidney. The kidneys often lie somewhat obliquely; therefore, in order to obtain an adequate long-axis view the transducer may need to be rotated slightly from the coronal plane. The transducer may be rotated 90° from the coronal position in order to obtain a transverse view. The kidney should be visualized in its entirety from the superior pole down to the inferior pole and from anterior to posterior surfaces.

BLADDER

Images of the bladder are best obtained with the patient supine and when the bladder is full. The bladder should be imaged in two planes, both sagittal and transverse, to ensure that the entire structure is appropriately visualized. The transducer should be placed just above the pubic symphysis and angled inferiorly to look down into the pelvis (Fig. 10-4). In the transverse position, the probe indicator should be pointed toward the patient's right side and fanned superiorly and inferiorly to evaluate the whole structure. In the sagittal position, the probe indicator should be pointed toward the patient's head and fanned to the left and right.

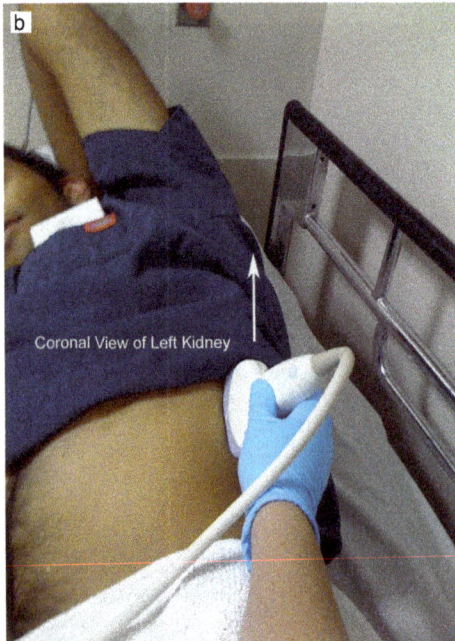

FIGURE 10-3(b) The proper positioning of patient and probe for left kidney imaging. The patient is in a lateral decubitus position with the probe in a coronal orientation with the indicator pointing toward the patient's head (arrow) in the posterior axillary line.

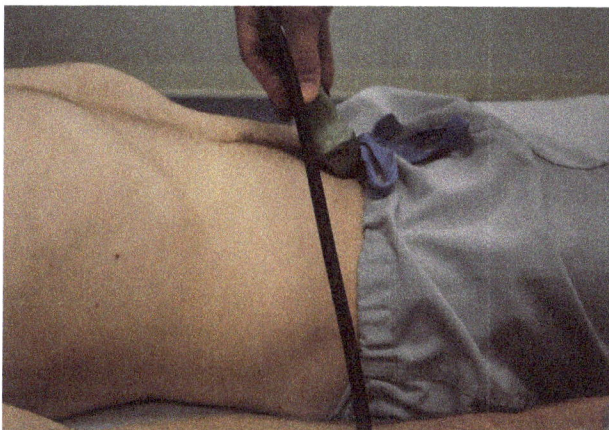

FIGURE 10-4 Proper positioning of the patient and probe to obtain a transverse view of the bladder. The probe is placed above the pubic symphysis in a transverse orientation with the indicator pointing toward the patient's right side. Notice the probe is angled inferiorly looking down into the pelvis.

PATHOLOGIC ULTRASOUND FINDINGS

HYDRONEPHROSIS

The most common indication for performing renal and urinary ultrasound is to evaluate hydronephrosis. Hydronephrosis is diagnosed when an anechoic area is noted within the renal sinus that is not vascular in origin. Color-flow Doppler can be used to differentiate between renal vasculature and true dilatation of the collecting system. When hydronephrosis ("hydro") is present, it is important to determine if the obstruction is unilateral or bilateral. While a patient with acute pain and hydro almost invariably has a kidney stone, there are other causes of unilateral hydro such as compression from a mass lesion or retroperitoneal lymphadenopathy. Bilateral hydro can occur with bladder outlet obstruction, pregnancy, and neurogenic bladder. Possible etiologies for bladder outlet obstruction include prostatic enlargement, bladder mass or clot, posterior urethral valves, or other forms of urethral obstruction. Simply not urinating, such as may occur in a trauma patient on a backboard after a few beers, may cause bilateral hydro. During pregnancy, maximal dilatation of the collecting system occurs at around 38 weeks' gestation, with hydronephrosis typically more prominent in the right kidney than the left. If hydronephrosis persists for greater than 2 weeks, permanent renal damage may occur. Hydronephrosis is graded as follows:

1. Mild or grade I: Prominent calyces and mild splaying of the renal pelvis (Fig. 10-5)
2. Moderate or grade II: Significant dilation of the renal pelvis into the calyces, typically causing a classic three-pronged anechoic area known as the "bear claw or paw" (Fig. 10-6)
3. Severe or grade III: The severely dilated collecting system causes cortical thinning (Fig. 10-7)

The grade of hydronephrosis does not correlate well with either the acuity or degree of obstruction. Hydronephrosis can be acute or chronic and comparison to

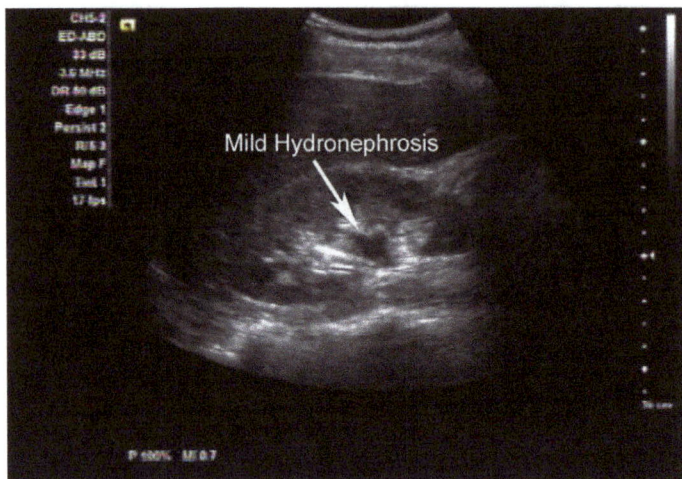

FIGURE 10-5 Mild hydronephrosis is characterized by prominent calyces and mild splaying of the renal pelvis.

prior imaging studies can be very helpful. In addition, both kidneys should be imaged and compared to one another.

In acute ureteral obstruction, forniceal rupture may occur, resulting in urine collecting around the kidney in the retroperitoneal space. This finding of perirenal fluid within Gerota fascia can easily be misinterpreted as a positive FAST exam (Fig. 10-8). Forniceal rupture occurs in up to 2%–3% of patients presenting with renal colic and accounts for up to 10% of perirenal abscesses; therefore, expedited urology follow-up is essential.

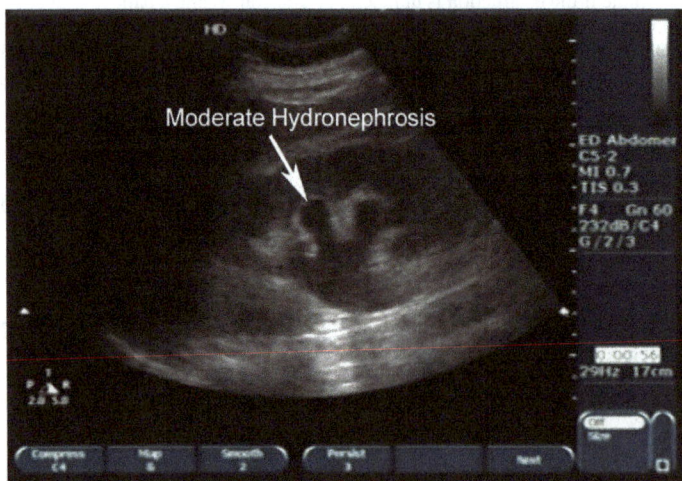

FIGURE 10-6 Moderate hydronephrosis is characterized by a "bear claw or paw" appearance of the collecting system.

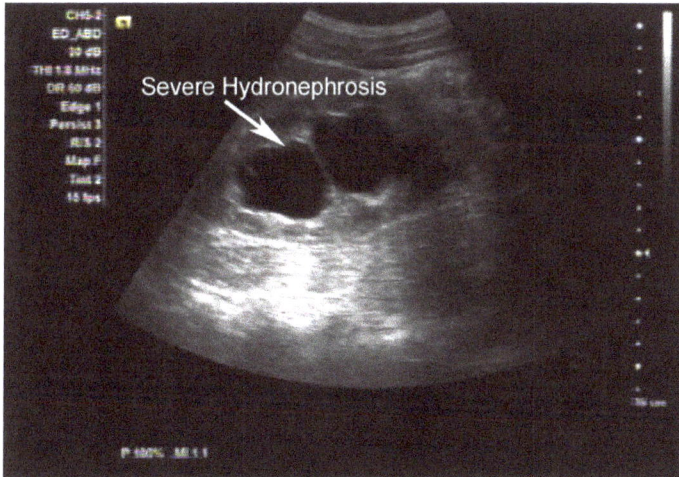

FIGURE 10-7 Severe hydronephrosis is characterized by dilatation that results in cortical thinning.

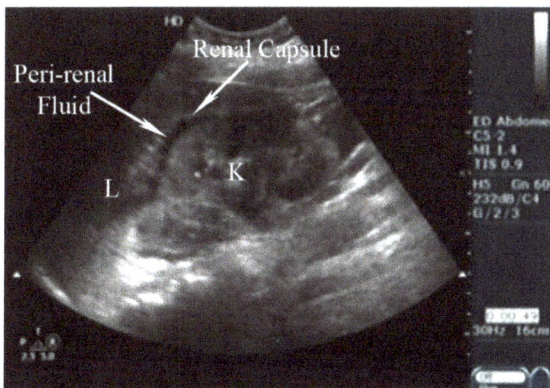

FIGURE 10-8 Hydronephrosis with forniceal rupture. This image illustrates perirenal fluid collection within the renal capsule. Note how the fluid traces the outline of the kidney and is within the hyperechoic renal capsule and does not lie in Morrison's pouch between the kidney (K) and liver (L).

NEPHROLITHIASIS

Renal stones are a common reason for patients presenting to the emergency department (ED). As much as 12% of the population experiences a kidney stone during their lifetime, and there are over a million ED visits per year for this problem in the United States. A non-contrast or "flank pain" CT is often a first-line test for suspected renal colic, but it is costly and involves ionizing radiation and may not be necessary in all patients.

As many as 80% of patients with significant renal colic may have hydronephrosis. While the presence of hydro and acute flank pain strongly suggests a kidney stone, hydro may be present with either small or large stones. While more than 95% of stones that are 6 mm or under will pass spontaneously, ones that are larger than 7 mm in size will likely need urologic intervention. If a large stone is suspected, a plain film (KUB) is likely to detect it, and may help follow its progress. CT scan may be avoided if the differential diagnosis does not include other high-risk abdominal pathology that must be ruled out.

In addition to identifying hydro, ultrasound can identify stones located within the renal parenchyma and may visualize stones located at the UPJ or UVJ. Renal stones can be identified by their hyperechoic appearance with associated posterior acoustic shadowing. While parenchymal stones are unlikely to be the actual cause of discomfort, they indicate that the patient is a "stone former" and may have a ureteral stone that is causing pain. The presence of a ureteral jet on the unaffected side and a lack of one on the side with pain typically indicates obstruction from a kidney stone. While the presence of obstruction in acute pain indicates ureterolithiasis, obstruction may occur with small stones that will ultimately pass and does not determine the need for intervention.

RENAL CYSTS

Renal cysts are a common finding in the kidneys, occurring in 25%–50% of people over the age of 50. Simple renal cysts typically arise from the renal cortex and are round, thin-walled, smooth, and anechoic (Fig. 10-9). They often will exhibit posterior enhancement artifact (brightness behind the cyst), similar to other cystic structures. On occasion, simple cysts can be problematic if they become so large that they distort the normal renal architecture. In contrast, complex renal cysts are characterized by thick walls, septations, and an irregular or heterogeneous appearance. Complex cysts require further imaging to rule out malignancy. The kidneys of patients with polycystic kidney disease (PCKD) have numerous cysts of varied sizes throughout the renal parenchyma (Fig. 10-10). Patients with PCKD often have cysts elsewhere, such as the liver (50%) or pancreas (5%), and

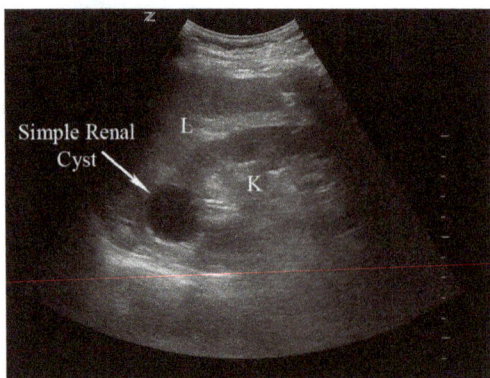

FIGURE 10-9 This image illustrates a longitudinal view of the kidney (K) and liver (L) showing a simple renal cyst. Notice that this cyst is regular-appearing, round, thin-walled, and anechoic.

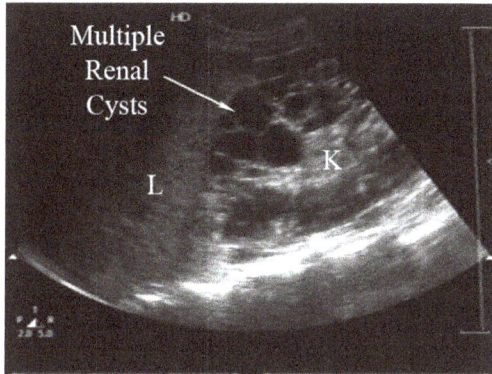

FIGURE 10-10 A longitudinal view of the liver (L) and kidney (K). This image illustrates multiple cysts within the kidney that have distorted the normal renal architecture, which is very typical of PCKD. Other organs, including the liver and pancreas, should be examined looking for similar findings.

imaging of these other organs may be helpful when multiple cysts are found in the kidneys. In addition, these patients are at risk for cerebral aneurysms (20%), and often progress to renal insufficiency and failure. As such, they need long-term follow-up and management. A patient who presents with unexplained hematuria and/or uncontrolled hypertension should have this diagnosis considered, especially when there is a known family history of the disease.

RENAL MASSES

The most common solid renal mass is renal cell carcinoma, which accounts for approximately 3% of adult malignancies and 90% of neoplasms arising from the kidney. Masses can be isoechoic in echotexture and without distinct borders or contours, making them difficult to detect by ultrasound. Because renal cell carcinoma has a variable sonographic appearance and is the most common solid renal mass, all renal masses should be considered malignant until proven otherwise. Discerning whether the mass arises from the kidney itself or from adjacent structures can be quite challenging. A common pitfall is mistaking an adrenal mass for a renal mass. Patients with suspected renal masses should undergo additional consultant-performed imaging (often with CT or MRI) and require follow-up.

Another type of solid renal mass is an angiomyolipoma, also known as a renal hamartoma. This is a benign tumor and usually asymptomatic. However, it may enlarge and bleed, resulting in flank pain, hematuria, and shock. Sonographically, angiomyolipomas appear as discrete, highly echogenic masses found in the renal cortex.

RENAL FAILURE

Ultrasound in new onset renal failure should be performed to determine if bilateral hydronephrosis is present from mechanical obstruction. Although uncommon (5% or less), bilateral ureteral obstruction or bladder obstruction is a treatable cause of renal failure.

Most renal failure is caused by dehydration or intrinsic kidney dysfunction. As renal failure progresses from acute to chronic, the echogenicity of the renal parenchyma will increase and the kidney may appear more echogenic than the adjacent liver or spleen. Patients with end-stage renal disease often have small, echogenic kidneys that are difficult to image sonographically.

BLADDER MASSES

Bladder masses can be visualized on ultrasound as projections from the bladder wall or as focal areas of wall thickening. Transitional cell carcinoma is the most common bladder mass. Bladder diverticulae, which are out-pouches of the wall, may appear similar to a bladder mass on bedside ultrasound. Typically, diverticulae are rounded, well-defined, thin-walled cystic structures located near the UVJ. These pouch-like invaginations can vary greatly in size and may become infected.

Bladder wall thickening can also be seen with prolonged or recurrent infection. In the developing world, schistosomiasis is a common cause of bladder wall thickening, and ultrasound may be used to diagnose and follow disease progression.

BLADDER VOLUME MEASUREMENT

Bedside ultrasound is useful for assessing bladder volume. Difficulties in voiding or decreased urinary output in a patient with a Foley catheter already in place are frequent complaints in the acute care setting. Pre- and post-void bladder volumes can be determined easily with minimal patient discomfort.

In patients with existing Foley catheters, bedside ultrasound can verify balloon location to ensure proper placement, assess for appropriate bladder decompression, and evaluate the presence of clot in the bladder (Fig. 10-11). The ability to accurately estimate bladder volume is particularly useful in pediatric patients where documenting a full bladder prior to catheterization can avoid an unsuccessful invasive procedure. If available, bladder volume can be measured utilizing the

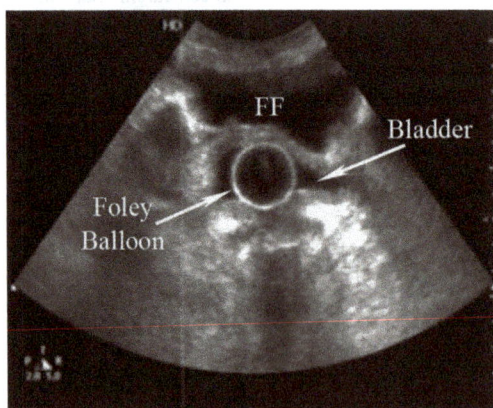

FIGURE 10-11 Transverse view of the bladder in a patient with ascites. This patient has a Foley catheter in place evidenced by the visualized inflated balloon and almost complete decompression of the bladder. Free fluid (FF) is also seen in the pelvis outside the bladder and could easily be mistaken as the bladder itself.

calculation tools provided by the ultrasound machine. If utilizing a machine without such software, the standard equation to estimate bladder volume is

$$\text{Length} \times \text{Width} \times \text{Height} \times 0.75$$

The length and width should both be obtained in a transverse image, while the height is measured in a sagittal view (see Fig. 10-12).

COMMON PITFALLS

INADEQUATE VIEWS OF THE KIDNEYS

Images may be impaired by poor patient positioning or obesity. It is important that the whole kidney is interrogated, including the inferior pole, which is often the hardest area to visualize. The inferior pole can be the site of a cyst or mass and is the first place where free fluid will collect due to gravity. When views of the kidneys are limited, consider asking the patient to maximally inspire and to then hold their breath. Alternatively, consider rolling the patient into the lateral decubitus position with the kidney being examined in the superior position. Both of these maneuvers shift the kidneys inferiorly and out from below the ribs.

In order to optimize technique, it is important to remember that the kidneys are retroperitoneal structures; therefore, the transducer must be directed and fanned posteriorly to bring them into view. The left kidney, given its more superior and posterior location, is often more challenging to image than the right. When rib shadows obstruct or limit the view, consider rotating the probe in a clockwise direction to move the transducer face into a more parallel alignment with the ribs. The same maneuver can be performed on the right kidney by rotating the transducer instead in a counterclockwise direction.

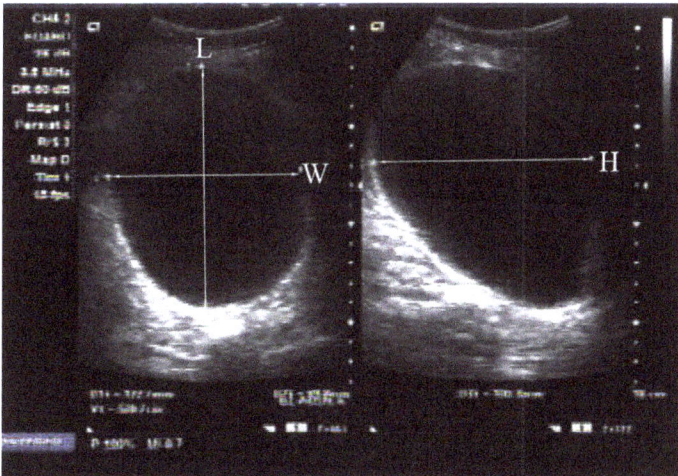

FIGURE 10-12 Image illustrating the calculation of bladder volume. The left panel shows a transverse image of the bladder with correct measurements of the width (W) and length (L). The right panel illustrates a sagittal view with calculation of the bladder height (H). The product of these three numbers multiplied by 0.75 provides a good estimate of total bladder volume.

If the kidneys are not visualized despite thorough interrogation and image optimization, consider scanning inferiorly as the patient may have an anatomic variant, such as a horseshoe kidney or ectopic pelvic kidney. Horseshoe kidney is the most common fusion anomaly and should be suspected when the inferior poles of the kidneys are difficult to image. When patients are obese, remember to decrease the frequency, which increases the penetration, and to increase the depth.

MISINTERPRETATION OF HYDRONEPHROSIS

The sonographer must be careful in diagnosing mild hydronephrosis as there are other findings that may resemble this entity on bedside ultrasound. Mild hydronephrosis may also be a normal finding, perhaps in a patient who needs to urinate. Examining the unaffected kidney first is always of great utility and may help avoid this error, as it provides a baseline image with which to compare the affected side. Use of the "split-screen" mode allows for direct side-by-side comparison of the kidneys on the ultrasound monitor. If findings of hydronephrosis exist only on one side, it makes the diagnosis more likely.

Other common false positives for hydronephrosis include dilated renal vessels, peripelvic renal cysts, or an extra renal pelvis. Color-flow Doppler can differentiate hydronephrosis from renal vessels. An extra renal pelvis is an anatomic variant and can be differentiated from hydronephrosis based on two findings: first, the area of dilatation will appear outside the renal parenchyma and renal sinus; second, the renal papillae will not be obliterated and the calyces will not be blunted. Similarly, a peripelvic cyst, while adjacent to the renal pelvis, will be completely encapsulated.

It is important to remember that the assessment for hydronephrosis may be limited by the patient's state of hydration. Patients who are obstructed but dehydrated will not always demonstrate the characteristic findings of hydronephrosis. Scanning after fluid resuscitation may help detect hydro.

MISINTERPRETATION OF RENAL MASSES AND CYSTS

Cysts should only be considered simple if all criteria are met: round, thin-walled, and completely anechoic. If a complex cyst or mass is discovered, consultant-performed imaging and urology consultation is essential.

The columns of Bertin can hypertrophy and extend into the renal sinus and mimic a renal mass. They can be differentiated from true renal masses, however, based on their similar echogenicity to the rest of the renal cortex and on their containing a renal pyramid.

MISTAKING FREE FLUID FOR THE BLADDER

The bladder forms a rectangular border to the pelvis. Significant free fluid in the pelvis may be mistaken for the bladder. It is important to scan all the way through the anechoic area, and to identify the walls of the bladder to make sure you are seeing bladder, and not free fluid, or vice versa. A somewhat full bladder or Foley balloon may help to identify this (see Fig. 10-11).

INTEGRATION OF BEDSIDE RENAL AND BLADDER ULTRASOUND INTO CLINICAL CARE

The use of bedside ultrasound in evaluating both the kidneys and bladder has increased substantially in the acute care setting. It has proven to be beneficial as a quick first-line evaluation for patients presenting with undifferentiated abdominal or flank pain, hematuria, urinary retention, or acute renal failure.

Bedside ultrasound not only helps to expedite the diagnosis and management of patients, but also helps in the decision to order higher-level testing, such as a CT scan or MRI, or in obtaining appropriate consultation. The routine performance of a bedside ultrasound on patients who present with abdominal or flank complaints can help to diagnose more serious conditions, such as an abdominal aortic aneurysm or internal bleeding. Likewise, it can prevent the patient from being exposed to unnecessary radiation when the condition is not life threatening, such as a patient with a presentation typical for renal colic who has hydronephrosis. If the pain is easily controlled, this patient can follow up with urology as an outpatient, perhaps with a KUB to rule out a large stone.

It is always important for the clinician to exercise caution before attributing patient's symptoms to the findings found on ultrasound. For example, renal stones are common, and parenchymal stones may not be the cause of the patient's symptoms. The sonographer must maintain a broad differential and incorporate the ultrasound findings into the entire context of the patient presentation. If interrogation of the kidneys and bladder is unrevealing, other abdominal and pelvic ultrasound exams should be considered in order to rule out life-threatening abnormalities. Consultant-performed imaging should be obtained for any uncertain or abnormal findings and follow-up care should be arranged as indicated.

Additional Reading

Chan H. Noninvasive bladder volume measurement. *J Neurosci Nurs.* 1993; 25(5):309.

Chapman JP, Gonzalez J, Diokno AC. Significance of urinary extravasation during renal colic. *Urology.* 1987;30(6):541-545.

Gaspari RJ, Horst K. Emergency ultrasound and urinalysis in the evaluation of flank pain. *Acad Emerg Med.* 2005;12(12):1180-1184.

Sheafor DH, Hertzberg BS, Freed KS, et al. Nonenhanced helical CT and US in the emergency department evaluation of patients with renal colic: prospective comparison. *Radiology.* 2000; (217):792-797.

Teichman J. Clinical practice. Acute renal colic from ureteral calculus. *N Engl J Med.* 2004;(350):684-693.

11 Hepatobiliary Ultrasound

Kristin Carmody

BACKGROUND AND INDICATIONS FOR EXAMINATION

Biliary tract disease exists as a spectrum that ranges from asymptomatic gallstones to biliary colic, cholecystitis, choledocholithiasis, and cholangitis. The incidence of gallstones is approximately 10%–20% and is dependent on several factors such as age, gender, fertility, race, ethnicity, and associated comorbidities. Only 1%–3% of individuals with gallstones report being symptomatic. Biliary colic occurs when a gallstone temporarily obstructs either the common bile duct (CBD) or cystic duct. Usually, biliary colic is self-limited and treated with analgesia and elective cholecystectomy. Cholecystitis results from prolonged obstruction of the cystic duct and causes inflammation of the gallbladder (GB), necessitating more urgent surgical removal. Complications of cholecystitis can lead to infection, empyema, gangrene, necrosis, perforation, and sepsis. Cholecystitis is usually caused by an obstructing gallstone, but acalculous blockage does occasionally occur.

Choledocholithiasis is a result of prolonged obstruction of the CBD. This disease can also occur post cholecystectomy when there are retained gallstones after surgery. Cholangitis is an ascending infection of the biliary tract. It can be due to prolonged obstruction from a gallstone and a resultant bacterial infection of the bile. It is a rare complication of cholecystitis, usually occurring in the elderly or in patients with associated comorbidities. Cholangitis has a high morbidity and mortality that increases with a delay in diagnosis.

Ultrasound is a rapid, noninvasive, well-tolerated, and sensitive modality in diagnosing both biliary colic and cholecystitis. Therefore, it is the first imaging modality of choice for suspected biliary disease in both the critical care and out-patient setting. The use of bedside ultrasound is important in order to rapidly identify this disease and prevent complications that result from diagnostic delays. The sensitivity of ultrasound has been reported to be as high as 95%. The four sonographic signs of cholecystitis (stones, sonographic Murphy's sign, wall thickening, and pericholecystic fluid) are highly specific when all four are present, although this is uncommon and any of the four signs may be nonspecific, particularly in isolation. The combination of a positive sonographic Murphy's sign and gallstones has been shown to have a positive predictive value for chole-cystitis as high as 96%. Hepatobiliary iminodiacetic acid (HIDA) scans (nuclear medicine scans) are used when ultrasound results are equivocal and the diagnosis is still suspected. HIDA scans have a reported sensitivity and specificity of roughly 95%.

Ultrasound is not highly sensitive for diagnosing choledocholithiasis. Although it may not be the best modality for diagnosing choledocholithiasis, the combination of a dilated common bile duct on ultrasound with lab abnormalities helps narrow the diagnosis. Endoscopic retrograde cholangiopancreatography (ERCP) and magnetic resonance cholangiopancreatography (MRCP) remain the gold standards for diagnosing this entity. Cholangitis is a clinical diagnosis (Charcot's triad: fever, right upper quadrant [RUQ] pain, and jaundice) associated with findings of cholecystitis or choledocholithias identified on ultrasound.

In addition to GB pathology, bedside ultrasound can be useful in evaluating for liver abnormalities, such as cysts, masses, abscesses, and hepatomegaly. A pancreatic pseudocyst or mass may also occasionally be diagnosed at the bedside. Finally, bedside ultrasound is ideal in the rapid diagnosis of new onset ascites in a patient who presents with abdominal pain and distension.

Bedside ultrasound evaluation of the hepatobiliary tract should be performed in:

- Any patient complaining of RUQ or epigastric pain
- Unexplained right-sided chest, shoulder, flank, or generalized abdominal pain
- The patient who presents with new jaundice
- The patient with abnormal liver or biliary function tests
- The patient who presents with abdominal distension or pain with suspicion of new ascites
- The sickle cell patient with abdominal pain
- Febrile or septic patients with an unidentified source, particularly the elderly

PROBE SELECTION AND TECHNICAL CONSIDERATIONS

CURVILINEAR PROBE WITH A FREQUENCY OF 3.5–5.0 MHz

A lower-frequency probe should be used for all hepatobiliary imaging. This probe provides better penetration, which is especially useful in obese patients who often have a higher incidence of GB disease.

DEPTH

Hepatobiliary scanning should begin at a greater depth in order to not miss pathology in the far field and to adequately image the portal triad (CBD, portal vein [PV], and hepatic artery [HA]). Once the area of interest is identified, the depth can be reduced so that the area of interest takes up approximately three-fourths of the screen.

FOCAL ZONE

The focal zone should be adjusted and placed at the depth of the structure being imaged. This improves the lateral resolution of the image. Focal zone may be particularly important when trying to elicit shadowing from suspected gallstones, and should be set at the level of the suspected stone.

GAIN OR TIME-GAIN COMPENSATION

The total gain, which increases the intensity or volume of the signal returning to the transducer and brightens the image on the screen, may need to be adjusted in hepatobiliary imaging. Often times, the near field is imaged adequately, but the far field (posterior GB or portal triad) is not visualized entirely. In this situation, time-gain compensation (TGC) can be adjusted in order to increase the far gain of the image. This produces an enhanced brighter signal returning from the far field and a resultant clearer image, but leaves the near field unadjusted. Adjustment of this control may be useful in obese patients with difficult anatomy.

COLOR-FLOW DOPPLER

Color-flow Doppler detects blood flow and is useful when attempting to differentiate ductal from vascular structures. The CBD lies just anterior to the PV. The CBD should not demonstrate flow, while the portal vessels and/or hepatics should light up when Doppler is turned on.

NORMAL ULTRASOUND ANATOMY

LIVER

The liver is located in the RUQ of the abdominal cavity just underneath the diaphragm. It is seen to the right of the stomach, superior to the intestines and overlying the GB. It is divided into four sections: the right, left, caudate, and quadrate lobes. The main lobar fissure (MLF) separates the liver into its right and left lobes and can be identified sonographically about 70% of the time, typically seen as a hyperechoic line between the neck of the GB and the portal vessels. The liver has two blood supplies, the hepatic artery (HA), which supplies blood from the aorta, and the PV that returns nutrients from the gastrointestinal tract and blood from the spleen. The normal liver should be less than 12.5–13.0 cm when measured from its superior border with the diaphragm across to the inferior tip. The falciform ligament attaches the liver to the anterior abdominal wall and can sometimes be visualized on ultrasound, especially in the presence of significant ascites.

The bile produced within the liver is contained within the intrahepatic biliary ducts. These intrahepatic ducts empty into the right and left hepatic ducts, which then merge to form the common hepatic duct. The common hepatic duct is part of the extrahepatic system as it exits the liver architecture. The common hepatic duct and the cystic duct from the GB merge to form the CBD, which joins the pancreatic duct to drain into the second part of the duodenum.

The normal liver on ultrasound appears homogenous with a medium echogenicity. The regular appearance of the liver and its large size allow it to be used as an important sonographic window for other structures, such as the right kidney, pancreas, and the heart in a subxiphoid view. The liver will contain regular-appearing anechoic structures within its architecture representing the portal and hepatic blood vessels and bile ducts (Fig. 11-1). These structures can be differentiated on ultrasound based on their different characteristics. Color-flow Doppler can be used to distinguish the vessels from bile ducts.

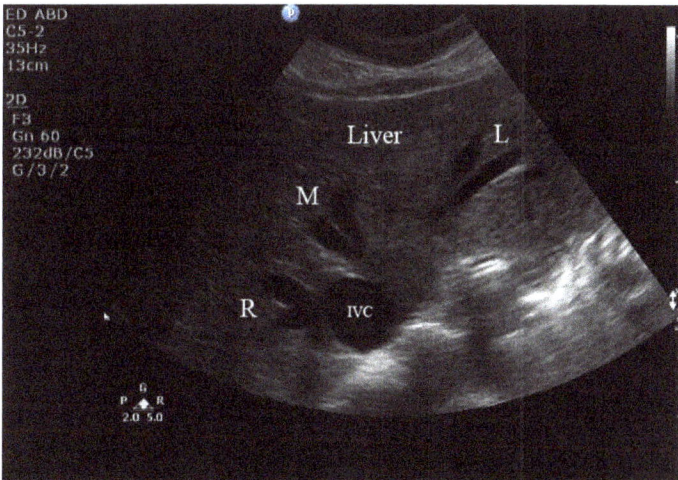

FIGURE 11-1 Coronal image of a normal liver with homogenous appearance. The hepatic veins (R: right, M: middle, L: left) can be seen coursing across the liver to drain into the inferior vena cava (IVC) at the posterior border.

The PV is formed from the confluence of the splenic and mesenteric veins. The portal vessels can be identified by their hyperechoic (white) border, a result of fatty tissue in the surrounding walls. The PV divides the liver into its superior and inferior segments.

The walls of the hepatic veins will appear thinner than the portal vessels and will not have the bright white hyperechoic border. The right, left, and middle hepatic veins drain the different lobes of the liver and converge as they drain into the inferior vena cava (IVC) (see Fig. 11-1). The IVC runs along the posterior border of the liver and empties into the right atrium of the heart. The hepatic veins divide the lobes of the liver into various segments: the right hepatic vein divides the right lobe into its anterior and posterior areas, the middle hepatic vein divides the liver into its right and left lobes, and the left hepatic vein divides the left lobe into its medial and lateral areas.

GALLBLADDER

The GB lies in the GB fossa located on the undersurface of the liver between the quadrate and right lobes. The GB consists of three portions: the fundus, body, and neck. The neck tapers into the biliary tree and connects to the cystic duct. The common hepatic duct drains the intrahepatic ducts and exits the liver to join the cystic duct and the two form the CBD (Fig. 11-2). The CBD then joins the pancreatic duct at the ampulla of Vater and drains into the second portion of the duodenum.

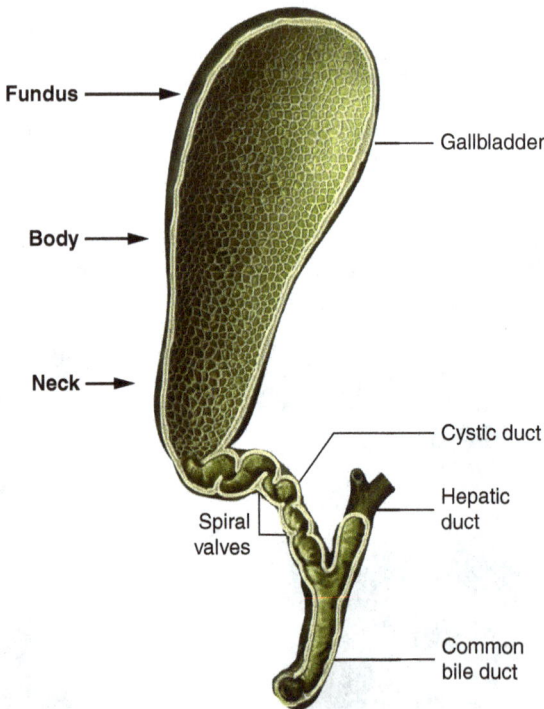

FIGURE 11-2 Normal anatomy of the gallbladder illustrating the fundus, body, and neck. The neck tapers down into the cystic duct and joins the common hepatic duct to form the common bile duct.

A normal GB measures about 3 cm wide × 8 cm long when it is fully distended. These measurements may vary somewhat depending on when the patient last ate a meal. A GB measuring over 10 cm in its longest dimension, particularly after a meal, is considered abnormally hydropic. The GB is a fluid-filled cystic organ and will appear as a round or elongated anechoic structure with thin walls on ultrasound. The normal GB wall is usually measured at less than 3 mm.

Landmarks   The landmarks of the GB include the MLF and the undivided right PV. The MLF divides the liver into its right and left lobes and can be identified on ultrasound in approximately 70% of all patients, but may be very short in some. It is visualized as a bright white hyperechoic line that extends from the portal triad up to the neck of the GB. The PV is formed by the union of the superior mesenteric vein and the splenic vein and divides just before entering the liver into the right and left PVs. It is the right portal vein (RPV) that constitutes the second landmark of the GB. In a sagittal image, with the transducer pointing cephalad, the RPV will be seen at one end of the MLF with the CBD and HA sitting just anteriorly to it, while the GB neck will be seen at the other end (Fig. 11-3).

When viewed in a transverse or short axis, the portal triad is often called the "Mickey Mouse sign" with the PV forming the face and the HA and CBD forming the ears (Fig. 11-4). The CBD is measured from inner wall to inner wall, and is typically 2–3 mm. The normal CBD diameter varies based on the age of the patient. The general rule is that the CBD is 1 mm by the age of 10 and increases by 1 mm for every decade after this. The upper limit of normal is considered to be around 7 mm in an older patient.

PANCREAS

Ultrasound is usually not the modality of choice for pancreatic imaging. Bowel gas causes significant gas scattering and resultant artifacts and can obscure normal pancreatic anatomy. Oftentimes, the pancreas is identified only when it contains abnormalities, such as pseudocysts, calcifications, or masses.

The vascular landmarks for the pancreas are the splenic and portal veins and the superior mesenteric artery (SMA). The head of the pancreas can be seen

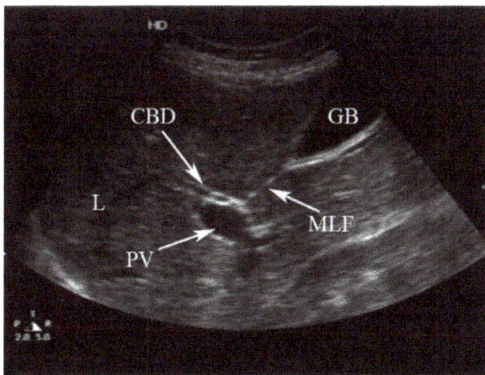

FIGURE 11-3 Sagittal image of the gallbladder (GB) with its landmarks, the undivided right portal vein (PV) and the main lobar fissure (MLF). The common bile duct (CBD) is seen with white hyperechoic walls just anterior to the portal vein. L: liver.

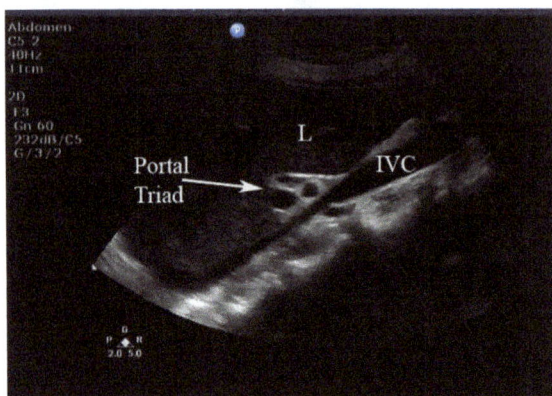

FIGURE 11-4 The portal triad seen as three round anechoic structures within the liver (L). The largest posterior structure is the portal vein. The hepatic artery and common bile duct sit anterior to the portal vein, seen as the ears of "Mickey Mouse." IVC: inferior vena cava.

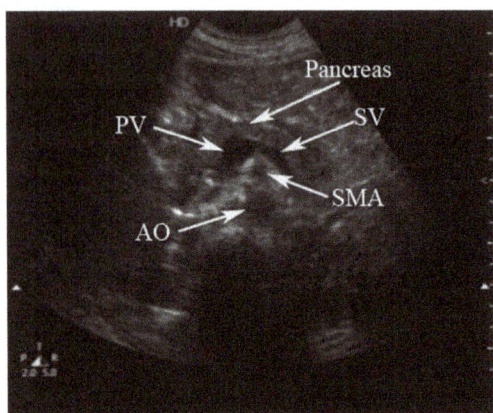

FIGURE 11-5 Transverse image of the pancreas. The body is seen anterior to the splenic vein (SV) and superior mesenteric artery (SMA). The head is seen anterior to the portal vein (PV). The SV is seen coursing along the posterior border of the organ. AO: aorta.

anterior to the PV and the body anterior to the splenic vein and SMA. The splenic vein runs posterior to the border of the pancreas in the epigastric region and can be seen draining into the portal vasculature (Fig. 11-5).

IMAGING TIPS AND PROTOCOL

Hepatobiliary imaging should include both longitudinal and transverse images in order to fully interrogate the RUQ. In the longitudinal approach, imaging should begin similar to the FAST scan in a coronal position with the probe in the midaxillary line in between the lower rib spaces pointing toward the patient's head. This view will allow the sonographer to evaluate the thoracic space and the RUQ for free fluid in addition to the hepatobiliary organs. The evaluation for free fluid is described fully in Chap. 9.

The liver is best imaged in this longitudinal axis from its superior pole down to the inferior tip. The probe should be advanced from the lateral position to the patient's anterior body surface as the liver echotexture is examined for abnormalities. The probe should be moved caudally until the inferior tip of the liver is fully imaged in order to not miss dependent free fluid that collects in this space. If there is an abnormality in the liver, the sonographer should be able to describe its location based on its relationship to the hepatic and portal veins, as described earlier.

The GB should also be imaged in both its long and short axes. There are two commonly used techniques in obtaining adequate GB images: imaging through the rib spaces or by using a subcostal technique. The most successful technique can depend on a variety of factors, including patient habitus and discomfort and the amount of bowel gas present. Imaging through the rib spaces is more successful in obese patients and in those that have too much bowel gas obscuring the GB. The subcostal technique is ideal in thinner patients without a lot of gas where the probe can be angled up toward the GB without much interference. A combination of these orientations may be necessary in order to adequately image the GB in both long and short axes.

There are certain aspects of hepatobiliary imaging that must be incorporated into every evaluation of the GB in order to have a complete exam. These include imaging the GB in two planes, fanning through the GB from the fundus down to the neck to not miss stones or other pathology, evaluating the anterior wall for thickness, and identifying and measuring the CBD.

IMAGING THROUGH THE RIBS

The probe can be placed as described earlier in a coronal lateral position and advanced anteriorly until the GB comes into view. The GB is located at the inferior border of the liver and therefore, on a longitudinal view, it will appear on the right side of the screen as a cystic, fluid-filled, anechoic structure. Because the probe is positioned over the ribs in this technique, it is important to make sure that rib shadows are not hiding parts of the GB and possible pathology. If a rib shadow is in the way, the probe can be angled just slightly oblique to bring the GB clearly into view. If the GB is not well visualized laterally, the probe should be slid anteriorly, again avoiding the ribs.

Once an adequate long-axis view is visualized, the probe should be fanned back and forth toward the patient's right and left sides in order to completely evaluate the lumen from the fundus down to the neck (Fig. 11-6).

The MLF (visualized in 70% of patients) should be used as a landmark if it is visualized. This will aid in identifying the GB and help to avoid mistaking other structures (bowel, renal, or liver cysts) as the GB. The MLF appears as a bright hyperechoic line that extends from the neck of the GB down to the undivided RPV and CBD (see Fig. 11-3). If this is located, the sonographer can follow this up to the neck of the GB.

The probe should then be rotated 90° counterclockwise (probe marker pointing toward the patient's right side) to obtain a transverse (short-axis) view. In this orientation, the probe should be fanned superiorly and inferiorly to visualize the whole GB fully and to make sure there are no impacted stones located in the fundus or neck (Fig. 11-7).

The anterior GB wall must be measured for a complete exam. The posterior wall will appear thicker and more brightly echogenic due to posterior enhancement

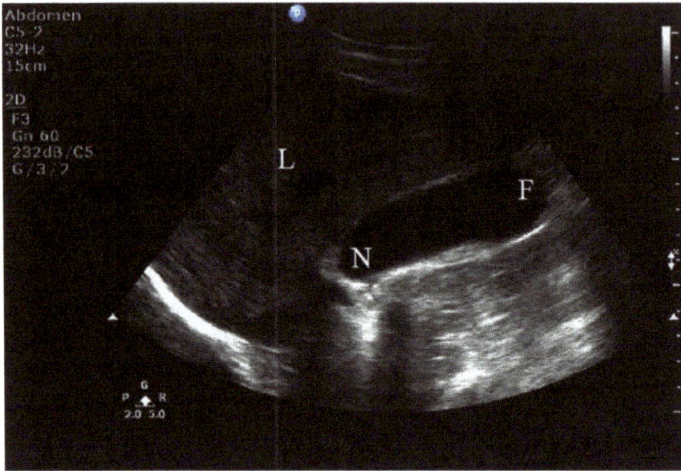

FIGURE 11-6 Normal sagittal (longitudinal) view of the gallbladder. The probe should be fanned medially and laterally in order to fully visualize the fundus (F) down to the neck (N). L: liver.

artifact that appears behind cystic structures; therefore, this wall should not be measured. The anterior wall will appear at the top of the screen, the image should be frozen, and calipers used to measure the thickness, which should be <3 mm (Fig. 11-7).

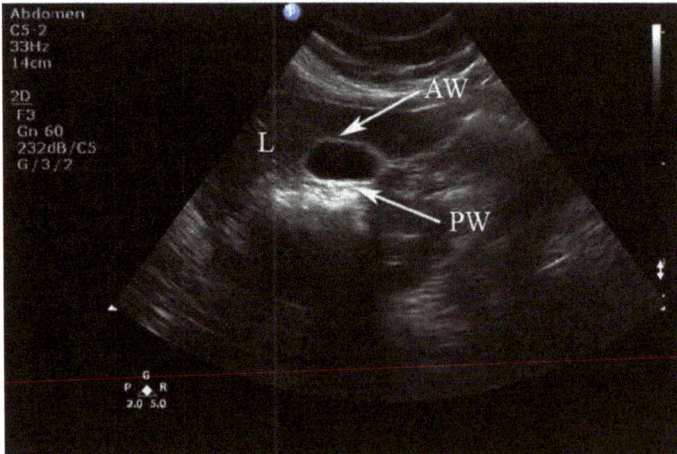

FIGURE 11-7 Normal transverse (short-axis) view of the gallbladder. The anterior wall (AW) will be visualized at the top of the screen and should be measured at <3 mm. The posterior wall (PW) is seen at the bottom of the screen and appears thickened due to posterior enhancement artifact and should not be measured. L: liver.

SUBCOSTAL IMAGING

With this technique, the GB is also imaged in both its short and long axes. The probe is placed in the sagittal position (on the anterior body surface pointing toward the patient's head) just below the subcostal margin. It should be angled slightly cephalad underneath the rib cage toward the liver. The GB will be seen at the inferior portion of the liver and should be fanned through as described earlier. The probe should then be rotated 90° counterclockwise (probe marker pointing toward the patient's right side) to obtain a transverse (short-axis) view. It should be angled upward underneath the rib cage and the GB should be fanned through from the fundus to the neck and the anterior wall measured, as described earlier. Subcostal imaging of the GB can often be enhanced by having the patient inspire and hold their breath while imaging.

COMMON BILE DUCT

The portal triad consists of the main PV, the CBD, and the HA. The CBD should be identified and measured if possible in all GB imaging. In a short-axis orientation, all three of these structures are viewed as the "Mickey Mouse sign," with the PV making up the face and the HA and CBD the ears (see Fig. 11-4). The PV is seen as a round anechoic structure most posteriorly with the HA usually sitting anterior and medial and the CBD sitting anterior and lateral, although the anatomy can vary. Color flow Doppler should be used to differentiate the CBD from the vessels and to ensure the duct is being measured properly (Fig. 11-8). In the longitudinal view, the PV will be seen as an anechoic-appearing tubular structure and the CBD coursing anteriorly to it with its bright white hyperechoic walls (Fig. 11-9).

The probe should be fanned down to the neck of the GB in order to locate the triad and CBD. The area surrounding the PV and CBD can be zoomed in on to make the measurement easier to obtain. When attempting to image and measure the CBD, color-flow Doppler should be used to identify the PV and to ensure that the sonographer is measuring the duct and not a blood vessel. It is important to

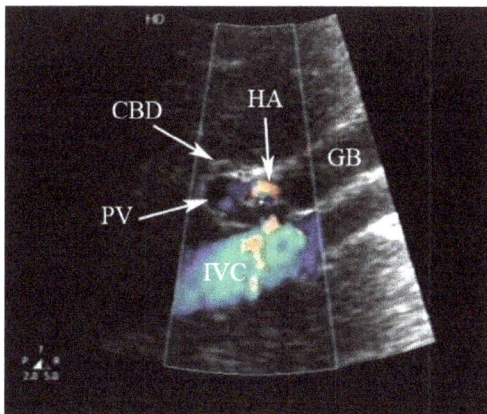

FIGURE 11-8 Short-axis view of the portal triad (PV: portal vein, HA: hepatic artery, CBD: common bile duct). The CBD is normally anterior and lateral and the HA anterior and medial to the PV. The use of color-flow Doppler, as seen in this image, helps to differentiate the vessels from the duct. IVC: inferior vena cava, GB: gallbladder.

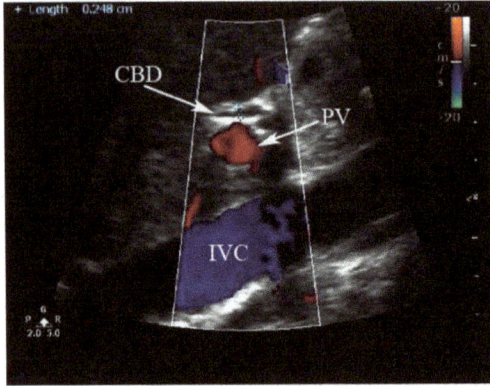

FIGURE 11-9 Longitudinal view of the portal vein (PV) and common bile duct (CBD). The CBD will have characteristic bright white hyperechoic walls and will be seen above the PV. Color-flow Doppler should be used to differentiate the vessel from the duct. The CBD diameter is taken from inside wall to inside wall and is measured at 0.248 cm visualized on the upper left corner of the screen. IVC: inferior vena cava.

angle the probe in order to avoid having the beam perpendicular to the blood flow, which will erroneously appear on the screen as a lack of color. The measurement of the duct should be from the inner wall to inner wall. The normal CBD diameter varies and naturally increases with age. Above the age of 40, the general rule is that the diameter will increase by 1 mm per decade and therefore a 70-year-old patient may have a normal CBD of 7 mm.

PATHOLOGIC ULTRASOUND FINDINGS

CHOLELITHIASIS

Cholelithiasis is the presence of gallstones within the GB. Cholelithiasis may be symptomatic or asymptomatic. Gallstones consist of two types: cholesterol and pigment containing. Cholesterol-containing stones are more common and are a result of the supersaturation of bile pigments. Pigment-containing stones are seen more commonly in the developing world and are due to chronic hemolytic states.

On ultrasound, gallstones will appear as echogenic structures that produce posterior acoustic shadowing (Fig. 11-10). When mobile, they are gravity dependent, and therefore if the patient is asked to roll into the lateral decubitus position, the gallstones should shift. If the stones are not mobile, particularly when found in the neck of the GB, this is a sign of impaction. Nonmobile hyperechoic structures adherent to the GB wall may represent a polyp or mass and not a stone. Stones are of different sizes and when they are less than 2 mm, they can be difficult to visualize. In particular, stones at the neck of the GB may be the most difficult to identify, but are more likely to cause symptoms. This stresses the importance of fanning through the entire GB from the fundus to neck to not miss small or impacted stones (Fig. 11-11).

WALL-ECHO-SHADOW SIGN (WES SIGN)

There are cases when a patient has multiple gallstones or one large stone contained within a contracted GB. This is important for the sonographer to recognize,

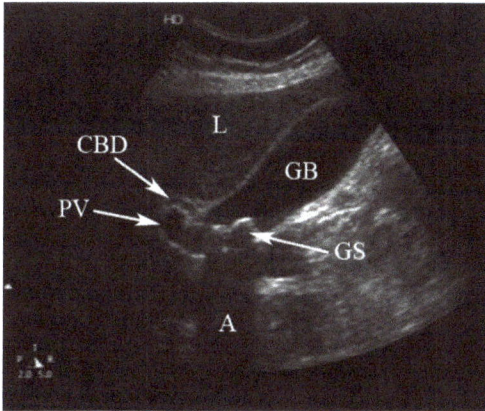

FIGURE 11-10 Cholelithiasis. Gallstones (GS) visualized in the body of the gallbladder (GB). The stones appear echogenic and produce posterior acoustic shadowing artifact (A). PV: portal vein, CBD: common bile duct, L: liver.

as the only clue may be the extensive posterior acoustic shadowing behind the contracted structure. This can make the GB and stones very easy to miss and the physician may just conclude it is contracted and overlook the pathology. This entity is called the "WES sign," which stands for the bright white hyperechoic **W**all that looks like an arch, the **E**chogenic stones inside the contracted lumen, and the posterior acoustic **S**hadowing due to the stones attenuating the ultrasound beam (Fig. 11-12). The "WES sign" is not always indicative of acute cholecystitis, which typically exhibits a dilated GB, but does indicate cholelithiasis.

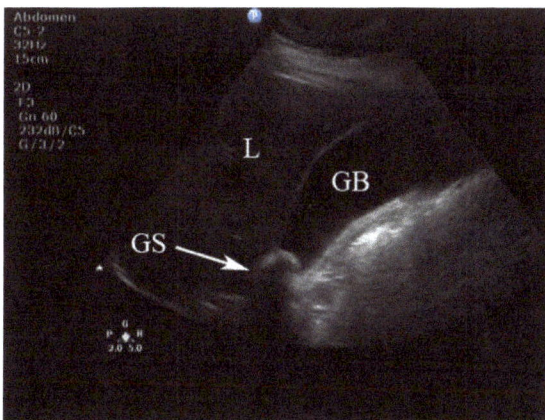

FIGURE 11-11 Large gallstone (GS) impacted in the neck of the gallbladder (GB). This finding was initially missed until the sonographer fanned the probe all the way down to the neck. L: liver.

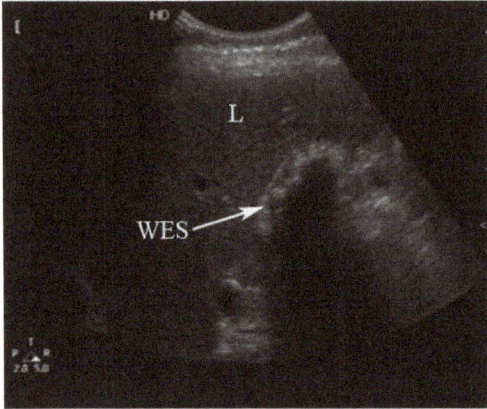

FIGURE 11-12 Wall-echo-shadow sign (WES). The wall is seen as a bright white hyper-echoic structure as the outermost arch. The gallbladder lumen is contracted and full of echogenic stones that are producing extensive posterior acoustic shadowing. L: liver.

ACUTE CHOLECYSTITIS

The sonographic signs of acute cholecystitis include (Fig. 11-13):

- The presence of gallstones or sludge
- Anterior wall thickening >3 mm
- Pericholecystic fluid (PCF)
- Sonographic Murphy's sign (SMS)

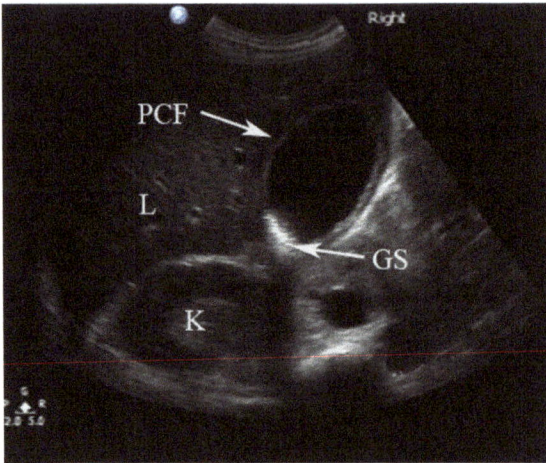

FIGURE 11-13 Acute cholecystitis. The gallbladder contains small stones (GS) close to the neck, has thickened walls and pericholecystic fluid (PCF) seen as black anechoic areas surrounding the outside walls. L: liver, K: right kidney.

All of these findings may not be present in cholecystitis, particularly in the early stages. Biliary colic with intractable pain (>4 hours) is typically indicative of cholecystitis and should prompt surgical consultation. The longer the patient's symptoms have been present, the more likely all four signs will exist on ultrasound as the GB inflammation increases. While gallstones are almost always present in cholecystitis, particularly in emergency department patients presenting from an outpatient setting, acalculous cholecysitis may occur in more chronically ill patients.

The appearance of gallstones on ultrasound has already been described earlier. In order to not miss smaller stones, the GB should be interrogated fully from the fundus down to the neck. In acute cholecystitis, there is often a stone impacted in the neck causing an obstructive picture. This emphasizes the need to fully visualize the whole GB in two planes and to ask the patient to roll over to one side to determine if the stone is mobile. In certain cases, acute cholecystitis can occur with sludge alone or with the combination of stones and sludge together. Small stones can be hidden within GB sludge and may not have the typical posterior shadowing present.

Sludge will appear as a layered out murky-appearing substance that will appear more echogenic than the GB lumen, but less than the liver architecture (Fig. 11-14a). Side lobe artifact (SLA) is an artifact that should not be mistaken for sludge. SLA is generated from the "side lobes" of the main ultrasound beam and when these lobes have enough energy, their echoes reflect back, become part of the main beam, and create artifact. This artifact occurs in cystic structures such as the GB and urinary bladder. It appears as wispy-looking hyperechoic lines that extend into the lumen with a similar echogenicity as sludge (Fig. 11-14b). The artifact and sludge can be differentiated from one another by fanning the probe throughout the GB. The SLA disappears with different angles of the probe, while sludge stays.

With experience, the clinician should be able to identify an inflamed GB wall from its appearance. When measured, the wall should be measured anteriorly

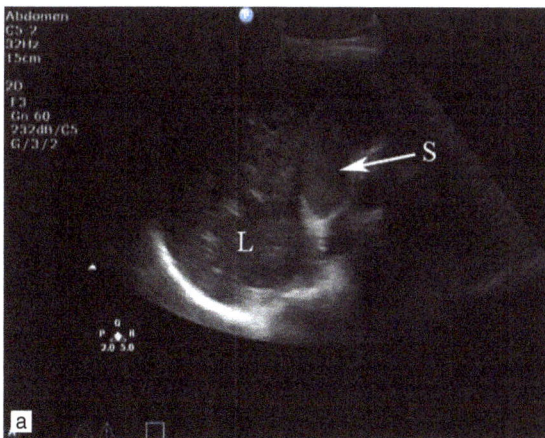

FIGURE 11-14(*a*) The appearance of sludge (S) within the gallbladder lumen. It has a thick murky layered out appearance with an echogenicity slightly less than the liver (L).

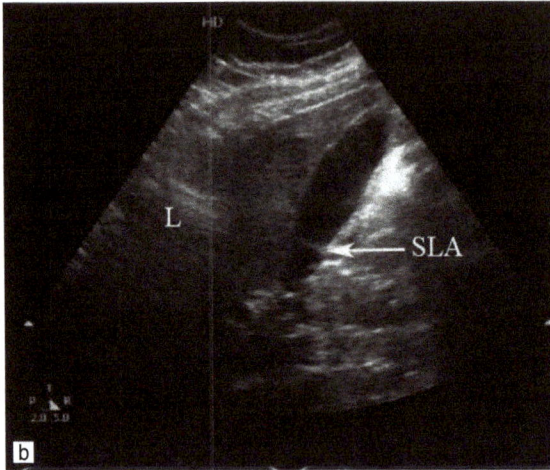

FIGURE 11-14(*b*) Side lobe artifact (SLA) appears as wispy lines extending into the lumen of the gallbladder and may be mistaken for sludge.

with the wall perpendicular to the beam of the ultrasound in the middle of the screen and should measure less than 3 mm. Acute cholecystitis causes circumferential wall thickening (see Fig. 11-13) and therefore, if there is only one area of focal thickening, another diagnosis must be considered. A noninflamed GB wall may appear thickened if visualized in an oblique plane. While GB wall thickening is typically seen in cholecystitis, it is not specific, particularly if gallstones are not present. Other conditions that cause wall thickening include congestive states (congestive heart failure, acute renal failure, cirrhosis), acute hepatitis, GB masses, or other inflammatory or infiltrative processes.

Pericholecystic fluid (PCF) appears as an anechoic (black) stripe that will follow the shape of and surround the outer walls (see Fig. 11-13). It is a result of the inflammatory changes that occur with cholecystitis. It is the least sensitive sign for acute cholecystitis, but very specific.

A SMS is elicited by placing pressure with the probe directly over the GB when visualized on ultrasound. This sign is the most sensitive for the diagnosis of acute cholecystitis and most often warrants a surgical consultation.

CHRONIC CHOLECYSTITIS

Chronic cholecystitis is due to repetitive episodes of acute cholecystitis that go untreated. This leads to a thickened GB wall and a contracted small lumen full of stones. This condition is more common in women over the age of 40. The major sonographic difference between chronic and acute cholecystitis is that the GB will appear much more shrunken and contracted after repetitive episodes of inflammation.

ACALCULOUS CHOLECYSTITIS

Acalculous cholecystitis is a serious condition that is associated with a high mortality. It accounts for approximately 5%–10% of cases of acute cholecystitis and usually results from prolonged bile stasis. It is most often diagnosed in the elderly patient who has multiple comorbidities or in the critical patient who has suffered burns, sepsis, recent trauma, or is on mechanical ventilation. The GB is inflamed similar to calculous cholecystitis, but without the presence of stones.

On ultrasound, acalculous cholecystitis appears as a distended GB with thickened walls minus the presence of gallstones. It is especially important to keep this diagnosis in mind in the ICU patient who keeps spiking fevers and has no source. In these situations, a bedside ultrasound can help narrow the diagnosis. These patients require an immediate surgical consultation and broad-spectrum antibiotic treatment.

EMPHYSEMATOUS CHOLECYSTITIS

Emphysematous cholecystitis is due to an infection of the GB wall with bacterial organisms. This infection is a result of multiple factors, including cystic artery vascular compromise, gallstone obstruction, immunodeficiencies (diabetes), and gas-forming organisms *(Clostridium, Escherichia coli, Klebsiella)*. This diagnosis carries a higher mortality rate than simple gallstone cholecystitis.

The diagnosis of emphysematous cholecystitis by ultrasound can be difficult. Due to the accumulation of gas within the walls of the GB, this can cause a lot of artifact and scattering of the ultrasound beam, which may make its appearance similar to bowel gas. This may result in enough artifacts that the GB may be obscured completely. These gas artifacts may produce "ring-down" or "comet-tail" artifacts emanating from the walls that are pathognomonic of this condition. These shadows are more irregular or "dirty" than comet tails seen with cholesterol deposits or adenomyomatosis.

This condition requires immediate surgical and possibly interventional radiology consultations as well as broad-spectrum intravenous antibiotics.

PORCELAIN GALLBLADDER

Porcelain GB is a term used to describe extensively calcified GB walls due to chronic inflammation. In most cases, cholelithiasis is present, but the true cause is not definitively known. The walls are chronically inflamed and develop internal calcifications, which lead to fibrotic changes and the typical appearance of the "porcelain" GB. These patients are usually asymptomatic and the diagnosis is discovered incidentally on radiographs or CT scans. An ultrasound will depict a calcified GB, but these findings may be mistaken as just gallstones and not necessarily a porcelain GB. A CT scan has better sensitivity at diagnosing this condition than an ultrasound. There is a controversial link between a porcelain GB leading to carcinoma; therefore, close follow-up is recommended even in asymptomatic patients.

CHOLEDOCHOLITHIASIS

Choledocholithiasis is a condition that occurs when a gallstone becomes impacted in the CBD. This condition can happen as a first presentation of RUQ pain in a patient with GB disease, but oftentimes occurs post cholecystectomy due to a retained stone in the ductal system. Patients will present with a similar complaint of RUQ pain and may have an obstructive picture on their labs with elevated liver enzymes, bilirubins, and alkaline phosphatase.

Ultrasound is not sensitive for locating CBD stones and most commonly only reveals a dilated CBD which, combined with the clinical scenario, may raise enough suspicion for the diagnosis. A dilated CBD alone should be considered with caution as it becomes enlarged in most patients post-cholecystectomy and is not necessarily a sign of pathology. Less commonly, a stone will be visualized within the lumen of the CBD and will exhibit posterior shadowing in a similar fashion as in cholecystitis (Fig. 11-15). If choledocholithiasis is suspected,

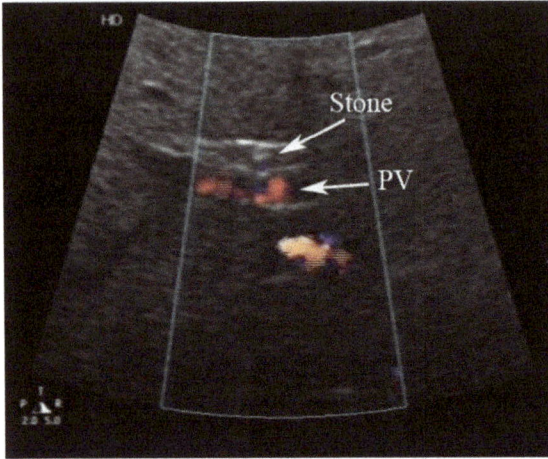

FIGURE 11-15 Longitudinal view of the portal vein (PV) with color-flow Doppler and the CBD lying directly anterior to the vessel. An echogenic stone can be visualized in the lumen of the CBD.

further imaging is warranted such as an ERCP or MRCP. In addition, both surgical and gastrointestinal consultations are needed in these cases for further intervention.

In certain situations, the CBD is dilated enough that it will be as large or even larger than the PV. In the longitudinal axis, this will be seen as two tubular anechoic structures overlying one another within the liver. This has been called the "double barrel shotgun sign," with the two tubular structures making up the barrel (Fig. 11-16).

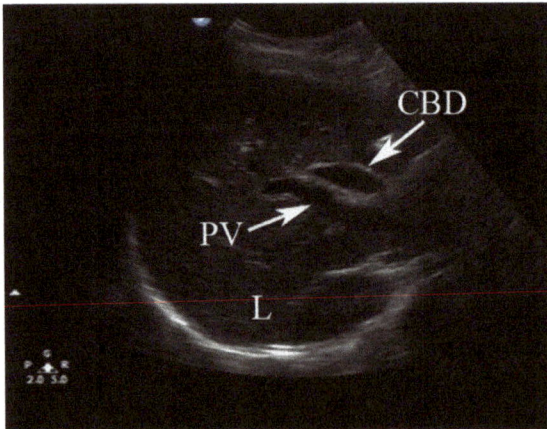

FIGURE 11-16 The common bile duct (CBD) is dilated and sits just anterior to the portal vein (PV). The two together resemble the double barrel of a shotgun. L: liver.

BILIARY DYSKINESIA

Some patients may present with classic symptoms of biliary colic (acute RUQ pain after eating, etc) but have no gallstones on thorough ultrasound examination. This may represent biliary dyskinesia. The most common type of biliary dyskinesia is when the GB cannot empty completely due to duct spasm. This is hypokinetic biliary dyskinesia, and may demonstrate a distended GB on ultrasound, sometimes with a sonographic Murphy's sign.

Hyperkinetic dyskinesia is less common and more controversial, but may be present when the GB empties too vigorously. While biliary dsykinesia is not dangerous, it may be very uncomfortable. Pain control and smooth muscle relaxants (eg, dicyclomine) may be helpful, although occasionally cholecystectomy is recommended. HIDA scan with cholcystikinin (CCK) stimulation may help delineate these conditions, although it may be difficult to obtain during an acute episode.

In hypokinetic biliary dyskinesia, the GB will not empty properly, while in hyperkinetic biliary dyskinesia the ejection fraction of the GB typically exceeds 90%, but this may also be seen in normal patients.

GALLBLADDER POLYPS OR MASSES

GB polyps are relatively common in all age groups and are usually benign and asymptomatic. They are small, oblong-shaped structures with smooth walls that extend off the GB wall into the lumen and have similar echogenicities as the walls themselves (Fig. 11-17). They can be mistaken as stones and there are a few differentiating characteristics that must be considered. (1) They do not appear as bright and echogenic as cholesterol stones; (2) they do not impede the ultrasound beam as they are soft-tissue structures, and therefore, do not produce posterior acoustic shadowing; (3) they are nonmobile and will stay attached to the wall even when the patient changes position. Once again, careful fanning of the probe through the GB in both orientations and having the patient roll to the lateral decubitus position will help in making the correct diagnosis.

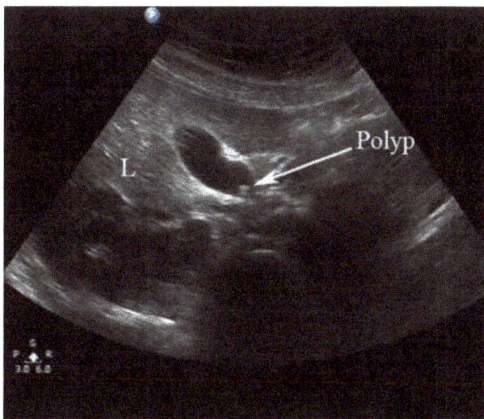

FIGURE 11-17 A polyp seen within the lumen of the gallbladder. Note the polyp has a similar echogenicity as the GB wall and the liver (L) and does not produce posterior acoustic shadowing.

GB masses are soft tissue masses that may be attached to the wall and extend into the lumen. They can have a similar appearance and characteristics as a polyp, but they are often more irregular-appearing and may have focal wall abnormalities, such as wall thickening, associated with them. These patients may complain of RUQ pain and develop an obstructive process if the mass is large enough, but the diagnosis is often not discovered until the disease is quite advanced.

ADENOMYOMATOSIS

Adenomyomatosis is a benign condition but one that appears very abnormal on ultrasound. Recognizing the characteristic features will help to not mistake it for acute cholecystitis. Adenomyomatosis causes GB wall thickening and the formation of diverticulae called "Rokitansky–Aschoff sinuses." The process can involve focal segments of the GB wall or can be diffuse. Its cause is unknown and patients are usually asymptomatic. It is usually diagnosed incidentally on ultrasound or CT scan.

On ultrasound, the GB wall will appear thickened with the presence of characteristic "ring-down" or reverberation artifacts coming from the sinuses seen in this condition. Also called "comet tails," these are closely spaced hyperechoic lines that taper as they go deeper, originating from the walls and extending into the lumen (Fig. 11-18). Other causes of comet-tail artifacts originating from the GB wall include cholesterol deposits and gas in the wall from emphysematous cholecystitis. The comet tails seen in emphysematous cholecystitis are much more "dirty" and irregular, and the patients are typically quite ill. While adenomyomatosis is typically benign, the findings may be difficult to distinguish from GB carcinoma, and the patient should have consultative follow-up.

LIVER MASSES OR CYSTS

Liver cysts on ultrasound are anechoic, round, and thin-walled, fluid-filled structures. They are usually asymptomatic and discovered incidentally. Liver (or renal) cysts may be mistaken for a GB with no stones, underscoring the

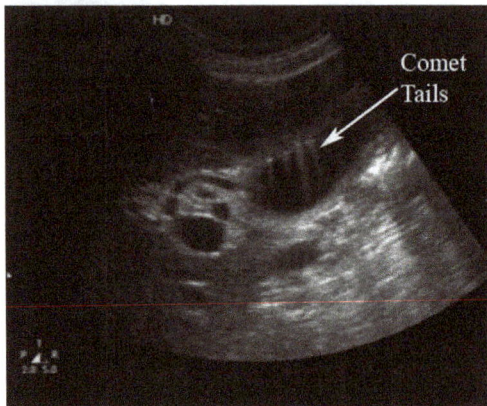

FIGURE 11-18 Adenomyomatosis diagnosed incidentally in this patient with abdominal pain. Note the comet tails (reverberation artifacts) emanating from the sinuses within the GB wall. This is highly specific for this condition.

importance of identifying the landmarks for the GB. If there are multiple cysts, this may involve other organs, such as the kidneys or pancreas and these areas should be imaged also. If multiple organs are involved, the patient will need a further workup.

Liver masses have different characteristics based on their composition. Hemangiomas are the most common benign liver tumor seen on ultrasound. Patients are asymptomatic and the diagnosis is usually made incidentally. These masses are composed of endothelial cells that line blood vessels and are surrounded by collagenous walls. On ultrasound, they appear as hyperechoic, homogenous, round, well-defined structures (Fig. 11-19a).

Hepatocellular carcinoma (HCC) is the most common malignant liver tumor. It is most common in patients who have preexisting liver disease, such as hepatitis C, alcohol abuse, or cirrhosis. These tumors on ultrasound will appear less well defined, relatively hypoechoic, and heterogenous structures that often contain calcifications (Fig. 11-19b). Their diagnosis on ultrasound requires further imaging and workup.

Liver metastases are typically described as "cannon ball" lesions in appearance. They are usually multiple foci of round hypoechoic (dark) structures that will appear throughout the liver parenchyma. The fact that they appear as multiple lesions is a clue to the sonographer that they are metastases from another primary source and not a primary HCC. If these are identified on ultrasound, the patient requires additional imaging and workup.

HEPATITIS

Acute hepatitis is a clinical diagnosis and not usually identifiable on ultrasound. Possible signs of this condition are an enlarged edematous liver with dilated intrahepatic biliary ducts. In addition, due to the congested liver, the GB wall may be thickened due to local inflammatory changes. Chronic hepatitis may also not be apparent on ultrasound, but if fibrotic changes have altered the architecture of the liver, it may appear shrunken and have a more heterogenous appearance.

CIRRHOSIS

End-stage liver disease or cirrhosis can be due to a variety of conditions, most often alcohol abuse and chronic hepatitis. The liver will appear shrunken,

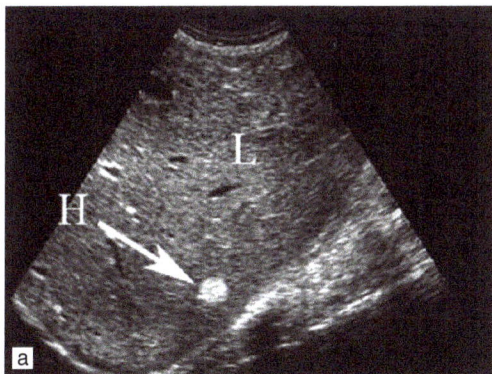

FIGURE 11-19(a) The typical appearance of a liver hemangioma (H). These benign masses are hyperechoic, round, well circumscribed, and asymptomatic.

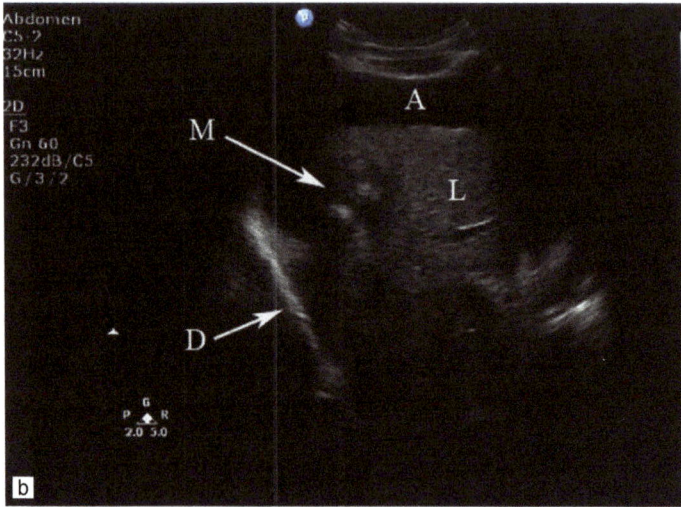

FIGURE 11-19(*b*) A primary hepatocellular carcinoma (HCC) appears as a less well-defined mass (M) that is heterogenous appearing. The HCC seen here contains calcifications producing posterior acoustic shadowing. Other signs that this patient has end-stage liver disease is the significant amount of ascites (A) present and the shrunken irregular appearance of the liver (L). D: diaphragm.

heterogenous, and irregular in appearance. There may also be signs of HCC visualized as a mass in the parenchyma. Oftentimes, cirrhotic patients will have free intraperitoneal fluid or ascites in the RUQ. This is seen as anechoic black areas within Morison's pouch extending around the inferior tip of the liver and above the dome anteriorly (see Fig. 11-19*b*).

PANCREATIC ABNORMALITIES

Although ultrasound is not ideal for pancreatic imaging, certain abnormalities may be visualized at the bedside. Acute pancreatitis results in an enlarged heterogenous-appearing pancreas, with hypoechoic areas throughout the architecture representing edema.

Chronic pancreatitis results in fibrotic changes and calcifications that may be seen on ultrasound. The calcifications will impede the ultrasound beam and produce characteristic posterior acoustic shadowing within the organ. In addition, this condition may cause pseudocyst formation, which will appear as rounded anechoic fluid-filled structures within the pancreas.

COMMON PITFALLS

PATIENT HABITUS AND BOWEL GAS

All structures in the abdomen can be difficult to locate in obese patients or those with excessive bowel gas. The curvilinear probe, with lower frequency and better penetration, should always be used in these patients. A significant amount of pressure may be needed in order to push bowel gas out of the way. Having the patient inhale and hold their breath may improve imaging from the subcostal approach. The GB may need to be imaged through the anterior or lateral intercostal spaces if the subcostal method is not adequate. Finally, if the patient is compliant, they can roll into the left lateral decubitus position, which can help to move the GB away from the ribs and bowel.

NOT PROPERLY IDENTIFYING THE GALLBLADDER

The sonographer may have difficulty identifying the GB for several reasons. As described earlier, patient habitus and bowel gas can be deterrents in identifying the GB. Proper probe selection, patient positioning, and pressure are tips to better visualize the RUQ structures.

A contracted GB can be difficult to find in certain patients. It is important to identify the GB landmarks, which include the undivided RPV and MLF and to follow these up into the neck of the GB. These landmarks are useful in visualizing the "GB bed" in cases where a patient is post-cholecystectomy. A contracted GB full of stones ("WES sign") may also be difficult to visualize and may be mistaken for bowel gas (or vice versa). The significant posterior acoustic shadowing that is produced by a GB full of stones is one clue that there are calcific structures blocking the ultrasound beam (Fig. 11-12). In comparison, bowel gas will also appear as bright white echogenic foci, but will scatter the sound beam and not produce posterior shadowing.

Gentle fanning of the probe in a medial-to-lateral position, while in the longitudinal orientation, and in a superior-to-inferior position, while in a transverse orientation, will also bring the GB into view. This can be further enhanced by asking the patient to take in a deep inspiration and to hold their breath for a few seconds, while searching for the GB.

MISSING GALLSTONES

This is probably the most common pitfall encountered in hepatobiliary imaging. There may be a stone impacted in one end of the GB, either in the fundus or neck, and if the structure is not interrogated completely, this pathology will be missed. Once again, it is important to fan through the GB completely to visualize the whole organ. Also, there may be very small stones present that are not readily visualized or sitting inside a pile of sludge. If there is enough suspicion, ask the patient to roll into the lateral decubitus position in order to move possible stones around so that they are more easily identified. In addition, adjusting the focus control so that it is at the level of a suspected gallstone will improve the lateral resolution and may help make the diagnosis.

MISTAKING FLUID-FILLED STRUCTURES FOR THE GALLBLADDER

Fluid-filled structures in the RUQ may resemble the GB and be mistaken for this structure. In particular, the duodenum is close to the inferior tip of the liver in close proximity to the GB. It is a fluid-filled structure that may have the same shape as the GB and therefore, can easily be mistaken for it. Gas in the bowel may cause hyperechoic echoes with shadowing that can be mistaken for gallstones. Correct identification of landmarks will differentiate the GB from bowel. The duodenum and other close-lying bowel may also exhibit peristalsis, which can help to differentiate the two.

The IVC courses along the posterior border of the liver also close to the location of the GB. It will appear anechoic and fluid-filled containing blood and sometimes can be mistaken as the GB by novice sonographers. The IVC will appear as more of a tubular structure, and following it will show the hepatic veins draining into the IVC inferiorly and the entrance to the right atrium superiorly. Color-flow Doppler can help to tell the two apart, as the vessel will pick up signal and the GB will not.

Other cystic structures in the RUQ can also be mistaken for the GB. These include liver and renal cysts and pancreatic pseudocysts. Careful fanning through these cysts can help to clarify which structures they are attached to. In the situation of liver cysts, properly identifying the GB landmarks and following these back into the bed of the GB can aid in telling the two apart.

INCORRECT MEASUREMENTS

It is important to measure the anterior GB wall in assessing for wall thickness. The novice sonographer will often measure the posterior wall that looks thicker due to posterior enhancement artifact. This will cause the erroneous conclusion that there is possible GB wall pathology. The wall is best measured in the transverse orientation at its anterior portion.

The CBD is often measured incorrectly and overestimated in size. Color-flow Doppler should be used to make sure that the CBD is being measured and not the PV or hepatic artery. The measurement of the CBD should be from the inside wall to inside wall in order to not mistakenly call it enlarged.

INTEGRATION OF BEDSIDE HEPATOBILIARY ULTRASOUND INTO CLINICAL CARE

Hepatobiliary bedside ultrasound should be an integrated part of the examination for patients who present with RUQ pain as well as undifferentiated, generalized, or epigastric pain of unclear etiology. It is also useful as a first look in patients with new onset jaundice or abnormal hepatobiliary lab values. It is also an important modality to use in the elderly or critically ill patient who may have unexplained fever or sepsis, without other symptoms. Ultrasound may be performed within minutes of arrival, in conjunction with other resuscitation measures. Ultrasound is very reliable in this situation for identifying hepatobilary abnormalities that require immediate interventions.

Bedside RUQ ultrasound can give the clinician valuable information that can expedite patient care. While gallstones and cholecystitis are often easily identified, it is also important to remember that in some patients hepatobiliary scanning can be among the most challenging of exams for the new sonographer. While the exam is typically specific for gallstones if the GB is easily imaged and stones are present, it takes more experience to reliably exclude gallstones. If there is high enough clinical suspicion for pathology, especially involving the GB, the most experienced sonographer should be performing or supervising the bedside ultrasound. In addition, if the results are unclear and the patient is ill, further imaging and consultation may be needed.

Additional Reading

Bassler D, Snoey ER, Kim J. Goal-directed abdominal ultrasonography: impact on real-time decision making in the emergency department. *J Emerg Med.* 2003;24:375-378.

Bennett GL, Balthazar, EJ. Ultrasound and CT evaluation of emergent gallbladder pathology. *Radiol Clin North Am.* 2003;41:1203-1216.

Gaspari RJ, Dickman E, Blehar D. Learning curve of bedside ultrasound of the gallbladder. *J Emerg Med.* 2009;37:51-56.

Summers SM, Scruggs W, Fox JC, et al. A prospective evaluation of emergency department bedside ultrasonography for the detection of acute cholecystitis. *Ann Emerg Med.* 2010;(56):114-122.

Wang HP, Chen SC. Upper abdominal ultrasound in the critically ill. *Crit Care Med.* 2007;35(5):S208-S215.

12 Ultrasound of the Female Pelvis

Cynthia Moon, Kristin Carmody, and Christopher L. Moore

BACKGROUND AND INDICATIONS FOR EXAMINATION

Pelvic ultrasound was first introduced into the acute care setting to answer simple yes or no questions such as "Is there an intrauterine pregnancy?" Pelvic ultrasound applications in the emergency setting have now expanded to include the nonpregnant patient. The improvement in skills now allows the clinician to evaluate for other pelvic pathology such as adnexal cysts or masses, ovarian torsion, fibroids, or tuboovarian abscesses.

The complaint of abdominal or pelvic pain in the young female patient comprises a significant number of the total emergency department visits throughout most institutions. Both transabdominal ultrasound (TAUS) and transvaginal ultrasound (TVUS) can help the physician diagnose the cause of these complaints and can guide clinical decisions and expedite patient care. While point-of-care pelvic ultrasound is a very useful tool in the acute care setting, it still remains focused and is not intended to examine all potential pathology.

Bedside ultrasound evaluation of the female pelvis should be performed in:

- The pregnant patient who presents with pelvic or abdominal pain
- The pregnant patient who presents with vaginal bleeding
- The pregnant trauma patient
- The nonpregnant patient who presents with pelvic or lower abdominal pain with suspicion for a gynecological cause

PROBE SELECTION AND TECHNICAL CONSIDERATIONS

CURVILINEAR PROBE WITH A FREQUENCY OF 3.5–5.0 MHz

A wide footprint curvilinear probe is appropriate for transabdominal pelvic imaging. This probe has a lower frequency with better penetration, which is suitable for imaging the pelvic organs through the abdominal wall. Smaller footprint or phased array probes may be used for transabdominal pelvic imaging but are not optimal.

ENDOCAVITARY PROBE WITH A FREQUENCY OF 8.0–13.0 MHz

The endocavitary probe has a higher frequency, which produces an image with better resolution. It also has a wider field of view and provides more detail. It is used for all transvaginal pelvic scanning, especially when the structure of interest is not visualized well using transabdominal imaging alone, such as in an early intrauterine pregnancy (IUP) or in evaluation of the adnexa.

DEPTH

In TAUS the sonographer should start with a deeper field and survey the areas surrounding both the uterus and bladder. This is important in the evaluation for free fluid, which will appear in the most dependent areas first, posterior to the uterus. Also, a deeper field allows the sonographer to better evaluate the adnexa for pathology. Once the far field is completely evaluated, the depth can be decreased so that the uterus appears more superficial and intrauterine structures better visualized.

ZOOM

The zoom control allows for magnification of a particular portion of the image being scanned. This becomes important when attempting to visualize small structures, such as obtaining the fetal heart rate (FHR) of an early pregnancy. The zoom function can sometimes distort the image, therefore the depth should be optimized first before the image is magnified.

GAIN OR TIME-GAIN COMPENSATION

The total gain can be adjusted in order to increase the signal returning to the transducer and brighten the image. In cases where only the far field needs to be brighter, the time-gain compensation (TGC) can be increased and the near field left alone. The gain should not be increased too high or the image can appear "washed" out and white, which can obscure free fluid in dependent areas, especially behind the uterus.

COLOR-FLOW DOPPLER

Color-flow Doppler identifies blood flow and is useful in the evaluation of the ovaries for torsion. Ovarian torsion demonstrates a decrease in blood flow compared to the unaffected side. Color flow also identifies blood vessels, such as the iliac artery and vein, which serve as landmarks for the ovaries. In addition, this modality can be used to diagnose retained products of conception (RPOC) after a pregnancy or abortion. The area in the uterus that contains debris will display more color flow compared to the normal endometrium. Unless absolutely necessary, Doppler should be avoided in the patient with early pregnancy due to the increased mechanical and thermal energy involved. M-mode should be used for FHR, as described below, not Doppler.

M-MODE

M-mode detects motion over time and is used to calculate the FHR of a pregnancy. Once the pregnancy is identified, the M-mode cursor can be placed over the fetal heart. The heart rate is then calculated graphically on one side of the screen depicting the motion of the heart over time.

CALCULATIONS

Gestational age estimations based on crown-rump-length (CRL), biparietal diameter (BPD), and other modalities are usually included in calculation packages supplied by the machine. In order to access these calculations, the sonographer must choose the obstetrical preset on the machine prior to scanning.

NORMAL ULTRASOUND ANATOMY

UTERUS

The uterus is located midline in the true pelvis superior and posterior to the urinary bladder and anterior to the rectum. The normal uterus is approximately 7–9 cm long, 2–4 cm thick, and 4–6 cm wide. The myometrium is the largest component of the uterus and has a uniform low-level echogenicity and appears hypoechoic relative to the endometrium. The endometrial stripe is composed of a canal surrounded by two layers of endometrium. The brightness and thickness of this stripe varies depending on the patient's menstrual cycle. The stripe is seen as a thin hyperechoic line, approximately 2–3 mm, at the end of the cycle (Fig. 12-1). At other points during the cycle, it will appear thicker and can be up to 15 mm during the proliferative phase.

The vaginal stripe is seen as an echogenic stripe that lies within the vaginal canal in between the anterior and posterior walls. Its presence indicates the lack of debris or foreign body within the vaginal vault. It is only visualized on a transabdominal scan and is best seen in the sagittal plane (Fig. 12-2).

The position of the uterus is described in terms of version and flexion, with version describing the orientation of the overall uterus, and flexion describing any bending within the uterus. The most common position is anteverted where the entire uterus, including the cervix, is tilted forward toward the anterior abdominal wall overlying the bladder (see Fig. 12-2). The uterus can be pushed slightly backward into a horizontal position when the bladder is full and distended. A retroverted uterus is tilted backward away from the bladder toward the posterior abdominal wall and spine (Fig. 12-3). Version of the uterus is best seen in a sagittal plane, and orientation is particularly important when using TVUS, as a normal uterus may appear retroverted (or vice versa) if the probe is turned over. The other common uterine variant described is flexion, in which the uterus bends on itself. The uterus can have any combination of positions mentioned earlier: anteverted-anteflexed, anteverted-retroflexed, retroverted-anteflexed, or retroverted-retroflexed.

The posterior cul-de-sac or "pouch of Douglas" is the space between the posterior wall of the uterus and rectum (see Figs. 12-1 and 12-2). It is the most dependent area in the female pelvis, the site where free fluid will collect first. This space can have a variable appearance depending on its contents. It may appear completely anechoic when containing new blood or may have a heterogeneous appearance if clots are present. The anterior cul-de-sac (retrovesicular or uterovesicular space) is the space between the urinary bladder and the anterior wall of the

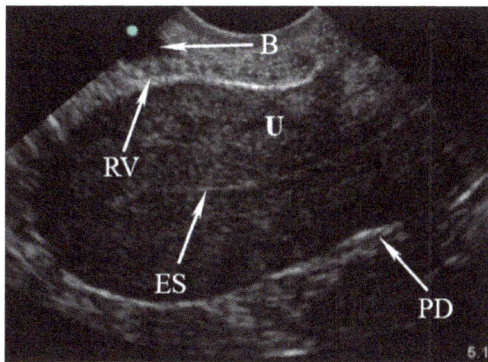

FIGURE 12-1 Transvaginal view of normal pelvic anatomy. The bladder (B) is visualized as an anechoic structure sitting anterior and inferior to the uterus (U). The endometrial stripe (ES) is seen as a hyperechoic line in the center of the uterus. RV: retrovesicular space, between the bladder and uterus, PD: pouch of Douglas, between the uterus and rectum.

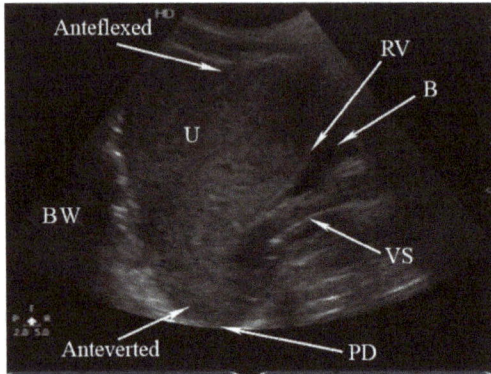

FIGURE 12-2 Sagittal transabdominal view of normal pelvic anatomy. The bladder (B) is visualized as an anechoic structure sitting anterior and inferior to the uterus (U). The vaginal stripe (VS) is seen as a bright white hyperechoic line within the vaginal canal. The pouch of Douglas (PD) lies between the uterus and the rectum, the most dependent area in the female pelvis, where free fluid collects first. BW: bowel, RV: retrovesicular space. The uterus is tipped forward toward the bladder and anterior abdominal wall (anteverted) and the fundus is tipped forward in relation to the cervix (anteflexed).

uterus (see Figs. 12-1 and 12-2). Due to its anterior position, it is less gravity-dependent and does not collect free fluid as quickly as the posterior space. If fluid collects in the uterovesicular space, it indicates a significant amount of fluid in the pelvis.

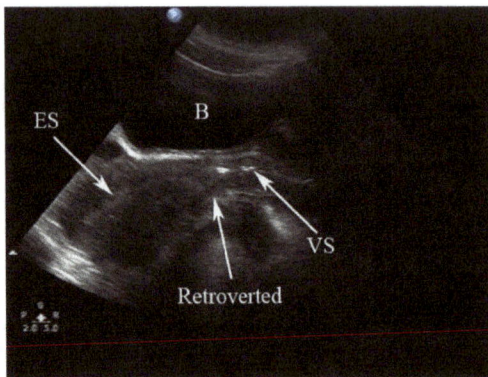

FIGURE 12-3 Sagittal transabdominal view of a retroverted uterus. The bladder (B) is visualized as an anechoic structure sitting anterior and inferior to the uterus. The vaginal stripe (VS) is seen as a bright white hyperechoic line within the vaginal canal. The endometrial stripe (ES) is seen as a hyperechoic line in the center of the uterus. The uterus is tipped backward away from the bladder toward the posterior abdominal wall (retroverted).

ADNEXA

The ovaries are usually found anterior and medial to the iliac blood vessels. These vessels are the primary landmarks for the ovaries, but they can be displaced according to the position of the uterus and can even be found in the cul-de-sac. Ovaries have a medium-level echogenicity with scattered anechoic follicles in the periphery, creating the "chocolate-chip cookie" appearance (Fig. 12-4). Ovarian size varies with age and with the menstrual cycle as the number and size of the follicles change. They are smallest at the time of menstruation and the largest at mid-cycle. The dominant follicle or corpus luteum can often measure up to 2 cm or larger in diameter. The ovaries are more readily identified in premenopausal women, as they tend to decrease in size with increasing age. In addition, they are usually more easily found using TVUS where the probe can be placed closer to the ovary.

Fallopian tubes, mesosalpinges, and broad ligaments may be difficult to identify sonographically unless pathology is present.

BLADDER

The urinary bladder lies anterior and inferior to the uterus. It appears as an anechoic structure with its sonographic size dependent on the urine volume present. It serves as a landmark for the uterus in TAUS scanning; therefore, it is preferably full during this exam (see Fig. 12-2). In TVUS, a full bladder can displace uterine and adnexal anatomy, thus an empty bladder is preferred (see Fig. 12-1).

NORMAL ULTRASOUND ANATOMY IN EARLY PREGNANCY

INTRADECIDUAL SIGN

The "intradecidual sign" is the earliest evidence of an IUP, although it is difficult to visualize by even expert sonographers. It consists of an embryo that is completely embedded within the uterine endometrium, but does not displace the endometrial stripe. On ultrasound, it appears as a simple anechoic area within the uterine cavity and can be seen as early as 4½ weeks' gestational age on a TVUS. It is not sufficient enough evidence to prove an IUP exists, therefore not routinely used by clinicians to make the diagnosis.

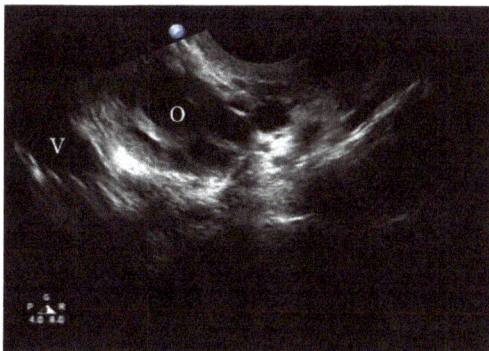

FIGURE 12-4 Transvaginal ultrasound of the adnexa. The ovary (O) has a typical "chocolate-chip cookie" appearance representing the follicles and lies anterior to the iliac vessels (V).

DOUBLE DECIDUAL SAC SIGN

The "double decidual sac sign" is more evidence that a true IUP exists, but it should also be relied on with caution. This sign is seen as two rings, the inner being the decidua capsularis and the outer the decidua vera that surrounds an anechoic area within the uterine cavity (Fig. 12-5). This sign can be seen on TVUS at about 5 weeks and on TAUS at 6 weeks' gestational age. Although its presence is good evidence that an IUP exists, the novice clinician can misinterpret this finding and it alone should not be used to make a secure diagnosis.

GESTATIONAL SAC

The gestational sac is an anechoic space surrounded by an echogenic rim that is visualized on TVUS at about 5 weeks and TAUS at 6 weeks' gestational age (see Fig. 12-5). The sac is usually visualized when it reaches a diameter of 5–6 mm.

There may be an anechoic area within the uterus that is not a gestational sac, but possibly free fluid or a pseudo-gestational sac. Visualizing the "double decidual sac sign," as described earlier, surrounding the anechoic area is good evidence that a gestational sac exists, but other criteria should be met to confidently make this conclusion. The presence of both a yolk sac with or without a fetal pole inside the anechoic area is more definitive proof that a true gestational sac exists. A normal gestational sac is located in the upper uterine body or fundus, and embedded in the middle of the uterine wall. In early pregnancy, the mean gestational sac diameter (MGSD) is used to estimate the gestational age.

YOLK SAC

The yolk sac is attached to the developing embryo and provides nourishment while the circulatory system is still developing. It usually disappears during early pregnancy as the circulatory system takes over. Its diameter in an early pregnancy is consistently 6-7 mm and is important in establishing a normal IUP. Its absence in the first trimester or an unusually large diameter may signify an abnormal pregnancy.

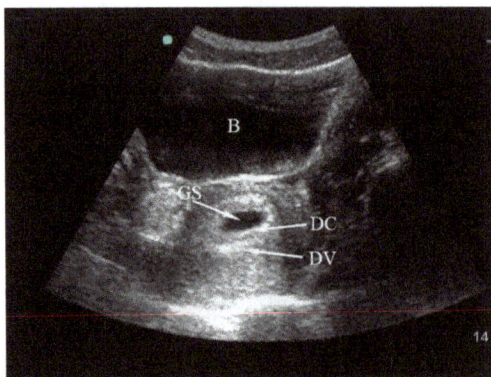

FIGURE 12-5 A transverse transabdominal pelvic view showing the "double decidual sac sign." The gestational sac (GS) will appear as an anechoic area surrounded by two hyperechoic rings, the decidua vera (DV) and the decidua capsularis (DC). B: bladder.

On ultrasound, the yolk sac is a round echogenic ring with an anechoic center that is often referred to as a "cheerio." It can be seen on ultrasound within the gestational sac at approximately 6 weeks on TVUS and at 7 weeks on TAUS. It is usually found eccentrically attached to one of the walls of the lumen (Fig. 12-6). A yolk sac visualized within the gestational sac is definitive evidence that a true IUP exists.

FETAL POLE

The fetal pole is the developing embryo that is first seen attached to one end of the yolk sac (see Fig. 12-6) within the gestational sac. It is usually visualized at 6 weeks on TVUS and about 8 weeks on TAUS. The fetal pole is usually identified when the CRL is approximately 2–4 mm. The FHR can often be seen flickering within the fetal pole when the CRL reaches 5 mm. The FHR is often better visualized on TVUS at this early stage and often is too small to assess properly with TAUS. The presence of both the fetal pole and yolk sac is more definitive evidence that an IUP exists.

LATER PREGNANCY

The yolk sac begins to disappear by the end of the first trimester and its remnants form the umbilical cord, which attaches the fetus to the placenta. The placenta grows throughout pregnancy, with the size of the placenta proportional to the age and health of the fetus. The thickness of the placenta can be used to approximate gestational age and is usually less than 3–4 cm at its maximum. In the early second trimester, the placenta should be easily visualized by TAUS as a homogenous structure that surrounds the gestational sac and fetus. A normal placenta will be visualized superiorly to the fetus close to the uterine fundus (Fig. 12-7). The different layers of the placenta will become more apparent in the third trimester. The amniotic fluid will begin to accumulate in larger amounts and will be seen as an anechoic area surrounding the fetus.

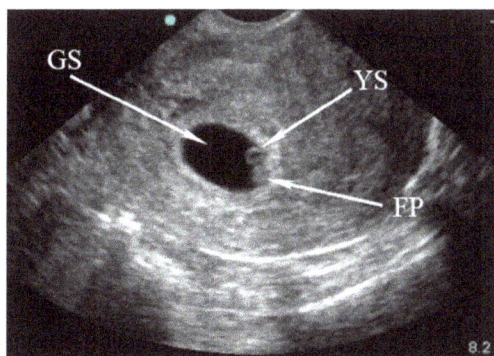

FIGURE 12-6 A normal early intrauterine pregnancy (IUP). The minimum criterion to establish an IUP is present in a gestational sac (GS) + a yolk sac (YS) +/– a fetal pole (FP). Although a fetal pole is not necessary to make the diagnosis, this illustrates the presence of all three structures.

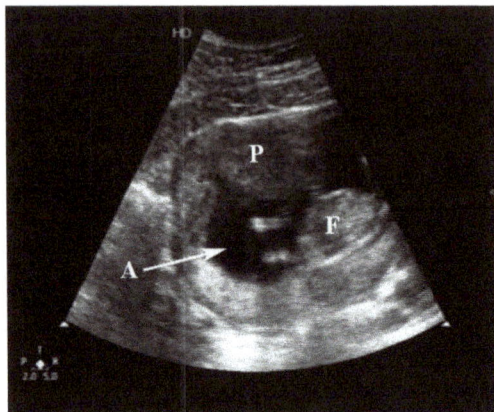

FIGURE 12-7 A normal second trimester pregnancy. The placenta (P) will appear as a homogenous structure that is visualized superior to the fetus (F) near the uterine fundus. Amniotic fluid (A) will continue to accumulate within the sac.

IMAGING TIPS AND PROTOCOL

TRANSABDOMINAL ULTRASOUND

Transabdominal ultrasound (TAUS) is the initial exam performed on any patient presenting with acute pelvic pain or bleeding (pregnant or nonpregnant). The curvilinear abdominal probe is used and the patient should be scanned in both the transverse (short-axis) and sagittal (long-axis) orientations.

The patient should be placed in the supine position, similar to other abdominal exams. In the sagittal view, the probe is placed midline on the patient's lower abdomen, just below the pubic bone, with the indicator pointed cephalad. The vaginal stripe and urinary bladder serve as landmarks in TAUS imaging, and therefore should be identified first. The patient should ideally have a full bladder as this cystic structure is used as a sonographic window in pelvic scanning. The monitor will show the patient's head on the left side of the screen, the feet on the right side, the anterior surface at the top of the screen, and the posterior surface at the bottom. The urinary bladder appears as a triangular or elongated structure with a thick wall around an anechoic area. The vaginal stripe appears as a bright white line within the canal. Once the landmarks are identified, the uterus will be seen superior and posterior to the bladder. The vaginal stripe can be followed up through the canal to the cervix and into the uterus (see Fig. 12-2).

Once an adequate sagittal image is obtained, the sonographer should interrogate the surrounding area by fanning the probe medially and laterally. In addition to surveying the organs for pathology, the anterior and posterior cul-de-sacs should be carefully examined looking for possible free fluid. This will appear as an anechoic or hypoechoic area outside the uterus, in between the bladder anteriorly, or rectum posteriorly.

While usually much better visualized with transvaginal imaging, imaging of the adnexa should be attempted to identify obvious pathology. When seen, the ovaries are anterior and medial to the iliac vessels (see Fig. 12-4).

In order to obtain a transverse view, the transducer is then rotated 90° counterclockwise with the indicator pointing toward the patient's right side. This image depicts the bladder and uterus both in their short axis with the bladder visualized anterior to the uterus (Fig. 12-8). The monitor will show the patient's right on the left side of the screen, the patient's left on the right side of the screen, the anterior surface at the top of the screen, and the posterior surface at the bottom. In this orientation, the uterus should be scanned from the cervix up to the fundus by fanning the probe in both superior and inferior directions. Once again, both the anterior and posterior cul-de-sacs should be examined for free fluid. The probe can be moved to the left and right in order to visualize the adnexa.

TRANSVAGINAL ULTRASOUND

Transvaginal ultrasound (TVUS) provides the sonographer with better resolution and image quality compared to abdominal scanning. It should be used in the evaluation of uterine and adnexal pathology when TAUS does not provide enough detail. The endocavitary probe, with its long shape and higher frequency, allows the sonographer to obtain a closer and more detailed view of the pelvic anatomy. In TVUS imaging, the patient should be scanned in two orientations, both sagittal and coronal.

The patient should be asked to empty their bladder before the exam because if it is full and distended, it can distort the anatomy, and interfere with visualization. The patient should be placed in a supine position with their legs abducted and bent at the knees at approximately a 45° angle. This is typically referred to as a "frog-legs position." A pelvic bed is extremely helpful in this exam. If not available, the pelvis should be elevated by placing a bedpan or blanket under the lower back to allow the tail of the probe to go low enough. The exam should be fully explained to the patient before starting the ultrasound. A sterile probe cover and gel should be placed over the endocavitary probe before beginning.

The TVUS is usually started in a sagittal orientation by inserting the probe into the vaginal canal with the indicator pointing toward the ceiling. The images produced on the screen in TVUS are more difficult for the novice sonographer to interpret. A full understating of the orientation of the transducer indicator in relation to the patient's body is essential before learning to use the endocavitary probe. In the

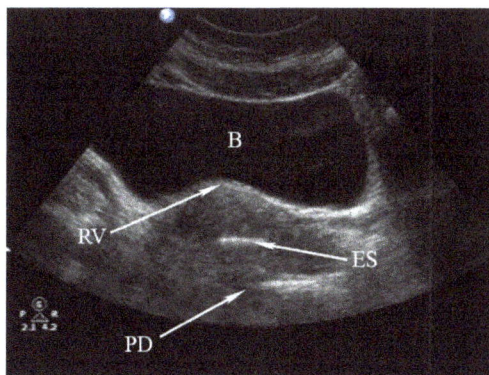

FIGURE 12-8 Transverse transabdominal view of normal pelvic anatomy. The bladder (B) is seen as an anechoic structure anterior and inferior to the uterus. The endometrial stripe (ES) is visualized as a hyperechoic line in the center of the uterus. Both potential spaces, the "pouch of Douglas" (PD) and the "retrovesicular space" (RV) are seen on the transverse view.

sagittal view, the left side of the screen is the patient's anterior body surface as the indicator is pointing toward the ceiling initially. The right side of the screen then represents the patient's posterior body surface, the top of the screen is the patient's feet (caudad), and the bottom of the screen is the patient's head (cephalad).

The uterus is usually easily identified when the probe is inserted and the full endometrial stripe should be visualized. If the uterus is not readily identified, the transducer may be angled up and down to help bring it into view. This is helpful in situations where the uterus has an extreme angle of version or flexion. The bladder will be more difficult to identify if it is emptied, but if seen will appear as a small anechoic structure anterior to the uterus (see Fig. 12-1). The vaginal stripe is not seen on these images as the probe is inserted into the vault up to the cervix. The uterine fundus will appear on the left side of the screen and the cervix to the right. The probe should be fanned anteriorly and posteriorly in order to fully view the pouch of Douglas and retrovesicular space. Once the uterus and cul-de-sacs are examined, the probe should be fanned to the left and right to identify the ovaries and possible adnexal pathology.

The probe is then turned 90° counterclockwise so that the indicator is pointing toward the patient's right side. This produces a coronal view of the pelvic structures (analogous to the transverse image obtained transabdominally). The image displayed depicts the patient's right on the left side of the screen, the patient's left on the right side of the screen, the top of the screen is the patient's feet (caudad), and the bottom of the screen is the patient's head (cephalad) (Fig. 12-9). Starting with the uterus centered on the screen, the probe should be fanned to visualize the cervix and cul-de-sacs through the uterine fundus, and then directed toward each side to fan through adnexal structures.

IMAGING PROTOCOL IN PREGNANCY

EVALUATION FOR INTRAUTERINE PREGNANCY

In transabdominal scanning, the landmarks of the bladder and vaginal stripe must be identified first in order to establish that a pregnancy is intrauterine. The vaginal stripe can be followed up through the cervix into the lumen of the uterus

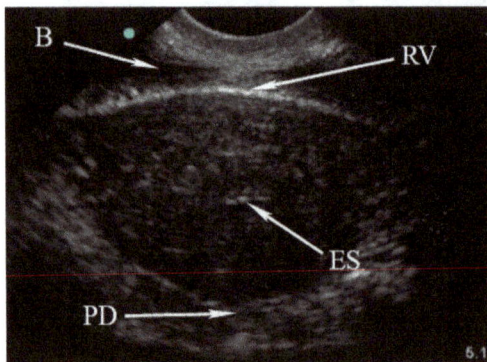

FIGURE 12-9 Coronal transvaginal view of normal pelvic anatomy. The bladder (B) is seen as an anechoic structure anterior and inferior to the uterus. ES: endometrial stripe, RV: retrovesicular space, PD: pouch of Douglas.

looking for an anechoic area that may represent the gestational sac. On transvaginal scanning the vaginal stripe will not be seen (this is where the probe is), but the uterus should be completely imaged to ensure that any contents are intrauterine. Once it has been established that the anechoic area is inside the uterus and not in the adnexa, it can be further evaluated to determine if it is a pregnancy.

The minimum criteria of an IUP are a gestational sac *with a yolk sac* or fetal pole. An anechoic area alone inside the uterus is not sufficient to diagnose an IUP, and should not be described as a gestational sac unless other signs of pregnancy are evident. An ectopic pregnancy may still have a fluid collection in the uterus, known as a psuedogestational sac.

GESTATIONAL AGE

There are numerous methods of measuring the gestational age of the fetus depending on the stage of pregnancy. In early pregnancy (12 weeks or less), the terms "mean gestational sac diameter" and "crown-rump-length" are most commonly used. In later pregnancy (over 12 weeks) BPD is recommended, although other methods may be used (femur length, abdominal, or head circumference).

Mean Gestational Sac Diameter   Mean gestational sac diameter (MGSD) is the earliest method used to estimate the gestational age (GA) of the fetus. MGSD is obtained by measuring the sac in three planes from the inner-to-inner edges, not including the walls. Once the three measurements are recorded, the GA is estimated based on the following formula:

$$GA +/- 4 \text{ days} = MGSD \text{ (mm)} + 30$$

A GA age of approximately 5 weeks will produce a MGSD of approximately 5 mm. A fetal pole should be visualized by the time the MGSD reaches 12–16 mm.

Crown-Rump-Length   Once the fetal pole is visualized, the CRL can be measured to determine the GA. The length of the embryo is measured using calipers and the GA is estimated based on calculation software packages that are included with most ultrasound machines. If this calculation is not included on the machine, the formula is:

$$CRL \text{ (cm)} + 42 = GA$$

The CRL should be measured from the crown of the head to the rump, not including the yolk sac or legs (Fig. 12-10). The CRL usually increases by approximately 1 mm per day.

Biparietal Diameter   The biparietal diameter (BPD) is measured across the skull from one parietal bone to the other. The most accurate GA is computed by taking the measurement through the third ventricle and thalami. One caliper should be placed on the outer edge of the near wall and the second caliper on the inner edge of the far wall, called the "leading edge technique" (Fig. 12-11). Most ultrasound machines contain calculation packages, which convert the BPD into an estimated GA.

FETAL HEART RATE

Cardiac activity can usually be visualized at about 6 weeks on TVUS and by 7–8 weeks on TAUS. FHR is determined using M-mode, which measures motion over time. Once the fetal pole is identified and the flicker of cardiac activity can be seen within it, the M-mode cursor is placed over the moving

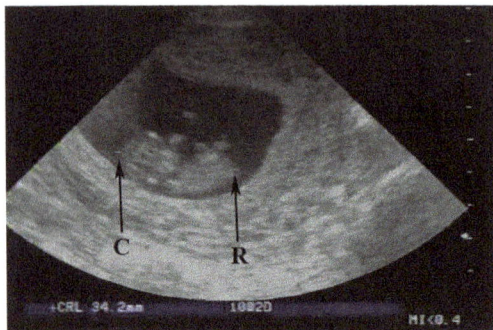

FIGURE 12-10 An illustration of where to properly measure the CRL in early pregnancy. The measurement should be from the crown of the head (C) to the rump of the buttocks (R) without including the legs or yolk sac. The machine will use software packages to convert this into an estimated gestational age.

heart. This produces a tracing, which will record motion on the y-axis and time on the x-axis (Fig. 12-12). Calipers are used to measure the distance between the cardiac beats, and most machines contain calculation packages that will translate this distance into a heart rate. Due to the high energy of Doppler, it should not be used to measure fetal cardiac activity during the first trimester.

PATHOLOGIC ULTRASOUND FINDINGS IN EARLY PREGNANCY

The primary objective of performing an ultrasound in a patient with early pregnancy and vaginal bleeding and/or pelvic pain is to determine whether an IUP is present or not. While it is possible to be both an intrauterine and extrauterine pregnancy

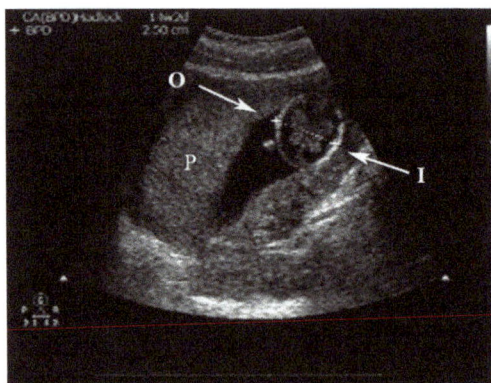

FIGURE 12-11 The correct technique to measure BPD in estimating fetal gestational age (GA). The measurement should be from one parietal bone to the other using the "leading edge technique." The cursor should measure from the outside edge (O) of the near bone to the inside edge (I) of the far bone. The machine software packages will convert this measurement into an estimated GA, seen at the top of the image. P: placenta.

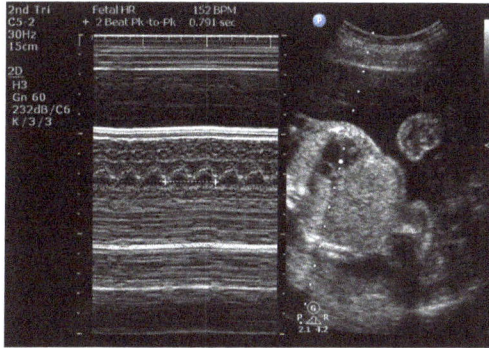

FIGURE 12-12 M-mode tracing calculating the fetal heart rate. The cursor is placed over the fetal heart on the right side of the image producing the graph on the left depicting motion on the y-axis and time on the x-axis. The measurement is then taken using the "two beat peak-to-peak" method and the machine's software converts this distance into a FHR of 152 bpm, seen at the top of the image.

(heterotopic), this is uncommon in a patient not undergoing fertility treatment. While the adnexa should also be examined in a patient with an IUP, if there is no significant free fluid or severe pain, an ectopic is extremely unlikely.

ABNORMAL INTRAUTERINE PREGNANCY

There are certain features on ultrasound that may indicate an abnormal pregnancy that is unlikely to be viable. Abnormal embryonic development can be seen as an enlarged gestational or yolk sac or one that has an irregular scalloped appearance (Fig. 12-13a and b). A gestational sac that is larger than 10 mm without a yolk sac, or a gestational sac above 15 mm without a fetal pole on TVUS, indicates an abnormal pregnancy. A yolk sac over 8 mm is abnormal. If a definite fetal pole is seen on TVUS, careful scanning should demonstrate cardiac activity. The absence of cardiac activity on TVUS when a fetal pole is clearly seen is evidence of fetal demise.

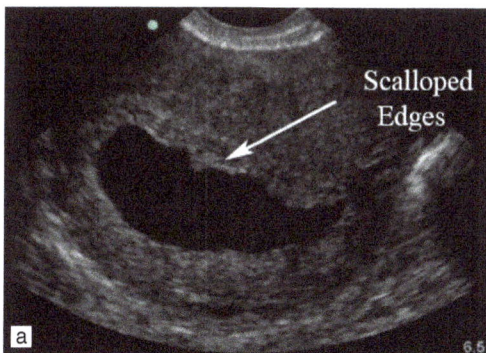

FIGURE 12-13(a) Illustrations of an abnormal IUP. The gestational sac is abnormally enlarged with scalloped edges. Both of these cases (a and b) went on to fetal demise.

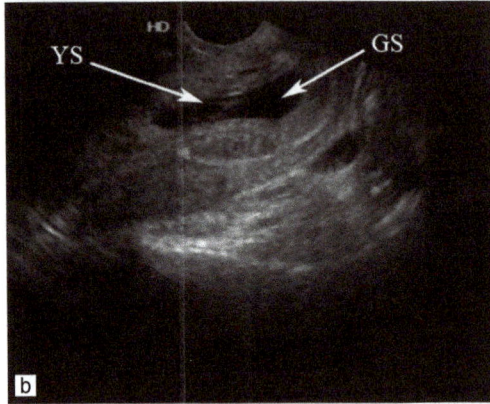

FIGURE 12-13(*b*) Illustrations of an abnormal IUP. The yolk sac (YS) appears enlarged and abnormally shaped. Both of these cases (*a* and *b*) went on to fetal demise. GS: gestational sac.

NO DEFINITIVE INTRAUTERINE PREGNANCY

The absence of an IUP on ultrasound in a patient with a positive pregnancy test may be broadly described as "no definitive intrauterine pregnancy" or NDIUP. NDIUP may include early pregnancy, ectopic pregnancy, miscarriage, or gestational trophoblastic disease, described later. Unless a diagnosis such as miscarriage is clinically evident, a sonographic diagnosis of NDIUP in a patient with vaginal bleeding or pelvic pain should generally prompt further evaluation, including quantitative beta-hCG and gynecologic consultation, particularly if the hCG is above the discriminatory zone.

An algorithm of how to approach the pregnant patient is outlined in Fig. 12-14.

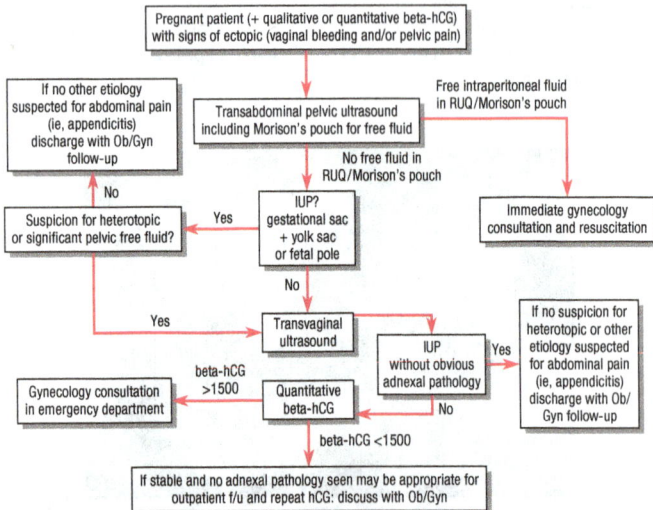

FIGURE 12-14 An algorithm of how to approach the pregnant patient.

THE DISCRIMINATORY ZONE

If an IUP is not identified, a quantitative beta-hCG is helpful in determining whether an IUP should be seen on TVUS. This is called the discriminatory zone, which may vary from institution to institution, but is generally between 1000 and 1500 mIU. If the beta-hCG is above this level, an IUP should be seen on TVUS. If the beta is above this level and there is not an IUP, an ectopic should be suspected and gynecology involved. If there is NDIUP, the beta-hCG is below the discriminatory zone, and there is no significant free fluid or evidence of adnexal pathology, the patient may be discharged with precautions and close follow-up, including repeat evaluation and repeat beta-hCG at 48 hours. The discriminatory zone does not apply to a TAUS. While the absence of an IUP on TVUS in a patient with a beta-hCG above the discriminatory zone (and no clear miscarriage) is highly suggestive of an ectopic, an ectopic may be seen and may rupture at lower levels (mean beta-hCG for ectopic rupture is 1000 mIU), so a low quantitative beta-hCG does not mean that an ultrasound should not be performed. Rarely, an ectopic may occur and rupture at beta-hCG levels so low that a urine pregnancy test is not positive; so a quantitative beta should be obtained if the suspicion for ectopic is high.

MISCARRIAGE

A miscarriage may show no definitive IUP with a beta-human chorionic gonadotropin (hCG) above the discriminatory zone. If products of conception are passed this may be diagnosed clinically. On ultrasound, the endometrial canal typically contains debris which may be blood or less commonly RPOC. The presence of color flow, seen with Doppler, within the material in the endometrial cavity may indicate RPOC rather than blood clot.

ECTOPIC PREGNANCY

An ectopic is an abnormally located pregnancy. This is most commonly outside of the uterus but may be in an abnormal location within the uterus (cornual/interstitial or cervical). The most common location of an ectopic is in the ampulla of the fallopian tube. Ovarian ectopics may occur but are unusual (1%–2% of ectopics), so a cystic area directly associated with the ovary is unlikely to be an ectopic and is more likely a corpus luteum cyst.

An ectopic pregnancy will take on a variety of appearances depending on its location and gestational age. Most commonly, an ectopic appears as a complex adnexal mass separate from the ovary. Occasionally, an extrauterine yolk sac or fetal pole (possibly with a FHR) may be visualized and this is definitive for an ectopic (Fig 12-15). Color Doppler of the adnexa may light up and show a "ring of fire" surrounding an ectopic in the adnexa. The appearance of the uterus may be normal or empty or may contain an anechoic area consistent with a pseudogestational sac. A pseudogestational sac is a collection of either fluid or hyperechoic material that distends the endometrial canal. It usually conforms to the shape of the endometrial canal and there is no associated embryo or yolk sac.

A cervical ectopic will be located in a low position in the uterus, almost appearing in the vaginal canal. A cornual (interstitial) pregnancy is located in an eccentric location high up in the fundus of the uterus. It appears to be intrauterine, but actually forms in the interstitium of the fallopian tube where it crosses over the uterine fundus. These pregnancies may appear to be intrauterine and can be mistaken as normal. The myometrium that surrounds the gestational sac in these situations will appear to be thinned out. The endomyometrial mantle, which is the area between the gestational sac and the wall of the uterus, should be greater than 8 mm in a normal IUP. If it is measured to be less than 8 mm, a cornual pregnancy

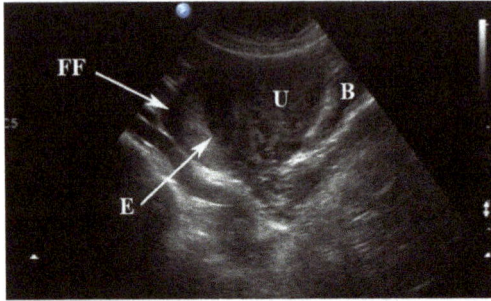

FIGURE 12-15 A sagittal transabdominal pelvic view illustrating an ectopic pregnancy. The ectopic (E) appears as a heterogenous structure in the adnexa adjacent to the uterus (U). Note the presence of free fluid (FF) in the pelvis also. B: bladder.

should be suspected (Fig. 12-16). These ectopics require more aggressive treatment, as they are associated with a higher risk of rupture than fallopian pregnancies.

The treatment of an ectopic pregnancy depends on several factors including the location and size. Oftentimes, a conservative approach is favored, which involves giving methotrexate and performing repeat ultrasounds and hCG levels afterwards in order to ensure success. Factors that predict which patients are not good candidates for conservative treatment include ectopics greater than 3.5 cm on ultrasound, those with a FHR present, hCG levels >5000, in patients where compliance is a concern, and in those who have already failed conservative treatment. In addition, an interstitial pregnancy should be considered higher risk and a more ideal candidate for surgical intervention.

The presence of significant amounts of pelvic fluid, in both the anterior and posterior cul-de-sacs, in a pregnant patient with abdominal pain is a ruptured ectopic until proven otherwise (Fig. 12-17). A RUQ coronal view is also beneficial in

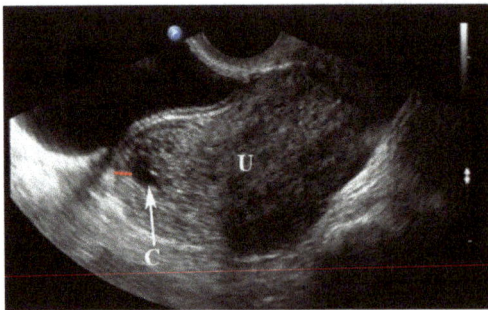

FIGURE 12-16 A sagittal transvaginal pelvic view showing a cornual (interstitial) pregnancy (C). The pregnancy appears to be within the uterus (U), but is actually in the interstitium of the fallopian tube as it crosses over the uterine fundus. Note the high-up appearance of the pregnancy. The red line illustrates the endomyometrial mantle, the distance between the fundus and the pregnancy, which is less than 8 mm, indicating an ectopic.

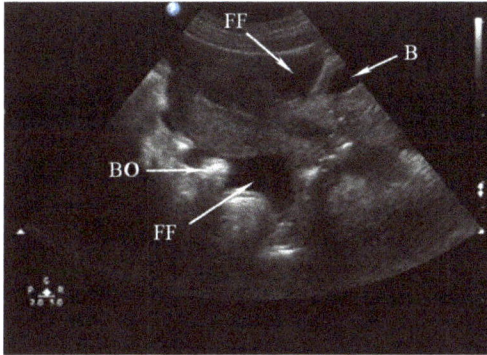

FIGURE 12-17 Sagittal transabdominal pelvic view showing pathologic free fluid (FF) in both the pouch of Douglas (in between the uterus and rectum) and in the retrovesicular space (in between the uterus and bladder) due to a ruptured ectopic. The free fluid is not limited to the posterior cul-de-sac and extends beyond one-third of the posterior-inferior uterine wall. B: bladder, BO: bowel.

these patients as free fluid in other quadrants leads to a high likelihood that the patient will go directly to the operating room. If there is fluid in Morison's pouch, gynecology should be called immediately.

SUBCHORIONIC HEMORRHAGE

A subchorionic hemorrhage (SCH) or perigestational hemorrhage is a bleed that occurs between the uterine wall and chorionic membrane when it becomes separated from its implantation site. SCH is the most common cause of vaginal bleeding in the first trimester. It usually appears as an anechoic crescent-shaped structure surrounding part of the gestational sac (Fig. 12-18). The prognosis of a

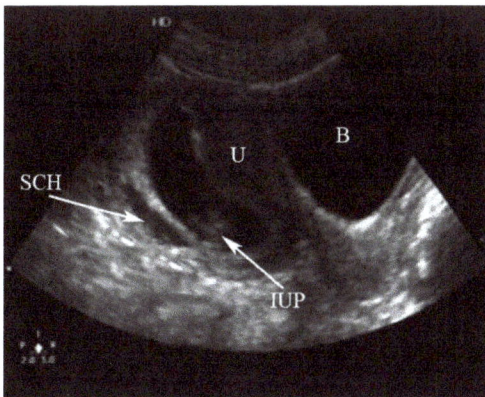

FIGURE 12-18 A sagittal transabdominal pelvic view showing a subchorionic hemorrhage (SCH). This patient had a confirmed intrauterine pregnancy (IUP) and presented with first trimester vaginal bleeding. This SCH is less than 20% of the gestational sac (GS) size and considered small. On repeat ultrasound it had completely resolved. B: bladder, U: uterus.

SCH depends on several factors, including the size of the hemorrhage, the age of the fetus and mother, and the stage of pregnancy. Asymptomatic small bleeds in the early first trimester usually reabsorb without complication and do not predict a poor outcome. Larger hemorrhages that cause vaginal bleeding, that occur in the late first trimester or second trimester, or ones that occur in older women carry a worse prognosis. A SCH is graded based on its size in relation to the gestational sac, large >50%, medium 20%–50%, and small <20%.

GESTATIONAL TROPHOBLASTIC DISEASE

Gestational trophoblastic disease (GTD) is a proliferative disease of the trophoblast that includes such entities as hydatidiform mole, invasive mole, choriocarcinoma, and placental site trophoblastic tumor. Hydatidiform mole is the most common form of GTD and can be either benign or malignant. These patients will often present with vaginal bleeding, an enlarged uterus that is out of proportion to the fetal age, a markedly elevated beta-hCG level, and hyperemesis. Sonographically, GTD can appear as complex heterogeneous structures filling the endometrial cavity that are described as having a "snowstorm" appearance or resembling a "cluster of grapes" (Fig. 12-19). In addition, a well-defined embryo is usually absent. Specialist consultation should be obtained if this is identified.

HETEROTOPIC PREGNANCIES

A heterotopic pregnancy is an IUP as well as an ectopic pregnancy. Heterotopic pregnancies are becoming more common due to the increased use of assisted reproduction and hormonal therapies. The occurrence rates have been noted to be approximately 3% in fertility-assisted pregnancies, and anywhere from 1/2500 to 1/30,000 in all pregnancies. These pregnancies can be misleading as the clinician may identify the normal IUP and not continue looking for an additional ectopic pregnancy. This illustrates the importance of thorough scanning of all the pelvic structures even when a normal IUP has been identified.

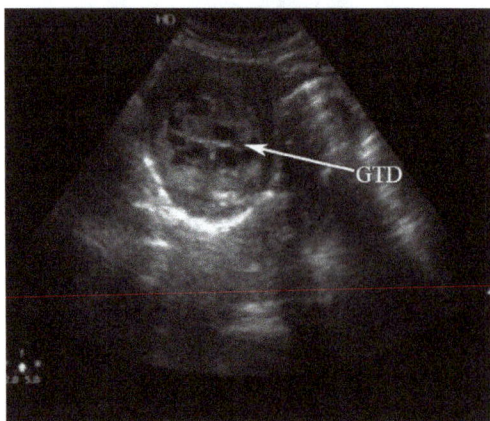

FIGURE 12-19 Gestational trophoblastic disease (GTD) appearing as a "cluster of grapes" or having a "snowstorm" appearance.

PATHOLOGIC ULTRASOUND FINDINGS—LATER PREGNANCY

PLACENTA PREVIA

Placenta previa refers to an abnormally low-positioned placenta, close to or completely covering the internal orifice (os) of the uterus. It is classified into four types depending on its location in relationship to the os. "Low-lying" is a placenta that is positioned in the lower segment of the uterus, close to the os, but does not come into contact with it. "Marginal" is when the placenta touches the internal os, but does not cover it. "Partial" and "complete" are defined by how much the inferior portion of the placenta covers the opening to the internal os. The exact cause is not known, but risk factors include previous previa, drug or alcohol abuse, previous abortions, younger and older maternal age, and the presence of twin gestations. These patients classically present with painless vaginal bleeding in the second or third trimester. In a patient with late pregnancy and vaginal bleeding, a placenta overlying the cervical os should lead to obstetrical consultation prior to pelvic examination or TVUS.

PLACENTAL ABRUPTION

Placental abruption involves bleeding in between the layers of the placenta that causes it to separate from the uterine wall. Abruptions are categorized by grades: Grade 0 is asymptomatic and only diagnosed after fetal birth; Grade 1 produces mild bleeding or pain, but no maternal or fetal distress; Grade 2 causes heavier bleeding, more maternal and fetal symptoms, but not shock; Grade 3 causes severe bleeding with maternal and fetal shock and possibly death. The main risk factors for abruption include maternal hypertension, cocaine use, previous abruption, extremes of maternal age, a short umbilical cord, or trauma. These patients will often present in significant pain with vaginal bleeding, although bleeding is not always present depending on the location of the abruption.

When identified, hemorrhage will be seen in between the placenta and uterus on ultrasound. Ultrasound is not sensitive enough to rule out placental abruption, and therefore, if it is suspected, obstetrics should be called immediately.

UTERINE RUPTURE

Uterine rupture usually occurs in the setting of trauma, but has been reported during active labor. Similar to other solid organ injuries, there will be free intraperitoneal fluid seen on ultrasound representing both blood and amniotic fluid. Examination of the fetus will usually reveal a lack of FHR activity. Uterine rupture is an obstetrical emergency and requires immediate cesarean section if the fetus is still viable.

SPECIAL CONSIDERATIONS: THE PREGNANT TRAUMA PATIENT

The pregnant trauma patient can be especially challenging to the acute care physician. This patient not only sustains similar injuries as a nonpregnant patient, but, in addition can have pregnancy and fetal-related injuries. Most critical care centers will triage patients who are in the second trimester directly to the obstetrical service on arrival to the hospital. The pregnant trauma patient is an exception to this policy, as the emergency physician must evaluate these patients for traumatic injuries first on arrival, although obstetrics should also be notified immediately for any pregnancy that may be viable. The standard FAST exam should be performed in these patients, as described in Chap. 9 and 24 looking for injuries that create free intraperitoneal fluid, similar to the nonpregnant trauma patient. A negative FAST exam on arrival may help the physician avoid performing a CT scan on these pregnant patients if they are at low risk. While ultrasound is not sensitive for some of the other conditions discussed earlier (abruption, uterine rupture), it may be able to expedite identification.

OTHER PATHOLOGIC ULTRASOUND FINDINGS (PREGNANT OR NONPREGNANT PATIENTS)

FIBROIDS

Fibroids are benign smooth muscle masses (leiomyomas) that originate from the uterine myometrium. Fibroids most commonly affect the body and fundus of the uterus, and more rarely are found at the cervix. While benign, they can cause pelvic discomfort, fullness, and excessive vaginal bleeding. Fibroids tend to enlarge with hormonal stimulation and regress after menopause. Fibroids are a very common cause of vaginal bleeding and pelvic pain in women presenting to the emergency department.

The sonographic appearance of fibroids varies and they usually appear as round or ovoid-shaped heterogeneous structures. These masses have variable echogenicities and will have areas that are hyper- and hypoechoic compared to the surrounding myometrium. They may contain calcifications which will appear as white, highly echogenic structures with posterior shadowing due to sound beam attenuation (Fig. 12-20). Fibroids can also degenerate and become necrotic causing worsening pain. Degenerating fibroids will have an irregular anechoic appearance on ultrasound.

Fibroids can mimic other pathological conditions, such as gestational trophoblastic disease, intrauterine device perforations, uterine or adnexal masses, or uterine duplications. If an unusual appearing mass is identified on ultrasound associated with the finding of ascites, a sarcoma or other malignant mass must be considered. In this situation, CT scan or other imaging modalities are recommended for further evaluation.

ENDOMETRIAL CARCINOMA

Although endometrial carcinoma is not routinely diagnosed in the acute care setting, there are certain warning signs that the clinician should be aware of.

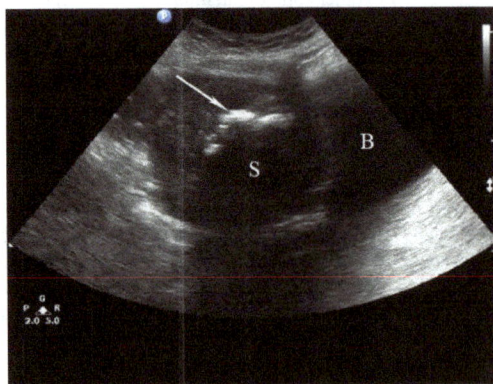

FIGURE 12-20 Sagittal transabdominal view depicting fibroids. Note the heterogenous appearance of the uterus and the arrow pointing at the calcifications within the fibroid that are producing posterior shadowing (S). B: bladder.

A postmenopausal woman who presents with vaginal bleeding is worrisome for carcinoma until proven otherwise. An obvious mass of variable echogenicity may be present on ultrasound evaluation. The endometrial stripe in these women should be less than 5-mm thick. An endometrial stripe measuring greater than 5 mm combined with a complaint of vaginal bleeding needs an evaluation by a specialist for a possible endometrial biopsy.

SIMPLE OVARIAN CYSTS

Simple ovarian cysts are termed "functional cysts" and include follicular, corpus luteum and theca lutein cysts. These cysts have particular appearances on ultrasound, which give them the definition of "simple." They consist of an anechoic fluid-filled center surrounded by a thin echogenic wall. They are usually unilocular, regular-appearing, well-defined structures ranging from 3 to 8 cm in diameter (Fig. 12-21). Simple cysts are normally benign in nature, but complications include rupture, bleeding, or ovarian torsion. Rupture may be associated with pelvic free fluid in the cul-de-sac. The finding of a simple cyst may not be sufficient to explain the patient's pelvic pain and other etiologies may need to be explored.

COMPLEX OVARIAN CYSTS

Complex cysts are irregular in their border or shape or are not completely anechoic (Fig. 12-22). A hemorrhagic cyst will commonly show a reticular pattern within the cyst and may cause significant bleeding, with free fluid on ultrasound and occasionally requiring intervention. Although most complex cysts are benign during the reproductive years, malignant tumors are still possible and any complex cyst should be followed closely.

PELVIC INFLAMMATORY DISEASE

Pelvic inflammatory disease (PID) is an inflammation of the upper female genital tract secondary to an ascending infection. The infection is usually a result of an untreated sexually transmitted disease and less commonly caused by local spread of an abdominal infection, such as appendicitis or diverticulitis. It is a broad term describing a pelvic infection that may include endometritis, salpingitis, salpingo-oophoritis, tuboovarian abscess (TOA), and peritonitis. Early diagnosis and treatment is important due to the associated morbidity, including widespread infection, chronic pain, ectopic pregnancy, and possible infertility.

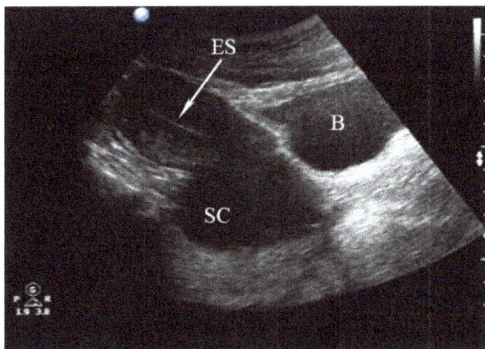

FIGURE 12-21 Sagittal transabdominal view illustrating a simple cyst (SC) in the adnexa. Note its regular, anechoic, thin-walled appearance. ES: endometrial stripe, B: bladder.

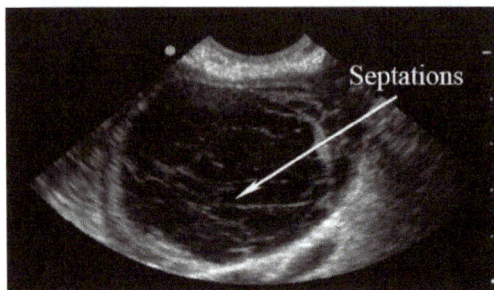

FIGURE 12-22 A complex cyst that appears more heterogeneous with thicker walls and septations. This requires further workup.

PID is usually a clinical diagnosis, but certain ultrasound findings can be helpful and may indicate the need for more aggressive treatment. The ascending infection of the female genital tract often results in dilated fallopian tubes (hydrosalpinx), which may be visualized on ultrasound (Fig. 12-23). The dilated tubes are usually due to postinflammatory obstruction. Hydrosalpinx can resemble the appearance of prominent blood vessels and it is important for the sonographer to distinguish the two. Color-flow Doppler is useful in this situation, as it will pick up blood flow in the vessels, but not in dilated fallopian tubes.

TOA is included in the spectrum of diseases that describe PID. It is an organized collection of pus and debris due to an ascending genital tract infection. It is most commonly found in the adnexa adjacent to the ovaries and fallopian tubes. These patients are usually more toxic appearing with systemic symptoms, such as a fever. Sonographically, a TOA appears as a well-circumscribed heterogenous cystic structure with internal echoes representing pus and debris (Fig. 12-24). This entity can resemble a complex cyst or mass; therefore, the clinician must take into consideration the clinical presentation of the patient. The young woman who presents with pelvic pain, vaginal discharge, and fever with a complex mass seen on ultrasound probably has a TOA until proven otherwise.

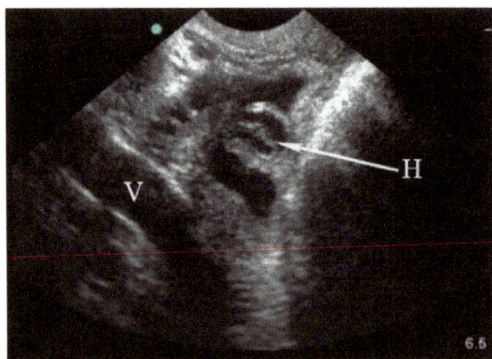

FIGURE 12-23 Hydrosalpinx (H) seen as dilated tortuous fallopian tubes due to PID. These dilated fluid-filled tubes may resemble the iliac vessels (V). Color-flow Doppler can help in differentiating these two adnexal structures.

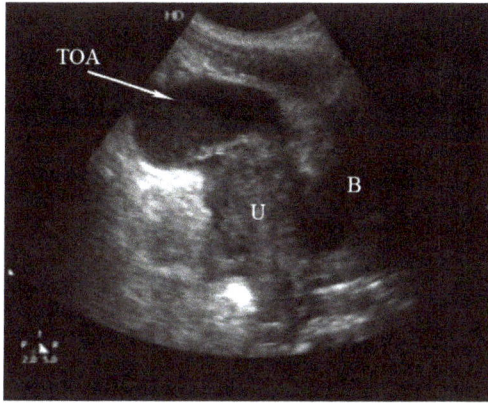

FIGURE 12-24 A tuboovarian abscess (TOA) in the adnexa as a result of PID. It appears as a well-circumscribed heterogeneous structure within the adnexa, separate from the uterus (U). Note the hyperechoic area within the TOA representing debris and pus. B: bladder.

OVARIAN TORSION

The diagnosis of ovarian torsion is difficult by ultrasound and is most often performed by experienced sonographers. Unlike the testes, the ovaries have a dual blood supply, which makes torsion possible even when blood flow is seen on Doppler. Ovarian torsion is frequently precipitated by a mass, especially the ones greater than 4 cm in diameter. Classically, the torsed ovary will appear enlarged with peripheral follicles. A normal size and regular-appearing ovary makes ovarian torsion extremely unlikely. However, ovarian torsion is a true clinical emergency therefore, if there is any suspicion of this diagnosis prompt gynecological consult should be obtained.

INTRAUTERINE DEVICE

The IUD is a contraceptive device that may contain copper or be hormone releasing. IUDs are usually identified based on their echogenic appearance relative to the uterine myometrium. They also produce characteristic artifacts such as shadowing and reverberation, which can help in situations where visualization of the device is uncertain (Fig. 12-25). If a patient presents with pelvic pain and gives a history of IUD use, the clinician must first verify that the device is intrauterine and in the correct location.

Although a displaced IUD is not always fully evaluated in the emergency department, it is helpful to understand the pertinent ultrasound findings. A malpositioned IUD is seen in a low position on ultrasound within the uterus or cervix. These patients will often have a longer string on pelvic examination and may complain of pain. The position of an IUD is determined by measuring the distance between the uterine fundus and the edge of the IUD closest to the fundus. It is correctly positioned when this distance is measured to be less than 2 cm or more specifically if it is no larger than 4/3 of the mean thickness of the uterine wall.

If an IUD is not visualized on ultrasound and the patient complains of pelvic pain they need to be evaluated for possible uterine rupture, peritoneal migration, and perforation. Other complications of IUDs that can be diagnosed by ultrasound include PID and ectopic pregnancy. If ultrasound is indeterminate and if there is high enough clinical suspicion, other imaging may be warranted and a prompt gynecological consultation is recommended.

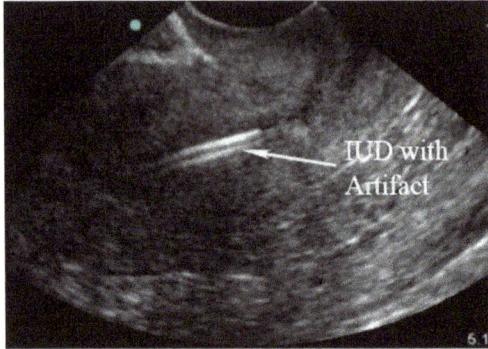

FIGURE 12-25 Sagittal transvaginal view illustrating an IUD. The top bright hyperechoic line represents the IUD overlying the endometrial stripe. The white line below it is reverberation artifact typically produced by an IUD.

ENDOMETRIOSIS

Endometriosis is a condition in which endometrial tissue is found outside of the uterine cavity. There are several locations where endometriosis occurs, including the ovaries, fallopian tubes, uterine wall, uterine ligaments, in the peritoneum, intestines, or urinary bladder. While endometriosis is often not evident on ultrasound, endometrial invasion of the ovary may produce an endometrioma or "chocolate cyst." These cysts take on a heterogenous debris-filled appearance similar to other complex adnexal structures (Fig. 12-26). These patients can experience pelvic pain and vaginal bleeding depending on hormonal changes. Although this diagnosis is not emergent, follow-up with a specialist is needed for definitive treatment.

FREE FLUID

Females will often have a small amount of simple free fluid in the posterior cul-de-sac (pouch of Douglas), which is considered normal and physiologic. A general

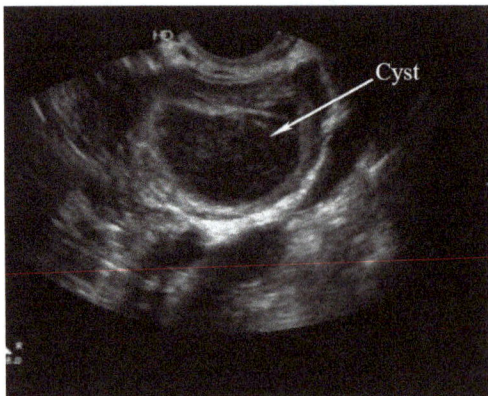

FIGURE 12-26 A "chocolate cyst" seen in the adnexa, typical of endometriosis of ovarian tissue.

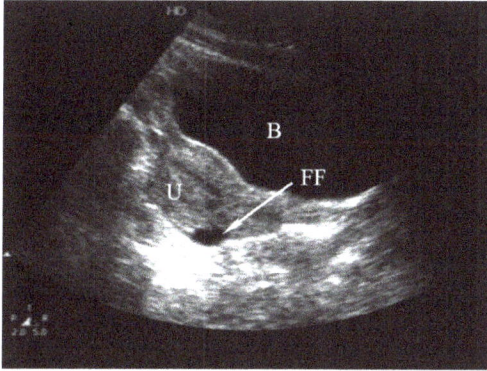

FIGURE 12-27 Sagittal transabdominal pelvic view showing physiologic free fluid (FF) in the pouch of Douglas or posterior-cul-de-sac. The free fluid is limited to the posterior cul-de-sac and does not extend beyond one-third of the posterior–inferior uterine wall. B: bladder, U: uterus.

rule is that if the fluid is contained within the posterior cul-de-sac or if it does not extend beyond one-third of the posterior–inferior surface of the uterine wall, it is most likely benign. This physiologic free fluid will appear as an anechoic black stripe in between the posterior uterine wall and rectum (Fig. 12-27).

If the fluid amount is large enough to track into the anterior cul-de-sac (retrovesicular space) or into other areas of the peritoneal cavity, then it is considered pathologic and further evaluation is warranted (see Fig. 12-17). If a considerable amount of fluid is found in the pelvis, a FAST exam should be completed to look at the other dependent areas in the abdomen. Significant free fluid can be seen in such conditions as trauma, ectopic pregnancy, PID, and ruptured ovarian cysts. Internal echoes or increased heterogeneity of the fluid is also another indication that there is a pathological process going on. Fluid that is not completely anechoic may represent clotted blood (Fig. 12-28). A pregnancy test should be performed

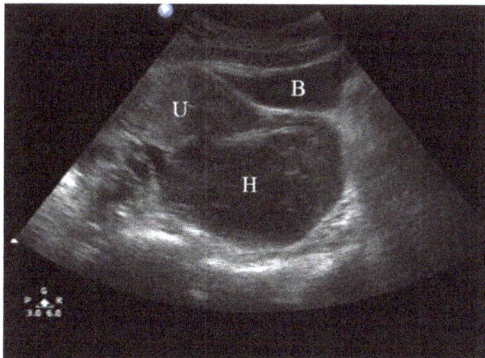

FIGURE 12-28 Sagittal transabdominal pelvic view illustrating clotted blood. This patient had a ruptured hemorrhagic cyst and resultant large hematoma (H), which can be seen in the adnexa. Note its appearance is more heterogeneous and organized compared to the appearance of an acute bleed, as illustrated in Fig. 12-15. B: bladder, U: uterus.

on all women of a reproductive age because the combination of a positive test with significant free fluid is highly indicative of an ectopic pregnancy, and fluid in Morison's pouch indicates a likely need for operative intervention. In a non-pregnant patient with significant free fluid, the most likely source is a hemorrhagic ovarian cyst, which may require operative intervention if severe.

COMMON PITFALLS

BLADDER VOLUME

In TAUS, a full bladder serves a sonographic window for imaging the female pelvis. If the bladder is empty, it may be difficult to identify pertinent female anatomy, especially in the obese patient. If the bladder is empty, the patient should be asked to drink something and rescanned after 20–30 minutes. The opposite is the case with TVUS. The ability of the TV probe to image closer to the object of interest and its better resolution obviates the need for a full bladder. A bladder that is too full can push on the uterus and falsely distort the anatomy and result in missed findings. The patient should be asked to empty their bladder and then rescanned.

NOT PERFORMING A TAUS FIRST

TVUS provides higher resolution and is much better for visualizing more subtle pathology. However, TVUS provides a close field of vision and may be confusing if there are large pathologic structures. Starting with a TAUS will ensure that you are oriented and that any large pathology is not missed.

MISSING IMPORTANT PATHOLOGY ON TAUS

While it may be diagnostic, a TAUS is not sufficient to rule out all relevant pathology when a patient presents with pelvic pain. If there is concern for any abnormalities that are not identified on TAUS, then TVUS should be performed. TVUS is the modality of choice for any adnexal concerns, especially if there is a suspicion of ovarian torsion.

MISINTERPRETING FREE FLUID

As discussed earlier, free fluid will collect in the pouch of Douglas or posterior cul-de-sac first. A small amount of physiologic fluid is normal in the female pelvis and this should not be identified as pathologic. The sonographer must be able to differentiate free fluid that is normal from abnormal and the clinical scenario must be considered in each case.

MISTAKING STRUCTURES FOR FREE FLUID

Fluid-filled structures in the pelvis may appear completely anechoic, similar to the appearance of free fluid. Fluid-filled structures in the pelvis include such things as the bladder, ovarian cysts, loops of bowel, and blood vessels. Free fluid will appear free flowing and will track around structures in the pelvis and appear between loops of bowel. Fluid-filled structures will appear more contained and have clearly defined walls. It is important to fan through and track all anechoic structures in order to properly identify them. The addition of color-flow Doppler can help to differentiate blood vessels from other fluid-filled structures.

MISTAKING LARGE FREE FLUID FOR THE BLADDER

Particularly on a transabdominal pelvic ultrasound, a large amount of free fluid may be contained by the pelvic walls and be mistaken for a distended bladder. The borders of any fluid collection must be clearly defined and the bladder should be definitively identified as a rounded, enclosed, fluid-filled structure.

PITFALLS IN EARLY PREGNANCY

VERIFYING AN INTRAUTERINE PREGNANCY

It is important to remember that when attempting to identify an IUP, the land-marks of the vaginal stripe and bladder in a sagittal plane must be located first. Then, the minimum criterion for an IUP must exist: a gestational sac (GS) + a yolk sac (YS) +/− a fetal pole (FP). The novice sonographer may incorrectly call an empty anechoic area inside the uterus a gestational sac and call it an IUP. If an empty anechoic area is seen in the uterus, it is not considered a GS or an IUP. If it is unclear if the findings are consistent with a GS or an IUP, a TVUS should be performed for better resolution.

MISSING AN ECTOPIC PREGNANCY

Any patient with a positive pregnancy test who does not have a clear IUP on TAUS should undergo a TVUS, regardless of the beta-hCG.

MISINTERPRETING AN INTERSTITIAL OR CERVICAL PREGNANCY AS AN "INTRAUTERINE PREGNANCY"

An interstitial (cornual) pregnancy is a dangerous entity. If a pregnancy is eccen-tric (particularly in the upper outer corner of the uterus) or if the myometrial mantle is thin (<8 mm), an interstitial pregnancy should be suspected. If there is concern about the location of a pregnancy within the uterus, consultation should be obtained prior to sending the patient home.

MISSING A HETEROTOPIC PREGNANCY

Although heterotopic pregnancies are rare, evaluation of the adnexa for patholo-gy and the pelvis for free fluid should be performed even if an IUP is identified. If fertility treatments are involved, the identification of an IUP in a patient with pain and/or bleeding should not significantly lower the suspicion for ectopic (hetero-topic) pregnancy.

COLOR-FLOW DOPPLER

Color-flow Doppler is a high-energy application and due to unknown fetal effects, should not be used in any pregnant patient.

INTEGRATION OF BEDSIDE PELVIC ULTRASOUND INTO CLINICAL CARE

Bedside pelvic ultrasound should be an integrated part of the examination for any female patient who presents with pelvic pain or vaginal bleeding. In an unstable patient, a quick bedside ultrasound that identifies free fluid obviates the need to transfer the patient to radiology and expedites the care of the sick patient.

Many patients present in early pregnancy with abdominal pain or vaginal bleeding. The serious concern in these cases is an ectopic pregancy. In a patient in whom the clinical concern for ectopic is not high, the rapid bedside identification of an IUP (particularly a live IUP) essentially excludes ectopic and can reassure the patient within minutes of arrival.

Pelvic ultrasound is the test of choice for evaluating other pathology in the pregnant or nonpregnant patient. While this ultrasound may be challenging and is often outside of the scope of point-of-care ultrasound, it may help to guide diagnostic evaluation and disposition. Ultrasound of the pelvis may also be combined with ultrasound of other areas that may help diagnose conditions such as cholecystitis, appendicitis, or any renal colic.

Although women in late pregnancy do not present as often in the emergency setting, bedside ultrasound can help the physician evaluate the patient for pregnancy related abdominal pain or vaginal bleeding, such as placenta previa or abruption.

As in all patients, ultrasound remains pertinent in the evaluation of the pregnant trauma patient. An early FAST exam can help avoid unnecessary radiation and diagnose maternal and fetal injuries on arrival. It is an ideal first modality in the pregnant trauma patient for evaluation of both the mother and fetus.

Additional Reading

Chiang G, Levine D, Swire M, et al. The intradecidual sign: is it reliable for diagnosis of early intrauterine pregnancy? *Am J Roentgenol.* 2004;183:725-731.

Condous G, Kirk E, Lu C, et al. Diagnostic accuracy of varying discriminatory zones for the prediction of ectopic pregnancy in women with a pregnancy of unknown location. *Ultrasound Obstet Gynecol.* 2005;26:770-775.

DeWitt C, Abbott J. Interstitial pregnancy: a potential for misdiagnosis of ectopic pregnancy with emergency department ultrasonography. *Ann Emerg Med.* 2002;40:106-109.

Moore C, Todd WM, O'Brien E, Lin H. Free fluid in Morison's pouch on bedside ultrasound predicts need for operative intervention in suspected ectopic pregnancy. *Acad Emerg Med.* 2007;14:755-758.

Tayal Vs, Cohen H, Norton HJ. Outcome of patients with an indeterminate emergency department first-trimester pelvic ultrasound to rule out-ectopic pregnancy. *Acad Emerg Med.* 2004;11:912-917.

13 Testicular Ultrasound

J. Scott Bomann

BACKGROUND AND INDICATIONS FOR EXAMINATION

Bedside testicular sonography may assist with the diagnosis and treatment of any patient presenting with acute testicular pain. It can be performed within minutes of arrival and may save time in the diagnosis and treatment of testicular emergencies. It is noninvasive and emergency physicians have been shown to accurately diagnose patients with acute testicular pain using ultrasound.

Testicular torsion and rupture are true surgical emergencies and ultrasound is the diagnostic test of choice for both conditions. Ultrasound may also reveal less acute causes of testicular pain, such as torsion of a testicular appendage, epididymitis, orchitis, hydrocele, and varicocele. These conditions represent the vast majority of cases of nontraumatic testicular pain presenting to the acute care setting.

Bedside ultrasound evaluation of the testes may be performed in:

- The patient with nontraumatic testicular pain, swelling, or mass
- The patient with posttraumatic testicular pain, swelling, or tenderness
- The patient with complaints of penile discharge and found to have testicular tenderness on physical exam

PROBE SELECTION AND TECHNICAL CONSIDERATIONS

LINEAR PROBE WITH A FREQUENCY OF 7.5–10 MHz

The testes are superficial structures; therefore, probes with higher frequencies that provide better resolution are preferred.

COLOR-FLOW DOPPLER

Color-flow Doppler helps to detect the presence and direction of blood flow within the testes. By convention, the color is blue when blood is traveling away from the probe and red when it is flowing toward the probe. The color does not necessarily indicate arterial or venous flow, which must be determined by the character of the flow. The Doppler gain can be increased as needed in order to improve the sensitivity and to detect lower flow states. The pulse repetition frequency (PRF) or "scale" can also be lowered to increase Doppler sensitivity. The sonographer must keep in mind that decreasing the PRF or increasing the gain too much may create unwanted artifact that will erroneously appear as color flow across the testes and can result in a false-negative scan. In contrast, increasing the PRF or decreasing the gain too much (both of which lower sensitivity for flow) may miss blood flow that is actually present, resulting in a false-positive interpretation.

POWER DOPPLER

Power Doppler detects the presence of blood flow only without regard to direction. It appears as shades of red depending on the volume of flow. It is more sensitive and less angle-dependent than color-flow Doppler at picking up low-flow

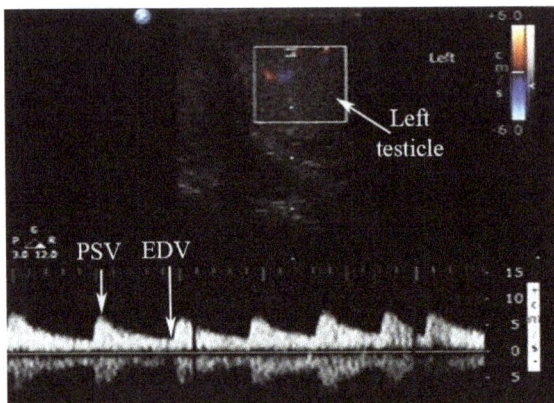

FIGURE 13-1 A transverse image demonstrating normal testicular blood flow. The top of the image shows the left testicle picking up normal color flow. Pulse-wave Doppler is being used to interrogate flow in the area bounded by the small double dashed lines within the box (the "gate"). The spectral image in the lower part of the screen shows velocity (on the y-axis) vs time (on the x-axis). PSV: peak systolic velocity, EDV: end diastolic velocity. The PSV and EDV in this image are approximately 5 and 2, respectively (corresponding to the numbers on the right side of the graph). This makes the calculated resistive index (RI) in this patient at about 0.6, which is considered normal.

states, and therefore is useful for structures such as the testes. But, due to its increased sensitivity, it is also more prone to motion artifact. The sonographer must be careful not to interpret this color artifact as a false-negative study.

PULSE-WAVE DOPPLER AND RESISTIVE INDEX

Pulse wave is a form of spectral Doppler that calculates flow velocity over time and produces a graphic waveform. Blood flow velocities are important to calculate for a particular sample volume. This graphic waveform typically shows a systolic and a diastolic peak (Fig. 13-1). With increasing resistance (due to torsion), the diastolic flow will decrease, ultimately reversing if the resistance is very high. The resistive index (RI) is defined by the following formula:

$$\frac{\text{Peak systolic velocity} - \text{end diastolic velocity}}{\text{Peak systolic velocity}}$$

A normal testicular RI is between 0.5 and 0.7. The RI will be lower in inflammatory conditions such as epididymitis or orchitis. The RI will be elevated in high-resistance states such as torsion. When there is no diastolic flow, the RI will be equal to 1, and may actually be greater than 1 if diastolic flow reverses.

NORMAL ULTRASOUND ANATOMY

The adult testicles are ovoid shaped; approximately $5 \times 3 \times 2$ cm and lie in a vertical position with a slight anterior tilt (Fig. 13-2). They have a homogenous, granular echogenic texture on ultrasound, similar to that of the liver. Immediately

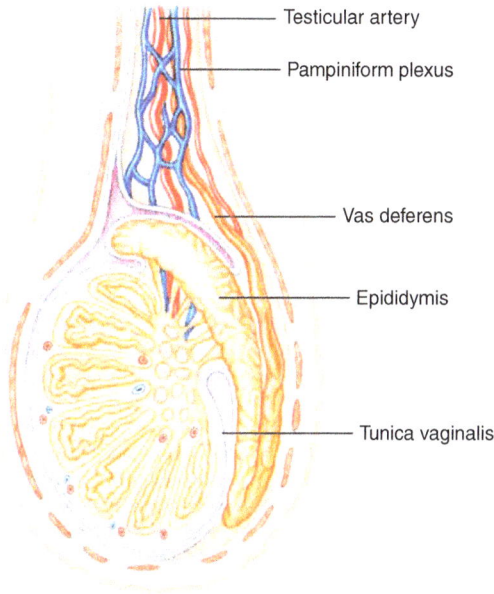

FIGURE 13-2 Normal testicular anatomy.

surrounding the testes is the thin, fibrous, hyperechoic tunica albuginea. The mediastinum testis is a band formed by the invagination of the tunica albuginea and can be seen on ultrasound as a longitudinal echogenic stripe within the testicle. In some patients, an embryologic remnant called the appendix testis can be visualized as a small extra-testicular nodule (2–7 mm) between the upper pole of the testicle and the head of the epididymis.

The tunica vaginalis is a remnant of the peritoneum that accompanies the testicles on their descent into the scrotum. It contains both visceral and parietal layers that envelop the entire testicle, except posteriorly, at the attachment of the epididymis. The "bell-clapper" deformity occurs when the tunica vaginalis completely surrounds the posterior testicle and epididymis, preventing its normal fixation and allowing for increased mobility within the scrotum. This is the main cause of torsion beyond the neonatal period.

The epididymis is 6–7 cm long and curves in a half-loop. Its head sits atop the superior-lateral aspect of the testicle and can be seen as a distinct structure of similar echogenicity. The body is 2–5 mm thick and runs caudally along the posterior testicle before coursing cranially to ultimately become the vas deferens. The epididymis may also contain an appendage, the appendix epididymis, and is seen attached to the head when visualized on ultrasound.

The spermatic cord contains the vas deferens, three arteries (testicular, cremasteric, and deferential), the pampiniform plexus of veins, nerves, and lymphatics. It is difficult to visualize on ultrasound, but an experienced sonographer may visualize the spermatic cord exiting the inguinal canal. The testicular artery supplies both testicles. The artery and all its branches have a low-resistance flow pattern with persistent diastolic flow.

IMAGING TIPS AND PROTOCOL

The patient should be placed in the supine position with a rolled towel beneath the scrotum for elevation. Each testicle should be scanned in two planes, both transverse and longitudinal, beginning with the unaffected side. The sonographer should start in a sagittal (longitudinal) plane with the indicator pointing toward the patient's head. The epididymis will be visualized superiorly on the left side of the screen. In this orientation, the probe should be moved both medially and laterally in order to interrogate the whole testicle and to not miss any irregularities in texture, size, and contour. The testicle should then be scanned in a transverse orientation with the indicator pointing to the patient's right. In this plane, the probe should be moved both superiorly and inferiorly to once again not miss any abnormalities. Once the anatomy has been fully evaluated, color flow to each testicle can be assessed. The Doppler settings should be adjusted, as described earlier, in order to accurately visualize blood flow and to minimize artifacts.

Once color flow is identified, pulse-wave Doppler can be used to record the spectral waveform. The sonographer should place the focal point of the cursor onto an area of color flow within the central testicle in order to obtain both the systolic and diastolic velocity (see Fig. 13-1). The waveforms will either appear above or below the baseline on the graph, depending on whether the flow is directed toward or away from the probe. The same technique should be used to evaluate flow to each epididymis. The resultant velocities are obtained from the spectral waveform graphs and on most machines, the RI will be calculated based on these velocities.

If color Doppler is not sensitive enough to provide evidence of blood flow, power (angio) Doppler, which is more sensitive to low-flow states, may be used instead. Power and pulse-wave Doppler can be used simultaneously. The sonographer should then repeat the whole process on the affected testicle.

For completeness, a grayscale and a Doppler study should also be performed in the transverse plane at the level of the mid-scrotum. The images obtained of each testicle should be compared side by side on the screen. This can help to highlight subtle differences in texture and flow.

PATHOLOGIC ULTRASOUND FINDINGS

TESTICULAR TORSION

In testicular torsion, the twisting of the spermatic cord initially causes blockage of venous drainage followed by a gradual obstruction to arterial inflow and ultimately testicular ischemia. The ability to salvage testicular function depends on the duration of torsion and the degree of twisting, with rescue rates decreasing substantially after 4 hours. Therefore, if there is any suspicion of testicular torsion, it should be treated as an emergency and urology should be consulted immediately.

In early torsion, the grayscale images may appear normal. With further ischemia, the testicle and epididymis will then become enlarged, edematous, and appear heterogenous over the course of hours. In addition, a reactive hydrocele and scrotal thickening may develop. In complete torsion, there will be an absence of blood flow on both color and power Doppler studies (Fig. 13-3). The RI in low-flow states, such as torsion, will begin to rise as the diastolic flow will decrease first, until it approaches zero. Therefore, torsion states will often have RI above 0.7. It is important to not mistake artifact for true blood flow as this can delay the diagnosis (Fig. 13-4*a* and *b*).

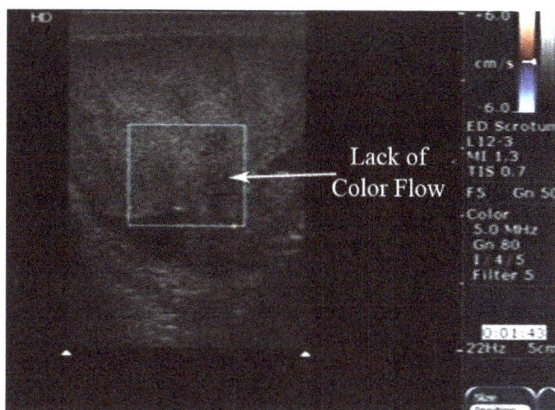

FIGURE 13-3 This image illustrates complete testicular torsion. The color Doppler box is placed over the testicular tissue and a lack of blood flow is visualized. The testicle also appears heterogeneous and edematous, seen as hypoechoic areas throughout the normal architecture. Note that the scale (PRF) is set very low, at +/− 6 cm/s (very sensitive).

Some patients may present with partial torsion, where low-pressure venous flow is absent, but arterial flow may still be present. The resultant spectral waveform will either resemble a slightly pulsatile venous form, an arterial form with reversed diastolic flow, or it may actually appear as a typical arterial wave. The RI may be normal or high. In order to fully evaluate torsion in these cases, both venous and arterial waveforms should be recorded.

The clinician must be aware of patients who present with a history of sudden onset of testicular pain that has since resolved on its own. This may be a sign of transient torsion (torsion-detorsion). In these cases, the affected testicle has regained arterial blood flow and the ultrasound may show a reperfusion hyperemia (Fig. 13-5). This will appear as an increase in flow to the affected testicle when compared to the other side. The flow pattern is similar to other high-flow states such as epididymitis or orchitis and can be differentiated by the absence of pain. The RI in these cases will be low. If torsion-detorsion is suspected, urology should be involved regardless of ultrasound findings.

TORSION OF THE APPENDIX TESTES OR APPENDIX EPIDIDYMIS

This is usually a self-limited condition that is found much more commonly than true spermatic cord torsion. The appendages are best visualized when a reactive hydrocele is present. In appendix torsion, there will be no appendage Doppler signal, but the testicle will have normal flow patterns. The epididymis may be swollen and hyperemic, similar to findings in epididymitis.

EPIDIDYMITIS

Epididymitis is an infectious process of the epididymis due to an upward migration from the urethra, bladder, or prostate. It affects all age ranges and is usually unilateral. Epididymo orchitis is a progression of the disease that affects both the epididymis as well as the testicle. Pure orchitis is uncommon, usually bilateral, and has a viral etiology, most commonly seen with a primary mumps infection.

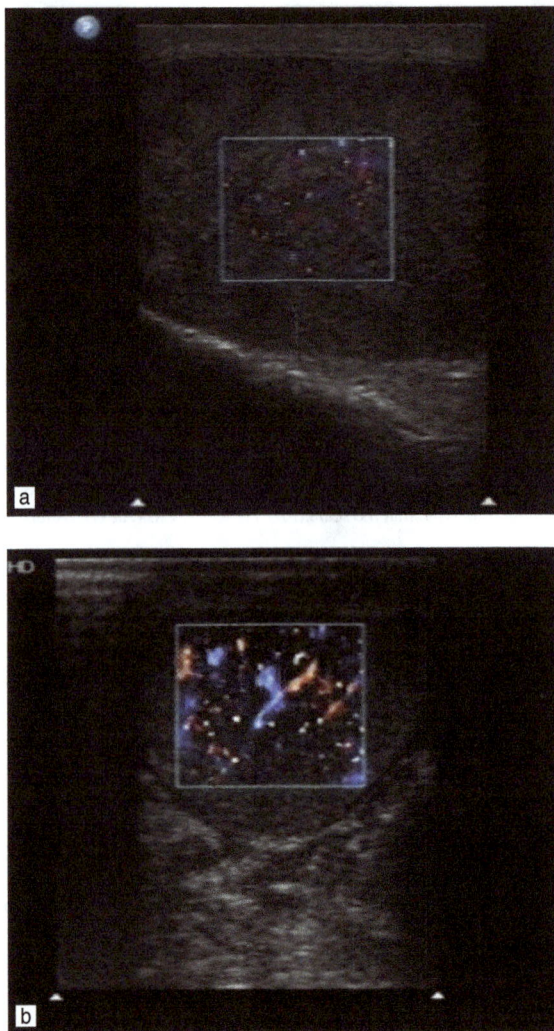

FIGURE 13-4 (*a*) A transverse image depicting torsion with artifact overlying the testicular image. This artifact can result in a false-negative study (ie, thinking there is flow when there is not). The Doppler settings need to be adjusted by turning down the color gain or increasing the pulse-repetition frequency (PRF) or scale on the machine. (*b*) A normal testicle with good blood flow. Notice the difference between the two images.

Grayscale ultrasound images of these conditions will show edematous swelling and decreased echogenicity of the testicular architecture. A reactive hyperemia is often present, represented by increased blood flow on Doppler imaging. Both the testicle and the epididymis should be fully scanned and interrogated with color-flow Doppler and compared to the unaffected side. The RI in these cases will often be low due to the increased blood flow (Fig. 13-6).

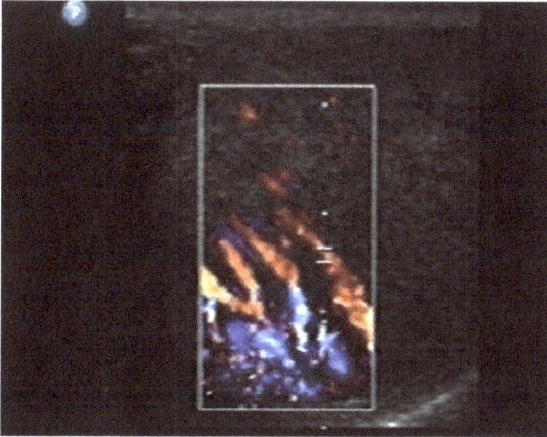

FIGURE 13-5 A detorsed testicle illustrating reperfusion hyperemia. Compare to Fig. 13-4*b*.

HYDROCELE

A hydrocele is an abnormal collection of serous fluid between the two layers of the tunica vaginalis. It is usually an idiopathic nonspecific finding, but may be caused by any pathological testicular condition. As it enlarges, it can become painful and leads to a compartment syndrome with testicular ischemia. In rare cases, if they are large enough, they can cause torsion. Hydroceles appear as

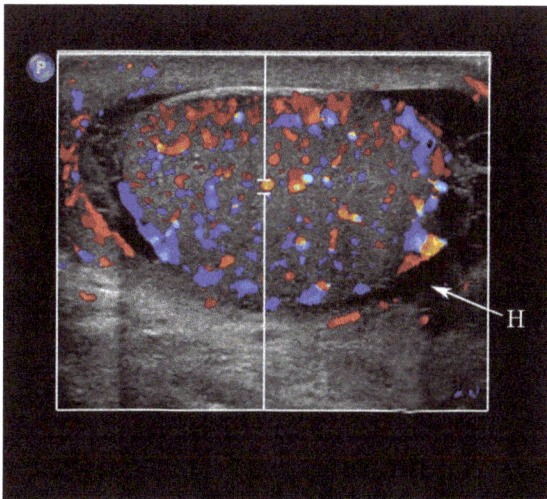

FIGURE 13-6 A transverse image depicting orchitis. The testicle in this image is hyperemic illustrated by enhanced color-flow Doppler signals across the parenchymal surface. A hydrocele (H) is also visualized, most likely a reaction to the infectious process.

anechoic collections that are usually found in the anterior portion of the scrotum, but can be elsewhere (see Fig. 13-6).

VARICOCELE

Varicoceles are dilated veins that appear around the testicles. They occur as a result of backward pressure due to incompetent valves within the spermatic veins. They can be found on either side, but more commonly appear around the left testicle due to higher surrounding pressures. They are usually asymptomatic unless they are large enough to cause compression on the adjacent testicle. On grayscale ultrasound they appear as dilated tortuous tubelike structures appearing either posteriorly or superiorly and lateral to the testicle (Fig. 13-7). The use of color-flow Doppler confirms the diagnosis.

TESTICULAR FRACTURE AND RUPTURE

A testicular fracture will appear as a hypoechoic line through the testicle while the testicular tissue remains encapsulated. It is usually treated conservatively as long as the blood flow remains intact. Testicular rupture occurs when the tunica albuginea is disrupted and testicular tissue extrudes into the scrotum. The grayscale images will show an ill-defined testicular edge with tissue freely leaking into the scrotal cavity. It may be difficult to distinguish from a hematocele (a collection of blood within the tunica vaginalis). Testicular rupture is a surgical emergency and requires emergent urology consultation.

OTHER FINDINGS

Other findings on a testicular ultrasound may include focal areas of hypo- or hyperechogenicity, including cysts and masses. Simple cysts (round, anechoic, thin walled) are likely to be benign. Other findings may represent a testicular malignancy or abscess and should involve consultant-performed imaging and urological follow-up.

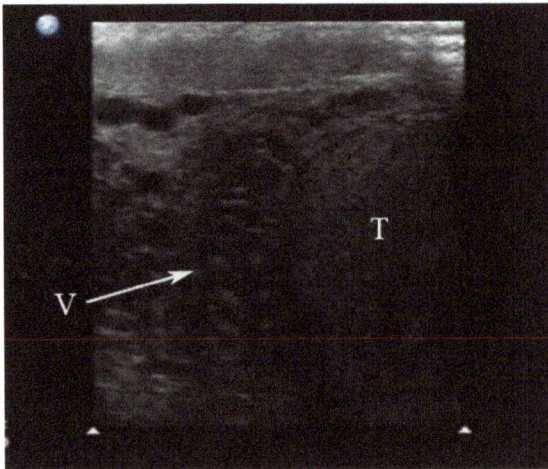

FIGURE 13-7 A grayscale image depicting a varicocele (V) lateral to the testicle (T). Notice the dilated tubular appearance of the veins.

COMMON PITFALLS

INCORRECT DOPPLER OR WAVEFORM INTERPRETATION

Testicular ultrasound requires the use of color and spectral Doppler in order to be complete. Misinterpretation of these results can delay the diagnosis. The sonographer must be careful to have the Doppler settings optimized on the machine. If the color gain is set too high, excessive color artifact overlying the image can be mistaken as normal testicular blood flow and result in a false-negative reading (see Fig. 13-4*a* and *b*). In contrast, if the color-gain setting is too low, a lack of color flow overlying a normal testicle may result in a false-positive diagnosis of torsion. In order to help avoid this pitfall, the examiner should begin with the unaffected testicle in order to visualize normal anatomy and to achieve proper machine settings. The PRF (scale) should be lowered until artifact occurs, and then raised slightly above this level. Similarly the gain should be raised until artifact occurs, and then lowered slightly. The affected testicle should then be scanned with similar settings for comparison.

In using spectral Doppler, both a venous and arterial waveform should be obtained when assessing testicular blood flow. In torsion, venous blood flow is interrupted first. A dangerous pitfall is mistaking the spectral arterial waveform for the venous waveform, leading the operator to a false sense of security. This mistaken venous waveform may actually be a muted arterial wave in partial torsion. Therefore, no study is complete without visualizing both arterial and venous waveforms.

MISDIAGNOSING TRANSIENT TORSION

The clinician needs to beware of the patient who presents with a history of testicular pain that has resolved prior to evaluation. This may be evidence of transient torsion and could result in testicular reperfusion hyperemia on ultrasound (see Fig. 13-5). This increased blood flow could be mistaken as orchitis or epididymitis. As stated earlier, both testicles should be evaluated for comparison. Unlike transient torsion, the pain does not resolve in orchitis or epididymitis. It is important not to mistake the diagnosis, as transient torsion requires emergent surgery.

MISSING OTHER DIAGNOSES

Testicular sonography can be a difficult study for the novice clinician. There can be irregularities found on bedside ultrasound that are difficult to interpret. For instance, there may be ill-defined hypoechoic, heterogenous, or solid lesions discovered at the bedside that require further evaluation. The contralateral testis should always be examined for comparison. In addition, a consultant-performed imaging study and urology consult should be obtained in any patient with abnormal findings on a bedside study.

INTEGRATION OF BEDSIDE TESTICULAR ULTRASOUND INTO CLINICAL CARE

Testicular pain is a common presenting complaint in the acute care setting. Ultrasound should be integrated into the clinical care of the patient. Testicular torsion may have a classic presentation—high-riding testicle with a transverse lie and absent cremasteric reflex. In these cases urology consultation should not be delayed, but bedside ultrasound may help confirm the diagnosis and guide detorsion. In less obvious cases, ultrasound may help confirm the diagnosis earlier and expedite definitive care.

Due to some of the subtleties of this exam, clinician-performed bedside testicular ultrasound should not replace consultant-performed ultrasound when one is immediately available; however, it can help to expedite the diagnosis and management. In general, bedside ultrasound should not be used to completely rule out the diagnosis of torsion. This is particularly important in the diagnosis of complete and partial testicular torsion as salvage rates vary with the degree and duration of the condition. However, prompt visualization of torsion with ultrasound may assist in rapid detorsion and definitive treatment. The same applies to testicular fracture and rupture which can benefit from urological intervention.

While less emergent, ultrasound may also expedite or help confirm the diagnosis of epididymitis or orchitis, allowing prompt initiation of antibiotics. Less serious cases of testicular pain, such as hydroceles, varicoceles, and torsion of the appendix testes or appendix epididymis, may be identified using ultrasound. Early identification of a testicular mass may help expedite the diagnosis and treatment of a testicular malignancy.

Additional Reading

Akin E, Khati N, Hill M. Ultrasound of the scrotum. *Ultrasound Quarterly*. 2004;20(4):181-200.

Blaivas M, Brannam L. Testicular ultrasound. *Emerg Med Clin N Am*. 2004;22: 723-748.

Dogra V, Rubens D, Gottlieb R, et al. Torsion and beyond: new twists in spectral Doppler evaluation of the scrotum. *J Ultrasound Med*. 2004;23:1077-1085.

Lee J, Bhatt S, Dogra V. Imaging the epididymis. *Ultrasound Quarterly*. March 2008:24(1):1-16.

14 Ocular Ultrasound

Edward Tham

BACKGROUND AND INDICATIONS FOR EXAMINATION

Ophthalmologic complaints comprise 2%–3% of all emergency department (ED) visits. Many of these complaints can be diagnosed by history and physical exam in conjunction with an ophthalmoscope or a slit lamp. Bedside ocular ultrasound may be used adjunctively with these traditional diagnostic methods in making the diagnosis and may add information that is difficult to obtain via other methods.

Ocular ultrasound has been performed by ophthalmologists for nearly half a century. Recently, due to increased access to machines and adequate training, emergency and critical care physicians have adopted this technology. While acute eye complaints are more common in the emergency department setting, ocular ultrasound may also be of use in evaluating intracranial pressure in the ICU setting.

The eye is a fluid-filled structure; therefore, ultrasound is an ideal diagnostic modality. Sonography provides a noninvasive method of evaluating the entire globe. It can be used in both traumatic and nontraumatic eye disorders.

Bedside ocular ultrasound should be performed in the following patients:

* The patient with an acute change in vision
* The trauma patient presenting with penetrating or blunt injury to the orbit or eye when globe rupture is not suspected
* The patient with atraumatic eye pain
* Patients with suspected increased intracranial pressure

The only absolute contraindication to bedside ocular ultrasound is suspected globe rupture.

PROBE SELECTION AND TECHNICAL CONSIDERATIONS

LINEAR PROBE WITH A FREQUENCY OF 7.5–15.0 MHz

Higher-frequency probes, which provide better resolution, are preferred for ocular ultrasound. These probes provide superior resolution for ocular imaging, as the eye is a superficial structure. In fact, while higher-frequency probes are typically not available in the ED or critical care settings, ophthalmologists may use probes with frequencies of 20 MHz or higher, which may provide superior images of the anterior chamber and retina.

DEPTH

Visualizing the small structures of the eye can be challenging. The sonographer should attempt to utilize as much of the screen as possible by adjusting the depth imaged. By decreasing the depth, the globe will take up most of the screen and this will allow the operator to better view the areas of interest.

ZOOM FUNCTION

The zoom tool may be used to help magnify the image and to better focus in on the area of pathology.

FOCAL ZONE

Adjusting the focal zone to the area of interest will improve the lateral resolution of the image and can aid in identifying abnormal structures.

GAIN

Initially, the overall gain on the machine should be turned down in order to better visualize the anechoic aqueous and vitreous humor. After interrogating the entire orbit at a lower setting, the overall gain should then be slowly increased. This adjustment in gain will increase the brightness of structures that are transmitted on the monitor and can help in picking up subtle abnormalities that may be missed on a lower setting. It is important to not increase the gain too much as this can create false artifacts that can be mistaken for pathology or may "wash out" true subtle abnormalities and result in a missed diagnosis.

MACHINE PRESET

If there is not an ocular setting on the machine, a "superficial" or "small parts" setting, which provides higher resolution, should be used.

GEL APPLICATION

While ultrasound gel is water soluble and generally not irritable to the eye, placing a Tegaderm layer over a closed lid prior to applying gel may improve patient comfort.

NORMAL ULTRASOUND ANATOMY

ORBITS

The eye is surrounded by the bony orbit. The orbital bones appear as hyperechoic structures that block the transmission of the ultrasound signal, and therefore produce a posterior shadowing artifact. Occasionally, it may be possible to visualize orbital fractures which appear as a hypoechoic disruption of the hyperechoic cortex.

ANTERIOR STRUCTURES

Structures that are anterior to the lens, including the cornea, sclera, iris, pupil, ciliary body or muscle, and anterior chamber containing aqueous humor, are well visualized with ultrasound (Fig. 14-1). The normal cornea appears as a round, thin echogenic stripe at the anterior surface of the eye. The lens surface is hyperechoic and is represented by a horizontal line that is attached to the peripheral globe by the echogenic ciliary body and iris. It is difficult to detect pathology of the small anterior eye structures without the use of specialized higher-frequency probes that are usually not available in the acute care setting.

POSTERIOR STRUCTURES

Posterior elements compose the majority of the eye and include the vitreous body, the retina, the retinal vessels, the posterior wall, the optic disc, and optic nerve. The vitreous body is located between the lens and posterior wall and is

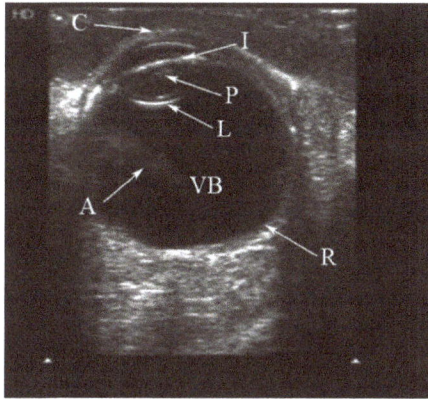

FIGURE 14-1 This image illustrates normal ocular anatomy using a high-frequency linear transducer. Artifact (A) is visualized inside the globe, which is typically seen in cystic structures. C: cornea, I: iris, P: pupil, L: lens, R: retina, VB: vitreous body.

normally anechoic. The posterior wall contains the retina and choroid and is normally adherent to the sclera (outside covering). The posterior wall will appear as an echogenic arc outlining the globe (see Fig. 14-1). The optic nerve and sheath are posterior to the globe and perpendicular to the posterior wall. The optic nerve is hypoechoic, while the sheath appears hyperechoic (Fig. 14-2). The ophthalmic artery branches into the central retinal artery and posterior ciliary arteries. The central retinal artery and vein are normally easily identified by their presence within the optic nerve sheath using color-flow Doppler.

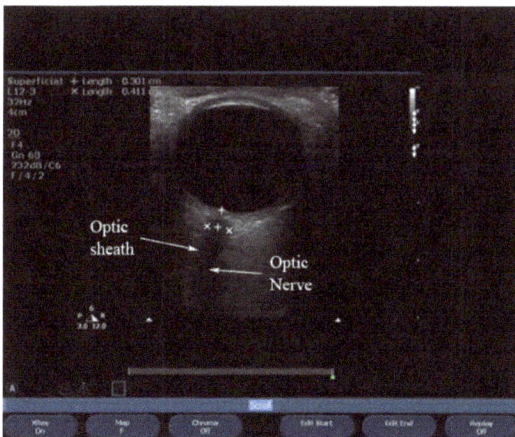

FIGURE 14-2 The optic nerve is the hypoechoic stripe directly behind the retina surrounded by the hyperechoic nerve sheath. By convention, the optic nerve sheath diameter is measured 3 mm behind the retina and should be less than 5 mm in width, illustrated by the numbers in the upper left corner of the image.

LANDMARKS

The sonographic landmarks of the eye are the lens, the posterior wall, and the optic nerve (see Figs. 14-1 and 14-2). These structures should be identified in order to help mark the axis of the eye. It is rare to mistake the eye for other cystic structures, but it is possible in the setting of massive lid edema, abscess, or enucleation.

IMAGING TIPS AND PROTOCOL

PATIENT POSITIONING

The patient should be placed in the supine position for optimal ocular imaging. If the patient is unable to lie flat or has a contraindication, such as increased intracranial pressure (ICP), imaging can be done in the upright position, if necessary.

COUPLING MEDIUM AND PROTECTIVE COVER

An adequate layer of ultrasound gel should be used in order to avoid direct contact with the eye and to reduce artifacts, thereby improving the quality of the image. Gel should be placed over the closed eyelid. Preferably, a sterile cover should be placed over the eyelid first, such as a Tegaderm™, before gel is applied in order to prevent irritation and infection.

PROBE POSITIONING

The sonographer can gently rest their scanning hand on the patient's face in order to keep the probe steady and to help avoid direct contact between the probe and the eyelid. The probe should be placed initially in the transverse position across the closed eyelid.

PATIENT COMFORT

Trauma to the eyes can be amongst the most painful complaints in an acute care setting. Appropriate topical or parenteral analgesia should be administered before starting any scan, when appropriate.

IMAGING PROTOCOL

Imaging of the eye should be done in two planes, both transverse and longitudinal. Scanning should begin in a transverse position with the probe indicator pointing to the patient's right side. Once the globe is fully interrogated the probe can be rotated 90°, with the probe marker pointing cephalad, in order to obtain a longitudinal or sagittal view. The key landmarks, the lens, posterior elements, and optic nerve, should be identified in a single view confirming a midline scan. The probe should be gently rocked from side to side in order to interrogate the entire eye in both planes.

In some patients, visualization of the entire globe or subtle abnormalities may be limited due to discomfort with the exam or noncompliance with the supine position. To help in these situations, the patient can be asked to move their eye while the lid is shut to facilitate visualization of the entire globe. These eye movements may help the sonographer visualize structures from an angle that would otherwise not be possible. For example, subtle lens subluxations may be diagnosed using this method. This technique also helps to differentiate pathology from artifact as abnormalities will remain with globe movements and artifacts usually disappear.

Although ocular vascular applications are usually beyond the scope of an acute care physician, color-flow Doppler evaluation may be utilized if there is concern for venous or arterial compromise. The vascular plexus is located behind the posterior wall and color-flow Doppler can be used to identify these vessels. Spectral pulsed-wave Doppler can also be used to verify arterial and venous waveforms. The probe should be placed in-line with the long axis of the vessel being measured.

PATHOLOGIC ULTRASOUND FINDINGS

INTRAOCULAR FOREIGN BODY

Intraocular foreign bodies (IOFBs) are usually diagnosed by history or physical exam alone. Occult IOFBs require specialized imaging in order to detect them. The patients at highest risk for occult IOFBs usually report a history of eye pain while drilling or hammering. Although the sensitivity of ultrasound for detecting these foreign bodies has been reported to be as high as 87%, computed tomography (CT) still remains the gold standard in making the diagnosis. Ultrasound may, however, provide better information about the extent of intraocular damage compared to CT scan.

Metallic IOFBs will appear echogenic on ultrasound and can be present at any level within the eye: anterior, posterior, or beyond. Therefore, the entire eye should be interrogated looking for irregular, asymmetrical, hyperechoic structures. Metallic IOFBs also produce a number of artifacts that may aid in the diagnosis, including posterior shadowing, reverberation, and ring-down artifacts.

Organic or plastic IOFBs will have variable degrees of echogenicity, depending on their composition. They are usually visualized as echogenic structures contained within the normally anechoic vitreous body. If the foreign body is more subtle-appearing, increasing the overall gain may help to improve visualization. In addition, radiolucent foreign bodies that are missed on CT scan may be more readily picked up on ultrasound.

In general, ultrasound should not be used to "rule out" a foreign body, but may help locate it. Clinicians should be aware of the possibility of a hyperechoic "focusing artifact" that may occur in the center of the vitreous body due to refraction as the ultrasound beam passes through the lens. This should not be mistaken for a foreign body. This artifact is typically seen in both eyes.

LENS DISLOCATION

Dislocation or subluxation of the crystalline lens is caused by a disruption of the zonular fibers and is most often due to blunt trauma. The lens normally appears as an oval echogenic structure with significant reverberation artifacts (see Fig. 14-1). The lens lies posterior to the ciliary body and often at an oblique angle that is not always in-line with the axis of the eye. Most dislocations will be obvious on ultrasound, but subluxations may be difficult to appreciate. In order to help accentuate abnormalities, the patient should be asked to move their eye, and the contralateral eye should always be scanned to compare for symmetry.

RETINAL DETACHMENT/VITREOUS DETACHMENT AND/OR HEMORRHAGE

Retinal and vitreous detachments can be both traumatic and nontraumatic. Spontaneous retinal detachment is most commonly associated with vitreous hemorrhage secondary to diabetic retinopathy. Retinal detachments appear as wavelike,

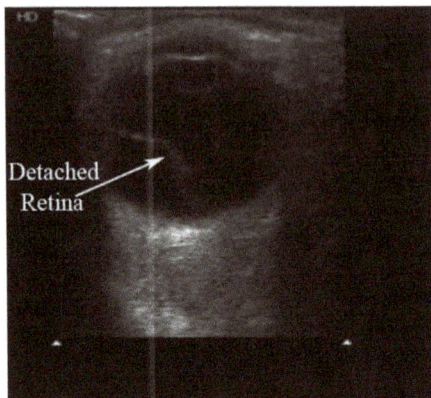

FIGURE 14-3 A retinal detachment is visualized as a hyperechoic linear structure within the normally anechoic posterior chamber.

echogenic flaps on ultrasound, which lie above the posterior wall of the eye (Fig. 14-3). A vitreous hemorrhage, which may occur with or without a detachment, will appear as echogenic material layering out within the normally anechoic vitreous body (Fig. 14-4). The above disorders can appear similar and be difficult to differentiate on ultrasound. In most situations, a consultation by a specialist is warranted if the patient presents with a clinical history consistent with retinal tear or detachment along with any of the ocular ultrasound findings discussed earlier.

OPTIC NERVE SHEATH DIAMETER

An enlarged optic nerve sheath diameter (ONSD) has been associated with an increased ICP. Studies that have evaluated ONSD have compared it to brain CT

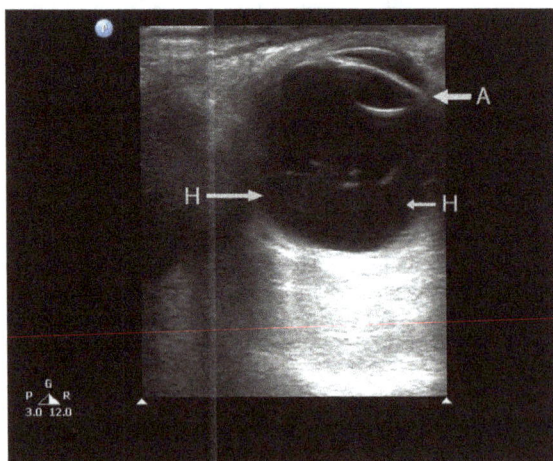

FIGURE 14-4 This image illustrates a large vitreous hemorrhage which is seen as an echogenic layer within the posterior vitreous body. A: anterior chamber, H: hemorrhage.

scan findings as evidence for increased ICP, as opposed to invasive intracranial monitoring. The ONSDs should be measured 3 mm behind the posterior wall of the globe where it is found to be the most porous (see Fig. 14-2). The normal measurement should be no more than 5-mm wide at this point. The ONSD should be measured in both eyes, in two planes, using an average of the four values in order to be most accurate. Care should be taken to try to measure the actual optic nerve sheath, as opposed to a shadowing artifact which can appear behind the optic cup.

Ultrasound does not replace CT scan in diagnosing increased ICP, but the measurement of the ONSD should be used in conjunction with other imaging studies. In a patient with intracranial hemorrhage, serial measurements of the ONSD may be used to detect increased ICP. If the repeat ONSD measurement increases to greater than 5 mm, this is an indication for repeat head CT, invasive ICP monitoring, or medications and maneuvers to decrease ICP. ONSD measurements may also be helpful in situations where resources are limited, such as in mass casualty events or when CAT scan is not available.

In addition to enlarged ONSD diameter, some preliminary work has shown that papilledema may be seen directly on ultrasound as a protrusion of the optic disc into the eye. In addition to traumatic increases in ICP, optic nerve sheath or disc abnormalities may help diagnose pseudotumor cerebri.

COMMON PITFALLS

INADEQUATE COUPLING MEDIUM

An adequate amount of gel should be applied to the eyelid before performing an ocular ultrasound. This helps in limiting the direct pressure applied to the eyelid, which is especially important in ocular trauma and for patient comfort. Also, without adequate coupling medium, unwanted artifacts may appear, obscuring pertinent pathology or leading to a false-positive result. In addition, an ultrasound friendly cover, such as a Tegaderm, should cover the eyelid first before gel application to maintain sterility and help prevent infection.

ARTIFACTS CONFUSED FOR PATHOLOGY

The eye is a cystic structure; therefore, there are ultrasound artifacts that may interfere with proper interpretation. Posterior enhancement artifact, commonly seen in cystic structures, originating from the back wall of the eye, may wash out posterior structures and can make visualization of the optic nerve difficult. Decreasing the total gain control or far gain by adjusting the time-gain compensation may help to attenuate this artifact.

Side lobe artifacts, often seen in cystic structures, may be confused for echogenic intraocular pathology (see Fig. 14-1). This artifact usually disappears with proper probe fanning, decreasing the gain setting or with eye movements. When the gain is turned down and the abnormality is still present, it is likely to be a pathological finding. In contrast, if the finding disappears at a lower-gain setting, it is most likely an artifact. Artifacts that do not disappear with maneuvers are most likely true pathological findings and require further workup.

A refraction or focusing artifact may be seen as a curved hyperechoic artifact in the center of the eye and should not be confused for a foreign body or other pathology. It is usually seen in both eyes.

INCORRECT OPTIC NERVE SHEATH MEASUREMENTS

ONSD measurements must be made at the widest point along the axis of the eye or its size may be underestimated. In addition, the measurement must be taken perpendicular to the axis of the eye. An oblique measurement can result in an overestimation of sheath diameter. Care should be taken to measure the actual optic nerve sheath rather than the shadow that may result from the optic disc.

OBTAIN SPECIALTY CONSULTATIONS AS APPROPRIATE

Retinal detachment, choroidal detachment, and vitreous hemorrhage may all appear similar; however, their treatments vary significantly. If signs and symptoms of a retinal tear or detachment are present, a normal-appearing ocular ultrasound does not exclude the diagnosis. Appropriate consultation with a specialist and rapid follow-up is recommended.

INTEGRATION OF BEDSIDE OCULAR ULTRASOUND INTO CLINICAL CARE

Patients presenting with acute visual changes, orbital trauma, or atraumatic eye pain are all potential candidates for a bedside ocular ultrasound examination. Although ultrasound does not replace the gold standard of CT scan in diagnosing injuries due to facial or head trauma, intraocular foreign bodies, or increased ICP, it has many advantages.

Ultrasound is especially helpful in the evaluation of head and orbital trauma for many of the same reasons as other trauma applications have been. The exam can be performed at the bedside with minimal discomfort and lack of radiation exposure. Ocular sonography is fast and can be easily repeated with serial examinations if needed. It helps in preventing the unnecessary transport of the unstable trauma or intensive care unit patient who needs continuous monitoring. It is also useful in patients who are unable to cooperate with a fundoscopic examination or for evaluation of the globe when severe lid edema, chemosis, or hyphemas are present and preclude direct visualization.

Additional Reading

Blaivas M. Bedside emergency department ultrasonography in the evaluation of ocular pathology. *Acad Emerg Med.* 2000;7:947-950.

Fischer Y, Nogueira F, Sallies D. Diagnostic ophthalmic ultrasonography. In: Tasman W, Jaeger E, eds. *Duane's Ophthalmology.* Philadelphia, PA: Lippincott Williams & Wilkins; 2008:chap 108.

Lyon M, Blaivas M. Ocular ultrasound. In: Ma J, Mateer J, Blaivas M, eds. *Emergency Ultrasound.* China: McGraw-Hill; 2008:chap 17.

15 Ultrasound for Deep Venous Thrombosis

Pierre Kory and Adolfo E. Kaplan

BACKGROUND AND INDICATIONS FOR EXAMINATION

Deep venous thrombosis (DVT) is typically caused by one or more of Virchow's triad: stasis, hypercoagulability, and/or endothelial damage. DVT may occur in ambulatory patients presenting to the emergency department (ED) with leg pain and/or swelling, and is also a frequent complication of critical illness due to multiple and often coexisting risk factors, including immobility, surgery, trauma, indwelling devices, malignancy, and inflammatory states. A vexing problem is the unreliability of the symptoms and signs of DVT in the critical care setting, which are often limited by obesity, edema, and surgical dressings. In the intensive care unit (ICU), 10%–100% of DVTs are clinically unsuspected, and pulmonary embolism is the most frequent incidental autopsy finding, directly contributing to death in approximately 5% of all cases.

The true incidence and prevalence of lower extremity DVT (LEDVT) in the critical care setting is unknown, and patients may often be asymptomatic. Based on screening studies using ultrasonography for the diagnosis, incidence rates vary considerably as a result of differences in patient population, adequacy of prophylaxis, sonographic technique, and sonographer skills. Reported incidences range from as low as 8% to as high as 18% for proximal LEDVT, with the majority of cases occurring within the first week of an ICU stay. In the ambulatory and ED setting a DVT is typically symptomatic, and ultrasound is a reliable way to exclude one.

Clinically, LEDVTs are classified according to their embolic risk. Proximal (popliteal and higher veins) DVTs present a significant embolic risk, while isolated calf vein thrombosis is unlikely to embolize. Given that only 20% of calf DVTs will extend proximally, anticoagulation may be held in the ICU setting to avoid unnecessary complications. Therefore, calf veins are not routinely examined by ultrasound in the ICU setting. In the ambulatory and ED setting, if calf veins are not imaged it is recommended that patients return in 5–7 days to be reimaged in case a calf vein thrombus has propagated proximally.

Bedside ultrasonography can play a pivotal role in the diagnostic algorithms of venous thromboembolic disease. In order for the clinician to incorporate ultrasound into the timely diagnosis of DVT, a thorough understanding of the strength and limitations, clinical applications, and technical performance of lower extremity sonography is necessary.

Given the rapid growth in availability of portable ultrasound units in many EDs and ICUs, there are an increasing number of clinicians performing bedside diagnostic venous sonograms. While the examination is the same, whether it is performed in the ED or ICU, the ability of ultrasound to reliably exclude a DVT depends on the prevalence and/or pretest probability of a DVT. Ultrasound tends to perform much better in patients who are symptomatic in either setting.

Accuracy studies of ED and hospitalist physicians with variable amounts of ultrasound training (2–30 hours) reveal sensitivities between 70% and 100%, and specificities between 76% and 100% when compared to the "official" radiology study. Although these results lend support to the accuracy of bedside compression ultrasound (CUS) examinations performed by clinician sonographers, the experience of the sonographer plays an important role in the accuracy of diagnostic vascular sonography.

Bedside ultrasound evaluation for LEDVT should be performed in the following patients:

- The patient with signs and symptoms of LEDVT
- The patient with undifferentiated hypoxemia or shock

PROBE SELECTION AND TECHNICAL CONSIDERATIONS

LINEAR PROBE WITH A FREQUENCY OF 5.0–10.0 MHz

A 7.5-MHz probe is usually sufficient for most lower extremity vessels. To image deeper vessels, probes utilizing lower frequencies may be helpful. Likewise, to image more superficial vessels, higher frequencies may be beneficial.

FOCAL ZONE

The focal zone should be adjusted and placed at the depth of the vessel being imaged. This improves the lateral resolution of the image.

COLOR-FLOW DOPPLER

Color-flow Doppler (CFD) detects blood flow and therefore is helpful in identifying a blood vessel and distinguishing it from other structures present in the lower extremity. CFD can be especially helpful in obese patients where imaging is more difficult and with smaller vessels, such as the popliteals.

TIME-GAIN COMPENSATION

Time-gain compensation (TGC) can be adjusted in order to increase the far gain of the image. Gain should be adjusted so that the image results in a uniform brightness and resolution in both the near and far fields. Adjustment of this control may be useful in obese patients with difficult anatomy.

DEPTH

The depth should be adjusted once the appropriate vessels have been identified. The structures of interest should make up approximately three-fourths of the screen. Inadequate depth, either too shallow or deep, can result in a misidentification of the proper blood vessels.

NORMAL ULTRASOUND ANATOMY

The LE veins are divided into deep and superficial vessels. The deep veins are paired with and accompany the arteries. The external iliac vein originates from the IVC and crosses the inguinal ligament to become the common femoral vein (CFV). The CFV is joined medially by the great saphenous vein (GSV), and approximately 1–2 cm beyond this point, the CFV divides into the deep femoral vein (DFV) and the superficial femoral vein (SFV). Recently, many have begun calling the SFV simply the "femoral vein" to avoid confusion—it is important to note that the "superficial" femoral vein is part of the deep venous system, just more superficial than the DFV. The DFV can usually be tracked for a short distance before it dives deeper and away from the acoustic window. The SFV runs anteromedially down the leg and through the adductor canal, where it then cours-es posteriorly into the popliteal fossa becoming the popliteal vein (PV). The PV then trifurcates into the anterior tibial, peroneal, and posterior tibial veins in the proximal calf (Fig. 15-1).

The vessels are imaged in a transverse position, starting just below the level of the inguinal ligament. At this level, the CFV should be visualized medial and adjacent to the common femoral artery (CFA) (Fig. 15-2). The GSV will be seen joining the CFV from the medial side, high in the leg. When the probe is slid down about 1–2 cm distally, the CFA can be seen dividing into the superficial femoral artery (SFA) and the deep femoral artery (DFA). As the probe is moved distally and medially down the leg, the SFV should be visualized until it enters the adductor canal.

The popliteal region should also be examined with the probe in a transverse orientation behind the patient's knee. In this view, the PV will be seen on top of the popliteal artery on the screen. Keep in mind that the PV is still deep to the artery (ie, closer to the bed in a supine patient). Classically, the popliteal vein and artery will form a "figure eight," with the vein being the upper part of the eight (Fig. 15-3). While the PV should be compressed to the trifurcation, calf veins are not routinely examined in most cases, unless there is a focal area of symptoms.

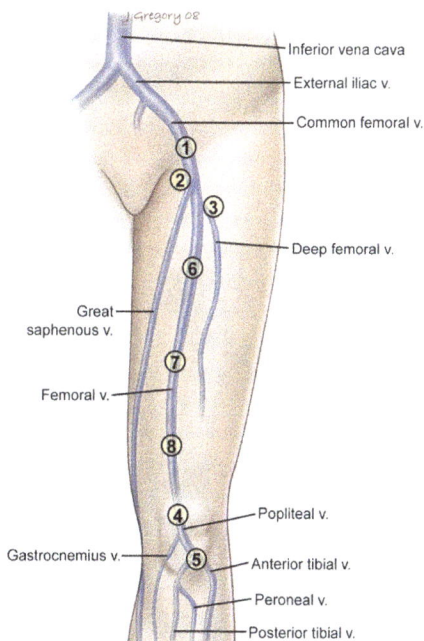

FIGURE 15-1 Depiction of normal lower extremity venous anatomy. A "two-site" or limited compression study involves interrogation of the upper and lower venous con-fluences alone (sites 1–5). A "complete" study includes areas 6, 7, and 8, which are performed only if thrombus is not found at areas 1–5.

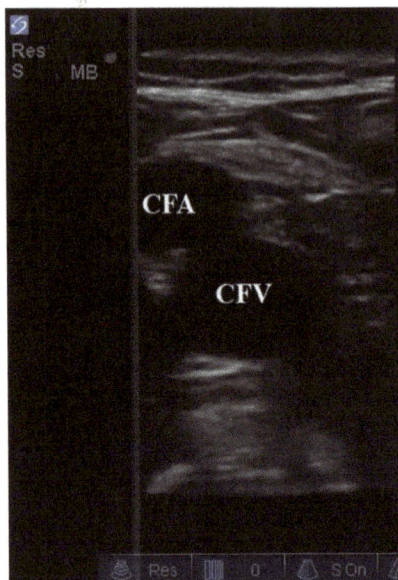

FIGURE 15-2 Normal common femoral vein (CFV) and common femoral artery (CFA). The CFV will appear medial to the CFA in the lower extremity. This image illustrates normal B-mode imaging of lower extremity vein and artery. The vessels appear anechoic signifying fluid (blood). Note the absence of echogenic material suggesting thrombus within the lumen of the vein.

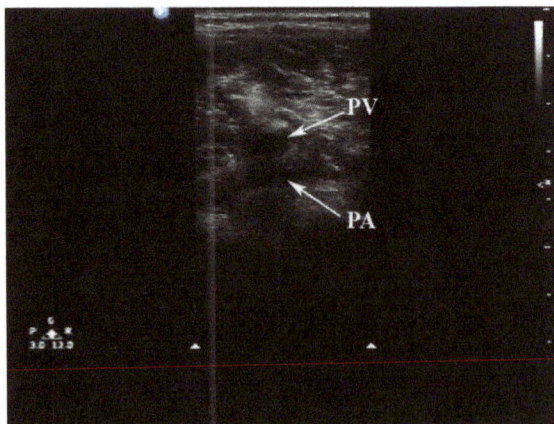

FIGURE 15-3 Normal popliteal vein (PV) and popliteal artery (PA). Notice the positioning of the vein in comparison to the artery. The vein appears to be more superficial, but is actually deeper as the probe is positioned behind the patient's knee in the popliteal fossa.

IMAGING TIPS AND PROTOCOL

PROBE ORIENTATION

LE ultrasound is performed in the transverse position with the probe indicator pointing toward the patient's right side. The femoral vein is medial to the femoral artery; therefore, the transverse orientation will result in the CFV and SFV appearing on the left side of the screen and the SFA and DFA appearing on the right when examining the left leg, and the opposite when the right leg is examined (ie, veins on right side of screen, arteries on left). As the veins travel distally, they will go deep to the artery. Only a few centimeters distal to the inguinal ligament, there is often complete overlap, worth noting when placing a femoral central line.

PATIENT ORIENTATION

In evaluating the femoral vessels, the patient should be placed in the supine position with the lower extremity fully exposed and externally rotated or in the "frog leg position" (Fig. 15-4). If the patient can tolerate it, reverse Trendelenburg positioning can be used to better fill the veins and improve ultrasound visualization. In evaluating the popliteal vessels, the patient may remain in the supine position with the knee in flexion, or the patient may lie on their stomach in a prone position. The probe should be placed in a transverse position at the back of the knee in the popliteal fossa (Fig. 15-5). As mentioned earlier, the PV will appear at the top of the screen and the popliteal artery will appear toward the bottom of the screen. The vein is still deep to the artery, but because the face of the probe is on the back of the leg, the vein will be seen closer to the probe (and on top of the screen).

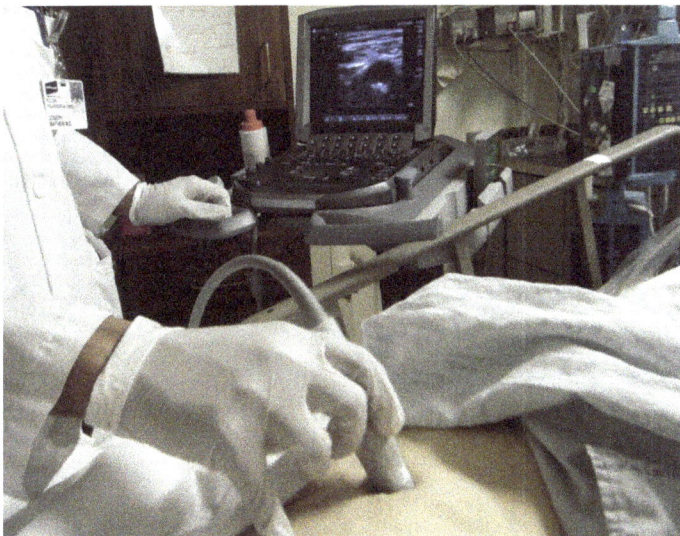

FIGURE 15-4 Demonstration of sonographer and probe positioning during compression of the common femoral vein. The leg is externally rotated with the probe held transverse to the vein.

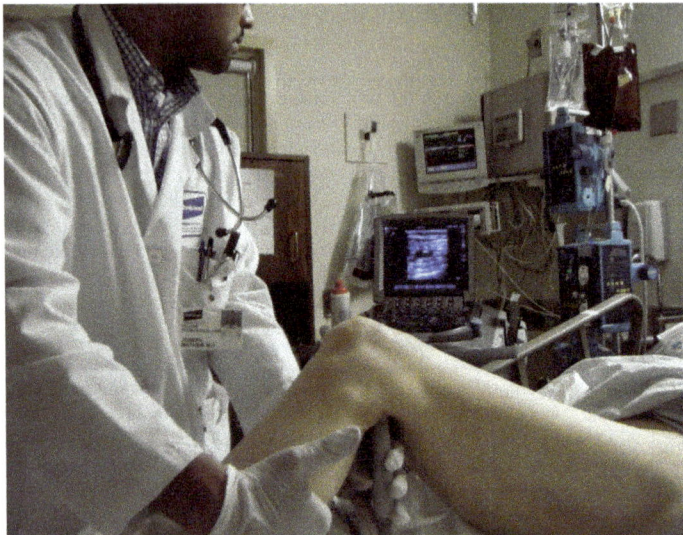

FIGURE 15-5 Demonstration of sonographer and patient positioning during compression of the popliteal vein in a supine patient. The leg is raised and slightly flexed and the probe is held posterior and transverse to vein in the popliteal fossa with upward pressure applied.

DEPTH

Once the vessels are identified, the depth should be decreased so that the lower vessel edge is visualized within one-fourth of the bottom of the screen.

IMAGING PROTOCOL

CUS alone is usually sufficient to diagnose or exclude a DVT in the area being interrogated. CUS uses B-mode (also known as 2-D) imaging to directly visualize the venous segment of interest. This technique allows real-time visualization of pressure-induced collapse of the vein of interest (Figs. 15-6a and b). If a vein does not collapse under pressure, it indicates a thrombus. Clots may also be seen directly as more hyperechoic (bright) than the rest of the vessel. Longstanding (chronic) clots are typically more hyperechoic than acute clots, although acute clots may also appear hyperechoic. It is important to apply enough pressure to completely collapse the vein. If enough pressure is being applied to deform the artery and the vein does not collapse, it indicates a thrombus.

- *Duplex ultrasound:* Adds Doppler (color or spectral) to the 2-D analysis modality, allowing for the visualization of blood flow within the vein (Fig. 15-7). Color-gain settings must be set appropriately in order to avoid over-saturation and not to obscure small intraluminal clots or areas of incomplete thrombosis. Although duplex is now typically a secondary method to CUS, the term duplex ultrasound is often used to describe a DVT ultrasound, as it was historically a primary method.
- *Triplex ultrasound:* Includes 2-D ultrasound, color-flow Doppler, and spectral Doppler.

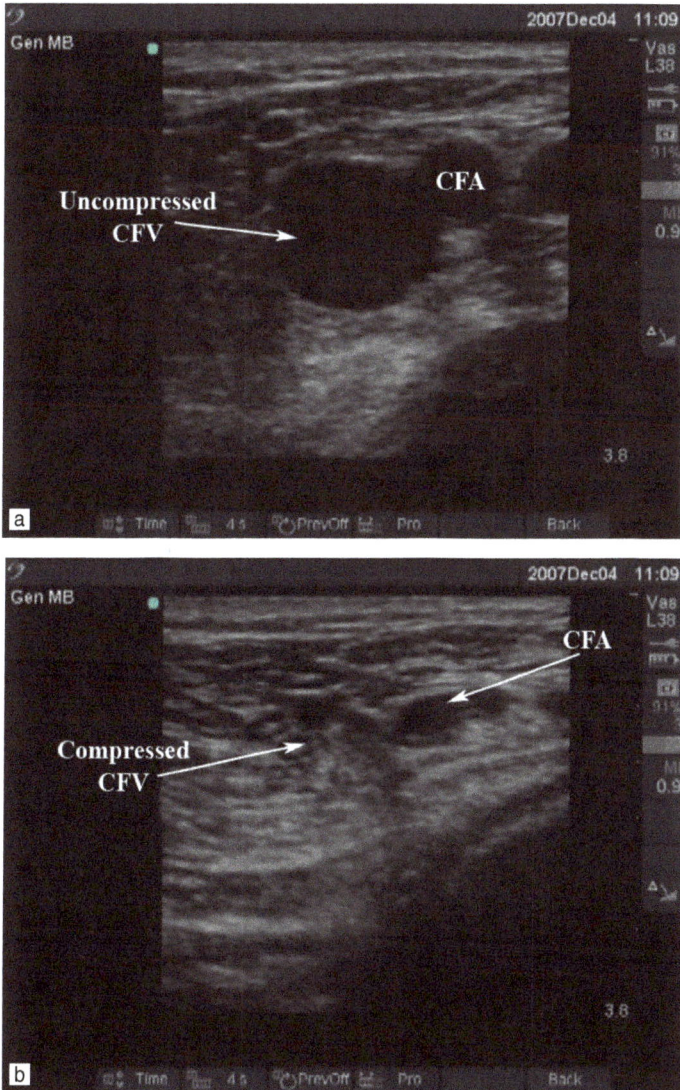

FIGURE 15-6   This image illustrates the full compression technique needed to demonstrate the absence of lower extremity deep venous thrombosis. (*a*) Shows uncompressed common femoral vein (CFV) next to common femoral artery (CFA). (*b*) Shows compressed CFV vein with obliteration of previously visualized anechoic lumen next to the CFA.

Traditionally, a diagnostic vascular exam employed a combination of the above modalities ("duplex" or "triplex" exams). A review of the literature has shown that using color-flow Doppler and spectral analysis does not improve the diagnostic accuracy of diagnosing DVTs; therefore, the compression technique is the only one described here.

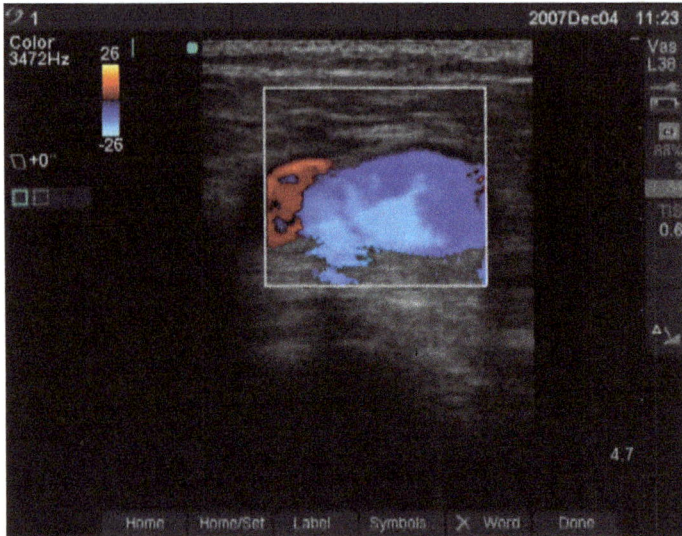

FIGURE 15-7 Color-flow Doppler allows for the identification of flow within blood vessels. Flow toward the probe is represented in red and flow away from the probe is represented in blue.

Prior to each compression, an assessment for intraluminal echoes should be performed, although their presence lacks specificity for thrombus. Acute thrombi may be hypoechoic and not directly visualized. However, the sonographer may encounter situations where an echogenic and well-circumscribed thrombus is found without compression.

Gentle but firm pressure is then applied with the transducer in the transverse axis. The pressure must be sufficient enough to completely collapse the vessel. Patent veins are fully compressible and the visible anechoic lumen should completely disappear, signifying that opposing venous walls have come into full contact (see Fig. 15-6a and b). With this technique, the inability to completely compress the venous lumen is the main criteria for the diagnosis of DVT (Fig. 15-8a and b). The amount of pressure applied needs to be lower than the pressure required to collapse the artery; therefore, only slight tenting of the adjacent artery should be seen. If the vein is not collapsible at this pressure, a venous thrombus is present. Adequate pressure is important since acute thrombi have jellylike consistency and may be frequently partially compressible. Excessive pressure can sometimes collapse the artery, especially in volume-depleted patients, while inadequate pressure can lead to the erroneous conclusion that a vein is noncompressible. A vein may be distinguished from an artery by partially compressing it and watching for pulsations, or using color-flow Doppler. The sonographer must ensure that the probe is transverse to the vessel and that downward pressure is applied directly over the vein. If the transducer is angled or positioned incorrectly, pressure is sometimes directed adjacent to the vein or the vein inadvertently slides away from the interrogation window, resulting in a false-positive finding.

A sonographic examination may be complete or limited. A complete exam consists of performing sequential compressions every 1–2 cm over the entire proximal venous system from the iliac vein at the groin to the distal popliteal

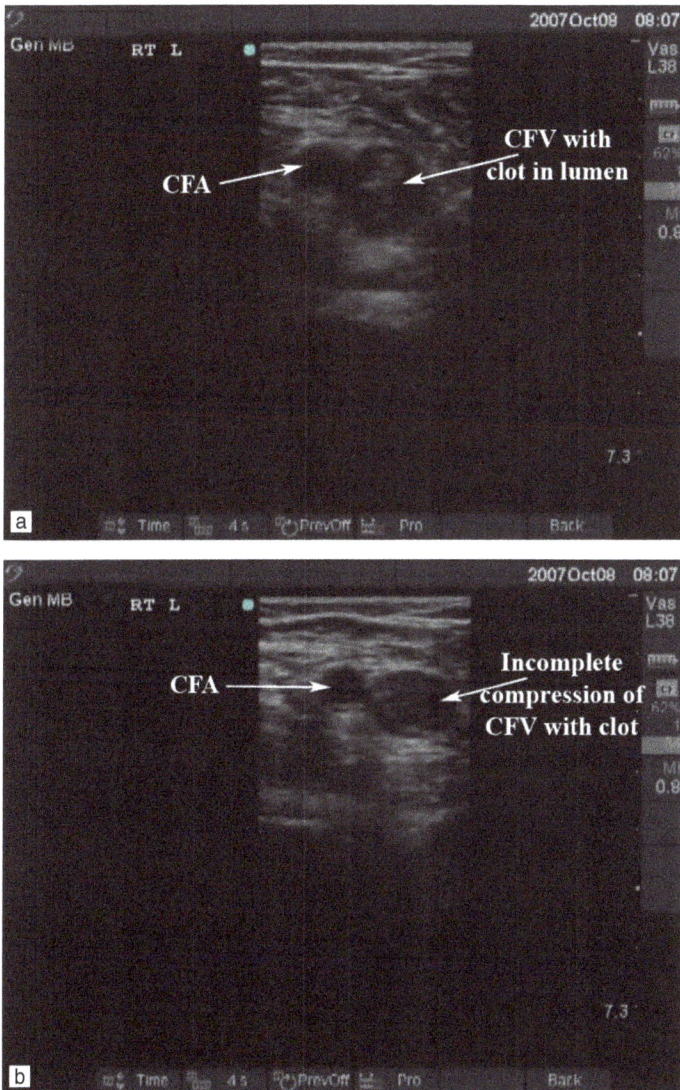

FIGURE 15-8 Incomplete compression of lower extremity vein signifying presence of thrombus. (*a*) Shows uncompressed common femoral vein (CFV) next to common femoral artery (CFA) (note the presence of echogenic material within the vein). (*b*) Shows the attempted compression of the CFV with clot (note lack of collapse of venous lumen) next to the CFA.

fossa. A limited or "two-point" exam consists of performing compressions at the two main venous confluences alone (see Fig. 15-1). While the majority of clots will be identified either in the CFV, proximal SFV, or PV, some studies have shown the limited exam to have slightly lower sensitivity.

When time permits, a more complete study of the lower extremity venous system evaluating the CFV, SFV, and PV down to the proximal portion of the calf vein trifurcation is recommended. This approach has been called the three-point compression technique; the two venous confluences are scanned first, and, if no thrombus is identified, the entire length of the SFV is interrogated down to the adductor canal.

Common Femoral Vein   The exam should begin with the transducer in the transverse axis at the origin of the CFV, just below the inguinal ligament and medial to the femoral artery. Sequential compressions should be performed, advancing 2 cm distally and medially along the vein before the next compression. At a short distance below the inguinal ligament, the GSV should be seen joining the CFV medially. The proximal portion of the GSV must be interrogated, as thrombus present at this level has a high risk for extension into the CFV and should be treated. Following the CFV distally, it will bifurcate into the deep and superficial femoral vein, also known as simply the femoral vein (being a deep and not a superficial vein). The examiner should continue to follow the CFV distally, compressing along the way, down to the popliteal fossa.

Popliteal Vein   Ideally, the patient should be in a prone position, which is not always possible in most critically ill individuals. In such patients, the knee is flexed approximately 45° or the patient is positioned in the lateral decubitus position (see Fig. 15-5). The paired popliteal artery and vein are located in a central position (see Fig. 15-3) (visualization of associated smaller vessels usually indicates that the transducer is positioned too low in the popliteal fossa). Compressions should be performed sequentially up to a point just distal to the trifurcation of the PV into the three calf veins.

Superficial Femoral Vein   As previously mentioned, if the above two-site technique is negative, the length of the SFV is then interrogated until it is lost medially in the adductor canal.

Important Junctions   Images should be recorded or printed at the following junctions:

- CFV proximal to GSV
- CFV-GSV junction
- CFV-DFV junction
- Mid PV
- PV-calf veins junction (trifurcation)
- Proximal SFV
- Mid SFV
- Distal SFV

PATHOLOGIC ULTRASOUND FINDINGS

ACUTE DVT

The inability to completely collapse the venous lumen signifies a clot. An acute DVT can sometimes appear as an echogenic structure within the lumen and be identified even before compression. More commonly, acute clots are hypoechoic and are sometimes only partially compressible, and therefore may not be as easy to identify.

CHRONIC DVT

Chronic clots are usually more easily identifiable before compressions due to their echogenicity. Chronic clots can sometimes recanalize and have a flow of blood through the center of them. In addition, the vessel walls surrounding a chronic DVT may appear thickened with scar tissue, which can also help the sonographer distinguish them from acute clots. Prior ultrasounds, if available, can be helpful in this situation for comparison.

SUPERFICIAL THROMBI

Clots present in superficial vessels are sometimes encountered when interrogating the lower extremity. These superficial vessels are not accompanied by an artery. It is important to distinguish a superficial clot from a DVT because the treatment, for the most part, differs.

COMMON PITFALLS

PATIENT HABITUS

Obesity is always a challenge when attempting any ultrasound study. Firm pressure needs to be applied in these cases in order to clearly visualize deeper vessels. In addition, the far gain may need to be increased by using the TGC controls, in order to enhance the signal returning from deeper structures. In the obese patient, positioning should be optimized. If possible, place the patient in reverse Trendelenburg position to increase flow to the venous vessels, and when interrogating the popliteal fossa attempt to have the patient in the prone position or flexed at the knee.

ACUTE VERSUS CHRONIC THROMBI

As discussed earlier, the distinction between acute and chronic DVT may be difficult. The ultrasound appearance of DVT changes over time: thrombi become progressively more echogenic as they organize, and the underlying venous wall in the area of thrombosis gets thicker, more echogenic, and resistant to compression. In this situation, a comparison with prior ultrasound studies may also be helpful.

INTERNAL ECHOES

Internal echoes ("smoke") are frequently encountered in patent veins in the presence of low-flow states. Smoke is more easily visualized in large veins (ie, internal jugular and subclavian in the upper extremities, and common, profunda, proximal superficial, and greater saphenous in the lower extremities). It should not be confused with true thrombi.

MISTAKING OTHER STRUCTURES FOR VESSELS OR CLOT

The novice sonographer will sometimes mistake other semisolid structures such as a lymph node or muscle band for a thrombosed vein. Lymph nodes usually have a hyperechoic center and a hypoechoic rim and muscle bands are rounded, well circumscribed with linear internal echoes. It is important for the examiner to pay close attention to the vascular anatomy, such as identifying the paired artery, which will not be present with other structures. In addition, scanning the structure of interest distally will help as blood vessels will continue and a lymph node will disappear. These techniques should assist the sonographer in not mistaking these structures for blood vessels.

Other fluid-filled structures can also easily be mistaken for blood vessels. For instance, an abscess, a simple soft tissue cyst, or Baker's cyst behind the knee can all resemble blood-filled vessels. The use of color-flow Doppler can assist in these situations as the blood vessels will pick up color flow and the other fluid-filled objects will not. These structures will also not be as easily compressible as a venous vessel will, so pressure over the suspected object of interest can help in differentiating the two.

DUPLICATED VENOUS SYSTEM

The presence of a duplicated venous system can cause the unsuspecting sonographer to miss the thrombosed segment. Conversely, a large collateral system could be mistaken for a patent venous segment while thrombosis is present in an underlying vein. This can be avoided by scanning the opposite extremity for comparison and also by referencing prior studies, if available.

THE ADDUCTOR HIATUS

As the (superficial) femoral vein passes through the adductor hiatus, it is surrounded by fibrous tissue that can make it difficult to compress directly, and may result in a false-positive interpretation of clot. This can be addressed by keeping the probe anterior and medial on the leg while compressing the vein and pressing with the other hand in the popliteal fossa.

PERFROMING A LIMITED EXAM

Because bedside ultrasound may be more limited and does not typically include the calf veins, ultrasound should be repeated in 3-7 days in a patient with continued symptoms or a high pre-test probability to avoid missing calf vein clots that may propagate proximally.

MISSING IVC OR PELVIC VEIN THROMBOSIS

Although isolated IVC or pelvic vein thrombosis are uncommon, they are not directly visualized with lower extremity compression, and diagnosis may be improved using Doppler waveforms or imaging beyond the scope of this chapter. Additional imaging or consultation should be obtained if a more proximal thrombosis is suspected, especially if the patient is post-partum or has just had recent pelvic surgery.

OTHER OBSTACLES TO THE EXAM

The presence of local tenderness, obscuring dressings, edema, burn areas, and local recent surgery may render the study difficult to perform or altogether unobtainable.

INTEGRATION OF BEDSIDE DIAGNOSTIC VENOUS ULTRASOUND INTO CLINICAL CARE

Based on extensive evidence in symptomatic outpatients, ultrasonography is currently the primary means of diagnosing DVT in the lower extremities. Although studies have suggested that the sensitivity of ultrasonography in asymptomatic, high-risk, inpatient populations is considerably lower, it remains the test of choice in acutely ill patients due to its accuracy, noninvasiveness, ease of performance, availability, low cost, and its ability to be repeated without restrictions. DVT can be confidently diagnosed when absence of venous collapse under sufficient pressure is present. Assessment of venous flow patterns can assist in confirming the diagnosis, but the significance of isolated abnormalities of spectral or color Doppler signal analysis should be questioned and alternative diagnostic tests should be considered (venography, CT venogram, MR venography). Color interrogation and maneuvers to augment flow help identify venous segments that are difficult to visualize with real-time sonography, but do not increase diagnostic accuracy.

Appropriately trained clinicians can perform bedside ultrasound to diagnose LEDVT, using CUS technique, with similar sensitivities and specificities as radiological exams. The benefits of this "point-of-care" exam are that it obviates the need for patient transport, venous access, and radiation exposure inherent in other diagnostic modalities. Further studies are required to better define the accuracy of ultrasound in the ICU population as well as the accuracy of bedside clinician exams in this challenging population of patients.

Additional Reading

American Thoracic Society. The diagnostic approach to acute venous thromboembolism: clinical practice guideline. *Am J Respir Crit Care Med.* 1999;160:1043-1066.

Blaivas M, Lambert MJ, Harwood RA, Wood JP, Konicki J. Lower-extremity Doppler for deep venous thrombosis: can emergency physicians be accurate and fast? *Acad Emerg Med.* 2000;7:120-126.

Frederick MG, Hertzber BS, Kliewer MA, et al. Can the US examination for lower extremity deep venous thrombosis be abbreviated? A prospective study of 755 examinations. *Radiology.* 1996;199:45-47.

Kaplan AE, Kory P. Use of ultrasonography for the diagnosis of venous thromboembolic disease. In: Bolliger CT, Herth FJF, Mayo PH, Miyazawa T, Beamis JF, eds. *Clinical Chest Ultrasound: From the ICU to the Bronchoscopy Suite.* Basel: Karger; 2009:96-109.

Tomkowski WZ, Davidson BL, Wisniewska J, et al. Accuracy of compression ultrasound in screening for deep venous thrombosis in acutely ill medical patients. *Thromb Haemost.* 2007 Feb;97(2):191-194.

16 Soft Tissue and Extremity Ultrasound

Fernando A. Lopez and Kenton Anderson

BACKGROUND AND INDICATIONS FOR EXAMINATION

Soft tissue and extremity conditions are common complaints encountered in the acute care setting. Traditionally, patient evaluation was performed using physical examination, radiographs, CT scans, MRI, and bone scans. More recently, these imaging modalities are now being augmented by the use of bedside ultrasound. Ultrasound has increasingly been shown to be useful in the evaluation of conditions such as cellulitis, abscesses, necrotizing fasciitis, foreign bodies, fractures, muscle and tendon inflammation, infection, or injury.

Bedside ultrasound evaluation of the musculoskeletal system should be performed in the following:

- Evaluation of presence, location, and extent of possible abscess or necrotizing fasciitis
- Identification of a suspected soft tissue foreign body not visualized on plain radiographs
- Dynamic assistance with removal of a foreign body visualized by ultrasound
- Assessment of muscles and tendons for inflammation or infection
- Evaluation of long bones for fracture and in guiding reduction

PROBE SELECTION AND TECHNICAL CONSIDERATIONS

LINEAR PROBE WITH A FREQUENCY OF 7.5 MHz OR HIGHER

Soft tissue and musculoskeletal structures are usually superficial, making a higher-frequency probe optimal for better resolution. In the case of deeper structures, a lower-frequency curvilinear probe may provide better penetration.

FOCAL ZONE

The focal zone should be adjusted and placed at the level of the structure being imaged. If the object of interest is too superficial, a standoff pad can be placed in between the probe and body part being imaged to increase the distance between the two and better the resolution. An IV fluid bag may be used as a standoff pad if a commercially produced one is not available. If possible, the body part being imaged can be submersed into a water bath, which also optimizes the focal zone and patient comfort.

DEPTH

Soft tissue and musculoskeletal injuries are usually superficial. The sonographer should decrease the depth in order to bring the area of interest into the center of the screen.

GAIN OR TIME-GAIN COMPENSATION

Total gain can be adjusted to optimize the strength of the signal returning from the object of interest. In deeper structures or obese patients, it may only be necessary to increase the far gain using time-gain compensation (TGC). Using too much gain can "wash out" the image and make it too bright; therefore, it should only be increased as necessary.

COLOR-FLOW DOPPLER

Color-flow Doppler detects blood flow. This is useful in differentiating blood vessels from surrounding structures. It helps prevent inadvertent injury to blood vessels when retrieving a foreign body under ultrasound guidance.

NORMAL ULTRASOUND ANATOMY

SKIN, MUSCLE, AND BLOOD VESSELS

The sonographer should be familiar with the appearance of normal soft tissue anatomy when evaluating for infections, injuries, inflammation, or foreign bodies (Fig. 16-1). The epidermis and dermis are seen most superficially with a more hypoechoic subcutaneous fatty tissue deep to the cutaneous layer. This adipose layer is highlighted with a reticular pattern of connective tissue between fat. The thickness of this layer varies with body location and habitus. Muscle is found deep to the subcutaneous fat layer and is also relatively hypoechoic with regular internal striations that will appear linear in long axis and punctate in short axis. Blood vessels are anechoic and have a circular appearance in short axis and a tubular appearance in long axis. They will display blue or red color patterns with Doppler, depending on the direction of blood flow relative to the probe. Veins are thin-walled and will collapse easily with pressure applied by the transducer, whereas larger arteries are thick-walled and remain patent and pulsatile with compression.

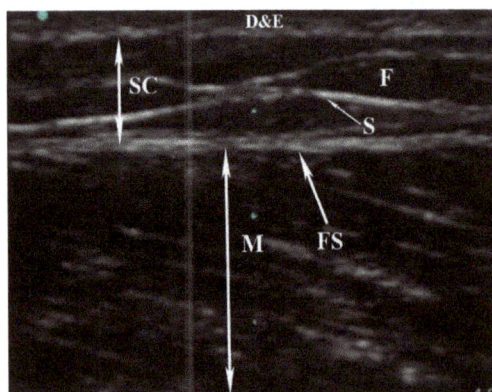

FIGURE 16-1 Normal longitudinal view of anterior thigh skin and muscle tissue. The top layer is the hyperechoic heterogeneous epidermis and dermis (D&E), which cannot be differentiated from each other at this frequency. The next layer is the hypoechoic heterogeneous subcutaneous layer (SC). Within the subcutaneous layer are fat globules (F) and the subcutaneous septa (S). The deepest layer is muscle (M), which has a hyper- and hypoechoic fibrinous pattern consistent with normal fascicles. The muscle fascia appears as a horizontal hyperechoic line (FS).

TENDON

Normal tendons are echogenic and have a characteristic fibrillar pattern in both the longitudinal and transverse axis (Fig. 16-2a and b). In a transverse orientation, the fibrils have a punctuate echogenic pattern which is best achieved when the probe is directed perpendicular to the axis of the tendon. The slightest angle away from the perpendicular axis will result in an artifact referred to as "anisotropy" of tendons (Fig. 16-3a and b). This is a result of the scattering of the ultrasound beam producing an apparent hypoechoic tendon. This artifact is important to identify as most tendon pathology will also appear hypoechoic on ultrasound and can result in the misinterpretation of findings. Anisotropy and the dynamic property of tendons are two unique characteristics that allow the sonographer to differentiate them from other surrounding structures that may have similar appearances, such as nerve bundles (see Fig. 16-3a and b).

Nerve bundles also demonstrate an echogenic fibrillar pattern on ultrasound; however, there are some differences that can help make the distinction between the two. Nerve axon bundles are also hypoechoic, but are much thicker than the fibrils that are visualized in tendons. On transverse scans, these bundles have a characteristic "honeycomb" appearance due to the presence of thick hypoechoic

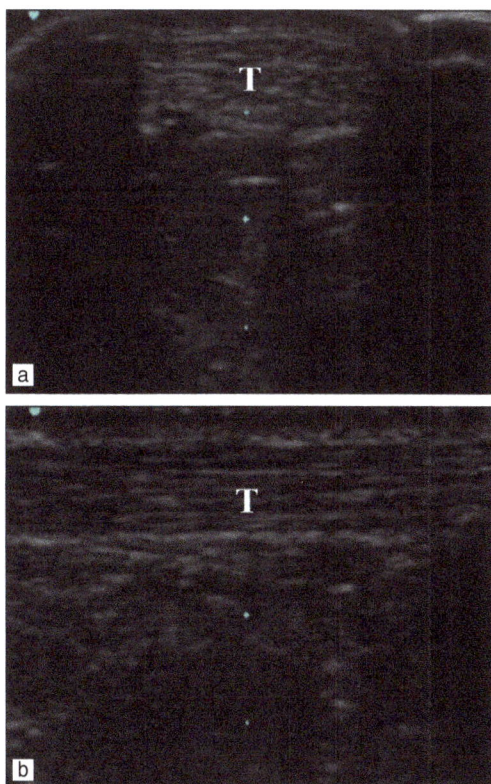

FIGURE 16-2 Normal transverse (a) and longitudinal (b) views of the Achilles tendon (T) with a classic fibrillar pattern.

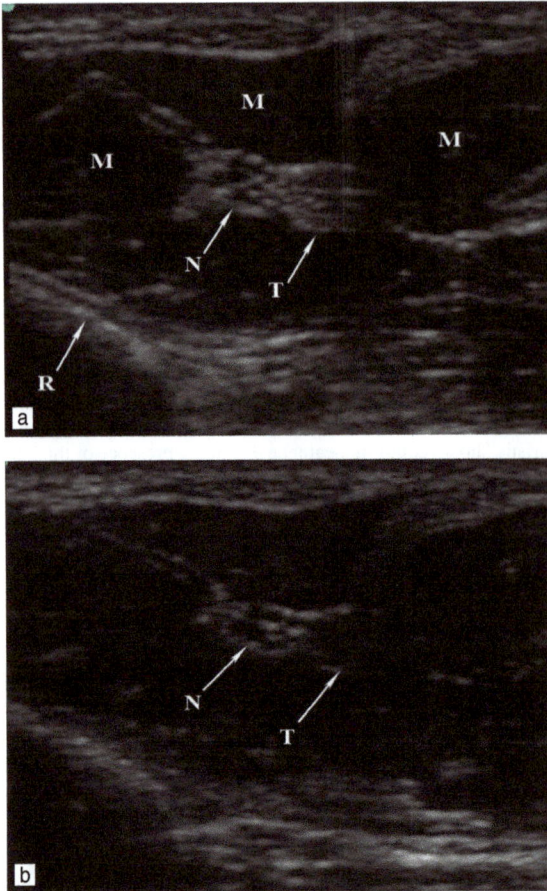

FIGURE 16-3 Transverse view of the mid-forearm illustrating the median nerve (N) and a tendon (T). The nerve has a more honeycomb appearance with distinct fascicles while the tendon has a more fibrillar pattern. In (*a*), the ultrasound beam is perpendicular to the nerve (N) and tendon (T) while in (*b*) the beam is at a 20° tilt decreasing the echogenicity of the tendon (T) but not the nerve (N). Also seen in (a) are muscle bundles (M) and the cortex of the radial bone (R).

axons that are found within nerves. Furthermore, as described earlier, tendons display anisotropy and nerves do not (see Fig. 16-3*a* and *b*).

BONE

Bones are visualized on ultrasound as thin, brightly echogenic cortex with a prominent posterior acoustic shadow and oftentimes reverberation artifact (see Fig. 16-3*a*). The shape of the cortex will reflect the contour of the bone in the plane that is being scanned. A long bone will appear as a bright curved line in a cross-sectional profile and as a straight line in a longitudinal profile. Although ribs are smaller and follow a curved path around the thorax, they have a similar appearance on ultrasound as long bones do. Ribs are superficial to the parietal and visceral pleura, which can be observed sliding back and forth between two ribs' shadows in cross-sectional profile (see Chap. 7).

IMAGING TIPS AND PROTOCOL

SUPERFICIAL SOFT TISSUE

Soft tissues and musculoskeletal structures should be scanned in both the longitudinal (sagittal) and short (transverse) axis. These structures are superficial, so high-frequency linear probes should be used. Lower-frequency curvilinear probes may be used in difficult patients or to identify deeper pathology. A hockey stick probe can also be utilized in small areas such as the fingers or for intraoral evaluation of a peritonsillar abscess. An endocavitary probe may also be very effective for intraoral evaluation. Even though this is not a sterile procedure, a probe cover or Tegaderm should be placed over the transducer for sanitary purposes. Any area of inflammation should be scanned from the outer edge to outer edge in order to not miss any underlying pus collection. Gentle pressure should be applied to the skin in order to evaluate for the typical appearance of pus flow signifying an underlying abscess or other debris. Color-flow Doppler should be used to differentiate an abscess from other surrounding structures such as a blood vessel, nerve bundle, or lymph node. A standoff pad can be placed in between the transducer and skin in order to improve the focal zone and resultant resolution. A standoff pad may be constructed with materials that are readily available such as filling an exam glove with water or gel or using an IV fluid bag. It is important to ensure that no air is introduced into the glove as it will impede the quality of the image by producing artifact. Commercially prepared standoff pads are also available and are often less cumbersome.

The water bath technique is easily performed by submerging the extremity in a basin of water. This helps to eliminate discomfort that may be caused by direct contact of the affected area with a transducer or standoff pad, and has been reported to provide superior images of tendons and foreign bodies when compared to more traditional methods.

PATHOLOGIC ULTRASOUND FINDINGS

CELLULITIS

Cellulitis on ultrasound has the appearance of a cobblestoning pattern representing edema within the subcutaneous fat layer secondary to engorgement of the lymphatic vessels (Fig. 16-4). This pattern is nonspecific and may also be seen in other disease processes such as congestive heart failure and deep vein thrombosis due to congestion. Cellulitis will not always have a distinct cobblestoning pattern and in some cases will appear as a homogeneous gray area with less distinction between the tissue planes. Color-flow Doppler may be used to further clarify the diagnosis of cellulitis where there may be signs of increased blood flow due to infection and inflammation. If the diagnosis is uncertain, the contralateral body part should always be scanned for comparison.

ABSCESS

Abscesses have a variable appearance on ultrasound, ranging from homogeneous and anechoic to heterogeneous with hyper- and hypoechoic regions (Fig. 16-5). In addition, an abscess may or may not be compressible depending on the presence of significant internal pressures and the patient's pain tolerance. If compression is

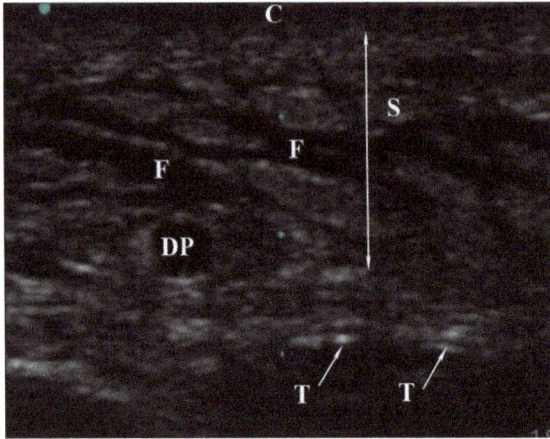

FIGURE 16-4 A transverse view of cellulitis of the foot. At the top is the cutaneous layer (C) containing epidermis and dermis. Note the cobblestoning pattern within the subcutaneous layer (S), which represents fluid (F) in between fat globules. The dorsalis pedis artery (DP) is seen in cross section as an anechoic structure. Also seen are hyperechoic lines with posterior shadowing that represent the cortical surface of the tarsal bones (T).

possible, swirls of pus and debris can often be seen moving around within the lumen. Posterior enhancement artifact is often visualized off the back wall of the abscess due to the ultrasound beam traveling through a cyst-like structure (see Fig. 16-5). When available, elastography (an ultrasound technique to measure tissue stiffness) has been shown to be helpful in delineating the abscess cavity and surrounding induration and may help to determine which abscesses may be successfully drained. Lymph nodes can also be inflamed with a hypoechoic appearance on ultrasound. It is important to differentiate the two as their managements are quite different. A lymph node is typically an ovoid structure with a

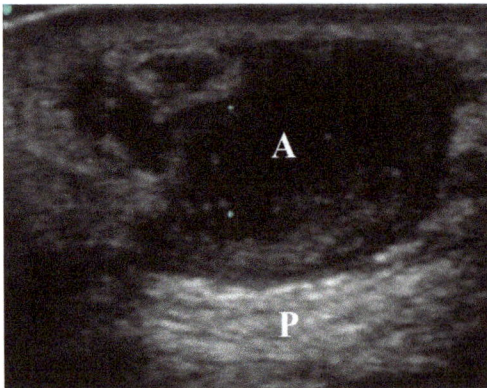

FIGURE 16-5 Transverse view of an abscess (A) in the lower leg. Note the lumen of the abscess is filled with heterogenous material typical of pus and debris. Posterior acoustic enhancement artifact is also seen off the back wall of the abscess (P).

hyperechoic center and a hypoechoic rim, with vascularity in the cortex that will demonstrate color-flow signals as opposed to an abscess. Therefore, if the structure is picking up color flow, further investigation is warranted before incision and drainage is attempted.

NECROTIZING FASCIITIS

The diagnosis of necrotizing fasciitis (NF) can be aided by imaging with plain radiography, CT, MRI, ultrasound (US), and ultimately confirmed by surgery. Although US is not as sensitive for NF as CT or MRI, it can be performed quickly at the bedside. On US, NF appears as a diffuse thickening of the subcutaneous tissue associated with a layer of >4 mm of fluid collection above the muscle fascial plane. Additionally, NF often involves organisms that form gas bubbles which may be seen as punctate hyperechoic areas on US, with "dirty" hyperechoic tapering comet-tail artifacts. In the evaluation for NF, images should be acquired in two planes and preferably in a gravity-dependent area. The fluid collection should be easily compressible, and it is important to note that if too much pressure is applied with the probe, the sonographer may interpret the exam as false negative. Applying less pressure and "floating" on the US gel over the affected area will help to avoid missing the diagnosis. If NF is suspected on US, surgery should be consulted immediately and additional studies performed to confirm the diagnosis.

MUSCLE PATHOLOGY

Complete and partial muscular tears can also be diagnosed by ultrasound. In complete tears, an anechoic region appears between the two muscle bodies that represents blood and edema. In partial tears, the muscle may only appear thinned. Other muscle pathology that may be seen with ultrasound includes myositis, in which the muscle fibers are inflamed and edematous, particularly when compared to a contralateral muscle.

TENDON INJURY

Complete tendon rupture is usually apparent on physical examination. Partial tears of a tendon are much more difficult to diagnose and ultrasound can be very useful. Complete tendon tears appear as an obvious full-thickness discontinuity of the fibers on ultrasound. The gap between the two ends of the tendon may be filled with hypoechoic blood if the rupture was recent and with hyperechoic clot or granulomatous tissue if the diagnosis is delayed (Fig. 16-6*a* and *b*). If there is an accompanying bone avulsion, a bright echogenic bony fragment with acoustic shadowing may be apparent. Incomplete tears will appear as hypoechoic defects in the regular fibrillar pattern or as a thinning of the tendon.

TENDONITIS AND TENOSYNOVITIS

Acute tendonitis is an inflammation of the tendon, most commonly as a result of an athletic or occupational activity. Acute tenosynovitis is a bacterial infection of the tendon sheath. Both inflammatory tendinitis and bacterial tenosynovitis may appear similar on ultrasound, although historical and clinical features should help to differentiate them. On ultrasound, tendon inflammation appears as a thickened tendon with decreased echogenicity and ill-defined margins. Anechoic fluid may be seen to surround the tendon. Suppurative tenosynovitis, a purulent infectious process, is a serious condition which can rapidly lead to tendon destruction if not treated immediately. The suppurative debris in this condition may be visualized as hyperechoic foci within the tendon sheath. The unaffected side should be scanned as a reference when evaluating tendons.

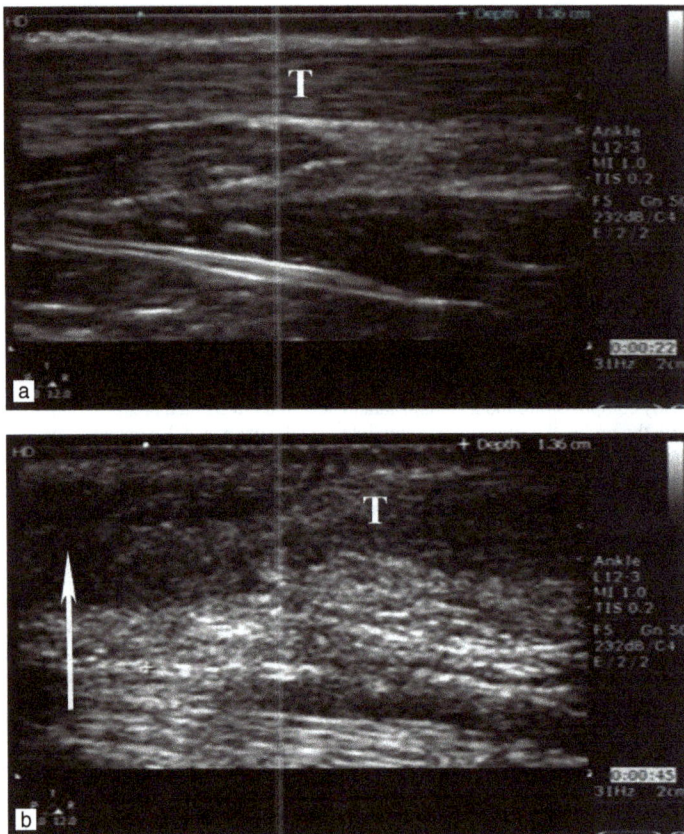

FIGURE 16-6 In (*a*) the probe is placed in the long axis over the patient's posterior ankle showing a segment of normal Achilles tendon (T). In (*b*) the probe is then slid more proximally up the posterior ankle overlying the area of tenderness, revealing a tendon (T) tear (arrow). Note the irregular appearance of the tendon and the hypoechoic areas most likely representing blood.

FOREIGN BODIES

Foreign bodies (FBs) exhibit a variety of sonographic appearances, depending on the composition, size, and length, as well as the amount of time it has been in the tissue. Most foreign bodies such as metal, glass, wood, and plastic are echogenic, but have different acoustic shadows depending on their size and shape. Wooden FBs are usually hyperechoic and cast a posterior acoustic shadow (Fig. 16-7*a* and *b*). Linear metallic FBs, such as needles, have a characteristic reverberation artifact which appears as bright, regularly spaced parallel lines distal to the metallic FB. Small or rounded metallic objects, such as ball bearings, may display a comet-tail artifact, which appears as a bright line projecting distally from the FB. Plastic typically has a prominent reverberation artifact, and gravel has a prominent posterior acoustic shadow, similar to gallstones. Glass FBs have less consistent findings, but some of these include

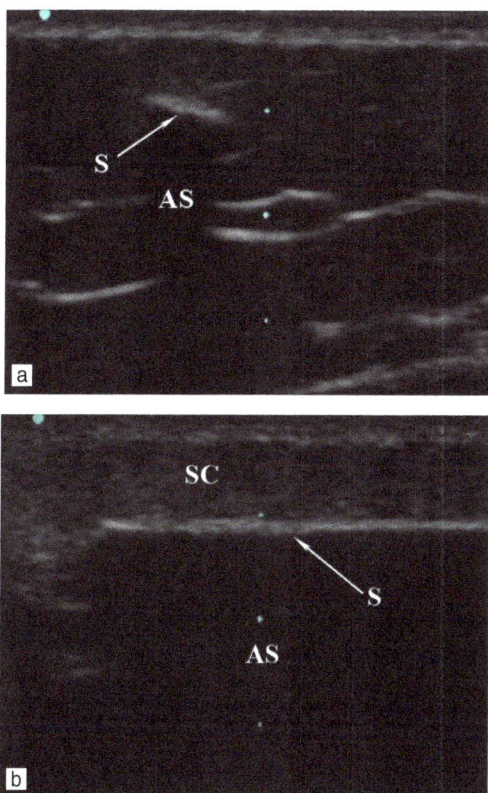

FIGURE 16-7 A wooden sliver (S) seen in short axis (*a*) and long axis (*b*) within the subcutaneous tissue (SC) of the buttock. Note the foreign body appears as a linear hyperechoic structure with posterior acoustic shadowing (AS).

acoustic shadowing, reverberation artifact, or diffuse beam scattering due to air trapping around jagged edges. If a FB has been retained for more than 24 hours, it may be surrounded by a hypoechoic "halo" which may represent surrounding edema, pus, or granulation tissue.

While ultrasound is often effective in visualizing FBs, it is not completely sensitive and should not be used alone to rule out the presence of a FB.

FRACTURES

A fracture is visualized as a disruption in the smooth echogenic linear cortex of the bone (Fig. 16-8). If a fracture is not readily apparent, but the patient has significant point tenderness, gentle pressure over the area with the probe may result in a widening of the cortex and visualization of a disruption that may not be seen on x-ray. Particularly in rib fractures, ultrasound may reveal minor cortical disruptions that appear with normal respirations that may not be seen on radiographs. The fracture is often associated with an anechoic region nearby representing blood or edema. Ultrasound has been shown to be helpful in guiding the correct cortical alignment of long bone fractures and may be used as an imaging adjunct during reduction.

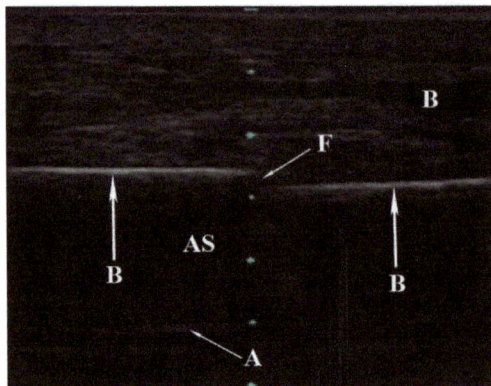

FIGURE 16-8 Fractured fibula. The normal cortex of the fibula in the longitudinal view appears as a horizontal hyperechoic linear stripe (B). A disruption in the cortex is visualized and represents a fracture (F). Note the hypoechoic region surrounding the bone, which is likely blood (B). Posterior acoustic shadowing (AS) is present due to bone impeding the ultrasound beam. Reverberation artifact (A) is also seen posteriorly.

COMMON PITFALLS

FAILURE TO RECOGNIZE NORMAL ANATOMY

If there is uncertainty as to whether the tissue is normal or pathologic, the unaffected extremity should be scanned and used as a control. The sonographer must be sure to scan the other side with the same probe and settings in order to ensure an adequate comparison.

MISTAKING OTHER STRUCTURES FOR TENDONS

Tendons may be mistaken for other similar-appearing structures such as nerves, muscle, or bone. Once again, both sides should be scanned to help identify normal tendon anatomy and pathology. In addition, the unique characteristic of anisotropy and the dynamic property of tendons are both important tools that also aid in this differentiation. The probe can be angled slightly away from the perpendicular axis in order to demonstrate the presence of anisotropy. The patient can be asked to move the body part in question to evaluate tendon function and to help distinguish it from other structures.

MISTAKING ANISOTROPY FOR TENDON PATHOLOGY

The ultrasound probe should be perpendicular to the tendon fibrils for optimal evaluation. As stated earlier, the more the probe is angled away from the perpendicular axis, the more hypoechoic the tendon will appear. This is anisotropy and is often mistaken for a tendon rupture or tear. Ideally, the transducer should be fanned in a proximal and distal motion, visualizing the whole tendon in order to identify true tears versus artifact. Anisotropy will disappear as the probe becomes more perpendicular to the tendon, while true tears will not.

DIFFICULTY IDENTIFYING TENDONS DUE TO LOCATION

Tendon fibrils are hyperechoic and usually easy to identify next to the relatively hypoechoic muscle fibers. However, when tendons are located next to more hyperechoic structures, such as adipose tissue, they can be more difficult to visualize. In this situation, the dynamic property of tendons is helpful. The sonographer can ask the patient to flex and extend the extremity in question and the resultant movement of the tendon can be scanned in real time.

THE DIFFICULT PATIENT OR DEEPER STRUCTURES

Most soft tissue applications are best studied with a linear high-frequency probe. In certain situations, such as in the evaluation of deeper abscesses, muscles, or hematomas, or in the obese patient, the use of a lower-frequency probe that allows for better penetration may be required. If the wrong frequency probe is selected, an ideal image may not be obtained and a pertinent finding may be missed.

PROBE PRESSURE

Applying too much pressure to a cellulitis, abscess, or necrotizing fasciitis may produce a false-negative result. The probe should be gently placed on the tissue of interest utilizing a thin layer of ultrasound gel as a coupling medium. This enables the viewing of the tissue in its true uncompressed state. If an abscess is suspected, gentle pressure may reveal the swirling motion of the pus within the cavity and help to not miss subtle fluid collections.

LYMPH NODES

Lymph nodes may resemble abscesses, and it is important to identify each and to avoid cutting into a node by accident. They can be differentiated by the use of color-flow Doppler as lymph nodes are highly vascular and abscesses are not. In addition, applying pressure to the lymph node may reveal a structure that is not compressible as opposed to an abscess, which may appear more fluid in nature.

INTEGRATION OF BEDSIDE MUSCULOSKELETAL ULTRASOUND INTO CLINICAL CARE

Bedside musculoskeletal US has become an integral part of acute care medicine. Traditionally, most of these conditions were diagnosed using conventional methods, including plain radiographs, CT scan, and MRI. The use of bedside US has been shown to be a convenient and accurate adjunct.

US is now regularly used in the evaluation of soft tissue infections and has been shown to accurately differentiate cellulitis from an abscess. In addition, although it is not extremely sensitive in diagnosing necrotizing fasciitis, if the findings are suspicious on ultrasound, the management can be accelerated and morbidity decreased.

Fractures are still mostly diagnosed on plain radiographs, but the use of US in the diagnosis of occult fractures will likely gain popularity. Using US decreases the radiation exposure associated with ordering an additional study, such as a CT scan. Also, US has gained momentum in diagnosing fractures in the pediatric patient, where radiation is even less desirable. In addition, US has proven to sometimes be more sensitive at diagnosing certain types of fractures such as in the ribs, sternum, or nasal bones that are often missed on x-rays.

The use of US in tendon evaluation has also increased due to its ease of use and accuracy at finding tears. This has become useful in settings where partial tears are suspected, the physical examination is unimpressive, and an expedient MRI is not available.

FB evaluation is also easily diagnosed by US. This is a quick, reliable modality that can be performed at the bedside without radiation exposure. US often identifies structures missed on radiographs and spares the patient complications from a retained FB.

The role of US is increasing steadily in musculoskeletal injuries, but it does still have its limitations. If a disease process is suspected and not found on US, then other modalities such as x-rays, CT scans, or MRIs should be performed and appropriate consultations utilized.

Additional Reading

Blaivas M, Lyon M, Brannam L, Duggal S, Sierzenski P. Water bath evaluation technique for emergency ultrasound of painful superficial structures. *Am J Emerg Med.* 2004;22(7):589-593.

Chau CL, Griffith JF. Musculoskeletal infections: ultrasound appearances. *Clin Radiol.* 2005 Feb;60(suppl 2):149-159.

Dean AJ, Gronczewski CA, Costantino TG. Technique for emergency medicine bedside ultrasound identification of a radiolucent foreign body. *J Emerg Med.* 2003;24(3):303-308.

Tayal VS, Hasan N, Norton J, et al. The effect of soft-tissue ultrasound on the management of cellulitis in the emergency department. *Acad Emerg Med.* 2006;13:384-388.

Yen ZS, Wang HP, Ma HM, et al. Ultrasonographic screening of clinically-suspected necrotizing fasciitis. *Acad Emerg Med.* 2002 Dec;9(suppl 12): 1448-1451.

17 Ultrasound for Venous Access

Frederick Korley

BACKGROUND AND INDICATIONS FOR EXAMINATION

The expeditious and safe placement of venous catheters is vital to the practice of acute care medicine. Venous access includes the cannulation of both superficial peripheral and large central veins, depending on the particular clinical scenario. Traditionally, venous access is performed blindly by palpation or with the use of anatomic landmarks. More recently, ultrasound guidance has become standard of care for most central venous access, and using ultrasound for difficult peripheral access may reduce the need for central access.

Obtaining venous access in certain situations may be difficult secondary to patient and operator characteristics. These factors include obesity, intravenous (IV) drug use, history of multiple prior attempts due to chronic illness, severe intravascular volume depletion, venous thrombosis, coagulopathy, operator inexperience, and operator anxiety due to the patient's clinical condition. There are clinical scenarios in which a patient must receive IV access expeditiously such as for the administration of fluids or medications, hemodynamic monitoring, transvenous pacemaker placement or hemodialysis.

Complications of central venous cannulation include multiple failed attempts, arterial bleeding, pneumothorax, loss of the guide wire, and catheter-related bloodstream infections. Recent studies have demonstrated that ultrasound-guided central venous access decreases the number of unsuccessful attempts and the complications when compared to the landmark technique. In addition, ultrasound reduces the time required to obtain venous access, which is critical in ill patients. With the possible exception of subclavian access in certain situations, ultrasound guidance is recommended for placing central venous catheters.

Bedside ultrasound-guided venous access should be performed in the following patients:

- The difficult patient who requires peripheral venous access
- Patients requiring central venous access

PROBE SELECTION AND TECHNICAL CONSIDERATIONS

LINEAR ARRAY PROBE WITH A FREQUENCY OF 7.5–10.0 MHz

A 7.5- or 10-MHz linear array probe should be used for vascular access. High-frequency probes provide higher-resolution images of superficial structures. Linear probes generate rectangular or square images, which makes it easier to follow the tip of the needle while visualizing the vessel.

FOCUS

The focus should be at the level of the blood vessel in order to maximize the lateral resolution of the image.

DEPTH

The depth should be adjusted so that the vessel of interest takes up approximately three-fourths of the screen. Most of the target vessels will be superficial; therefore, the depth should be decreased appropriately.

MACHINE PRESET

The machine should be used on the "vascular" setting for this procedure. This optimizes the resolution and clarity of the image.

GAIN

The total gain may be increased to brighten the signal returning from the walls of the blood vessel, making it easier to identify. The far gain or time-gain compensation (TGC) may be increased alone in order to enhance the signal returning from deeper vessels and is especially helpful in obese patients.

COLOR-FLOW DOPPLER

Color-flow Doppler identifies blood flow within a vessel. It is useful for the sonographer to use this modality to correctly identify blood vessels when they are difficult to locate. It also helps to differentiate blood vessels from other surrounding structures, which will not pick up color flow.

STERILE PRECAUTIONS

Although peripheral venous access is not a sterile procedure, it does involve exposure to patient body fluids. A probe cover, such as a Tegaderm, is recommended for this procedure to help keep the probe clean. Central venous access is a sterile procedure; therefore, typical precautions including a sterile probe cover and gel should be used.

STATIC VERSUS DYNAMIC APPROACH

The static approach involves using ultrasound to locate the target vessel and marking two places along the course of the vessel about 1 cm apart. The cannulating needle is inserted at the proximal mark and directed toward the distal mark without the use of real-time ultrasound guidance. This approach has a higher failure rate than the dynamic approach and is not recommended.

The more commonly used dynamic approach involves identifying and cannulating the vessel in real time with ultrasound guidance. The dynamic approach can be performed using one or two operators. In the case of two operators, one person can hold the probe and the other performs the procedure. It has the advantage of allowing the person performing the procedure to use both hands when inserting the needle and advancing the catheter. The procedure is more often performed with one operator who holds the probe in one hand and inserts the needle with the other. With this technique, the operator can make subtle adjustments to the orientation of the probe as needed without relying on an assistant.

LONG AXIS VERSUS SHORT AXIS

Ultrasound-guided venous access can be performed in either the short (transverse or "out-of-plane") or long (sagittal or "in-plane") axis. In the short-axis view, the probe is held perpendicular to the direction of the vessel, generating a transverse cross-sectional image (Fig. 17-1). This is the usual technique taught to the novice, as it is easier to puncture the vessel in the transverse axis. It also allows simultaneous visualization of neighboring structures, such as arteries and nerves. The disadvantage of this technique is that it is often difficult to judge how far the needle tip has advanced into the lumen of the vessel; therefore, it can be pushed in

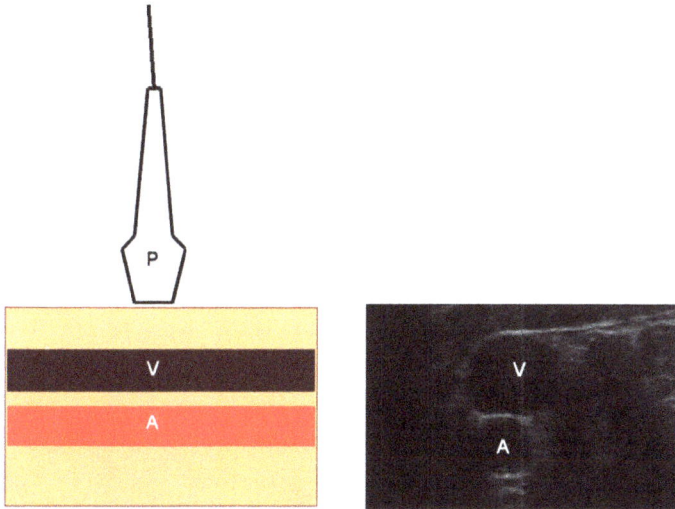

FIGURE 17-1 Short-axis (transverse) view of a vein and artery. In the illustration on the left, note the probe is held perpendicular to the direction of the vessel. The image on the right depicts the cross-sectional view of the vessels on the screen. V: vein, A: artery, P: probe.

too far and puncture the posterior wall. This can result in the vessel being "infiltrated" and the development of a soft tissue hematoma due to extravasation of blood, which renders the vessel unsuitable for IV access. It can also lead to injury of nearby vessels, such as an artery, especially in central venous access. With this approach, the cannulating needle is seen only when it crosses the ultrasound beam and appears as a hyperechoic dot on the screen. The needle punctures through the proximal wall of the vessel and produces a bright white hyperechoic artifact in the center of the anechoic lumen called the "target sign" (Fig. 17-2).

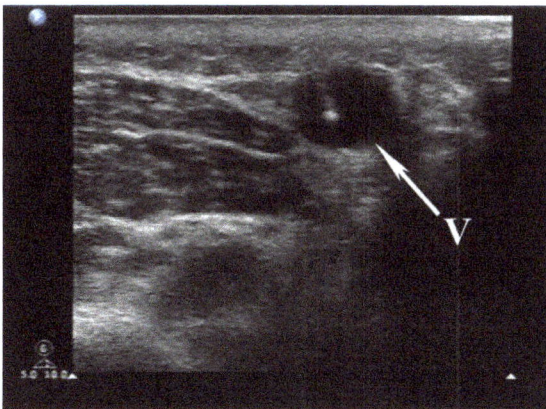

FIGURE 17-2 This image illustrates the short-axis approach to peripheral venous access. Note the blood vessel (V) in its cross-sectional orientation and the "target sign" seen as a bright white hyperechoic structure within the center of the lumen signifying the needle inside the vessel.

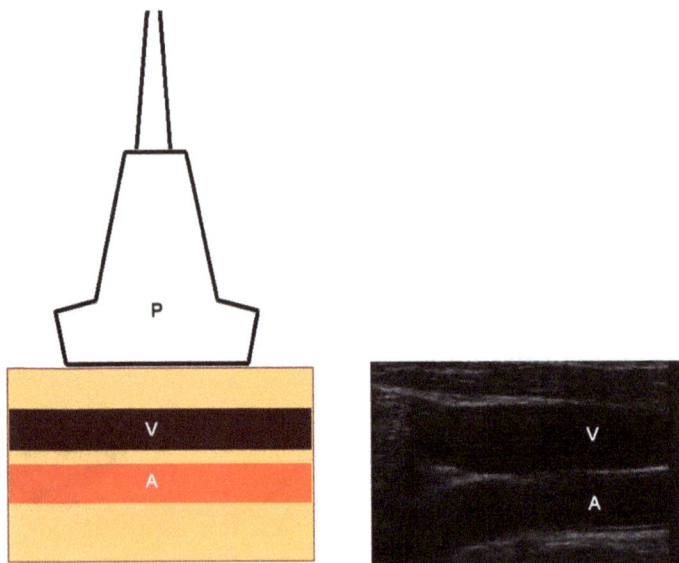

FIGURE 17-3 Longitudinal (sagittal) view of a vein and artery. In the illustration on the left, note the probe is held parallel to the direction of the vessel. The image on the right depicts the long-axis view of the vessels on the screen. V: vein, A: artery, P: probe.

Once this sign is visualized, the needle is inside the vessel, a flash of blood should be seen in the angiocatheter and the needle should not be advanced any farther.

In the long-axis approach, the probe is placed parallel to the vessel, generating a longitudinal cross-sectional image (Fig. 17-3). The advantage of this technique is that the full length of the needle may be visualized within the lumen of the vessel, making it easier to avoid puncturing the posterior wall (Fig. 17-4). A disadvantage

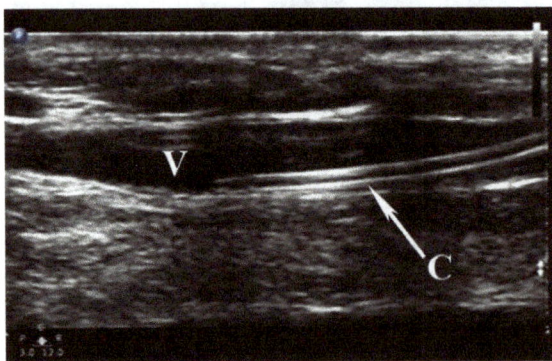

FIGURE 17-4 This image illustrates the long-axis approach to peripheral venous access. Note the blood vessel (V) in its sagittal orientation and the double bright white hyperechoic lines within the lumen representing the IV catheter (C). The full lengths of the needle and catheter are visualized in this axis, making it less likely to puncture the posterior wall and infiltrate the vessel.

is that the probe has a slender width in this orientation and the needle must be positioned directly underneath it in order to be visualized in its entirety. Subtle movements of the probe can cause the needle to fall outside the width of the ultrasound beam and no longer be visualized on the screen. Also, it may be difficult to simultaneously determine the location of the artery (except when the artery is directly below the vein). As a result, small movements of the needle outside the ultrasound beam may lead to undesired arterial puncture.

Oftentimes, it is recommended that the target vein be identified and punctured in the short axis and then the probe rotated 90° into the long axis to make sure the tip does not hit the posterior wall. The IV catheter can then be advanced in the long axis and can be seen in its entirety. Whichever method is selected, it is crucial to always follow the needle tip.

PERFORMING ULTRASOUND-GUIDED PERIPHERAL VENOUS ACCESS

EQUIPMENT

- *18- or 20-gauge angiocatheter:* A standard angiocatheter (1.25 in) is sufficient for superficial veins, but a longer one (1.88–2.5 in) is necessary for deeper vessels. In general, ultrasound is most helpful in identifying deeper (>5 mm) vessels and unless the vessel is very superficial, the longer angiocatheters should be used for ultrasound-guided peripheral access.
- Tourniquet
- Alcohol pads or chlorhexidine applicator
- A lidocaine syringe with a 25- or 27-gauge needle
- Gauze
- Dressing to secure IV and vacutainer/blood tubes/IV hookup and flush as needed

THE ANATOMY

The most common peripheral veins used for IV access are the cephalic, basilic, or brachial veins of the arm (Fig. 17-5). It is important for the sonographer to be familiar with the upper extremity anatomy before beginning the procedure. The cephalic vein is most lateral, coursing along the radial aspect of the extremity and best approached from the lateral surface of the upper arm. The brachial vein (or veins) runs with the brachial artery and is often cannulated in the antecubital fossa. There are often paired brachial veins on each side of the brachial artery. The artery should be identified by compressing the vessels slightly and looking for pulsations. The brachial nerve is also in close proximity and should be avoided. The basilic vein is the most medial, running along the ulnar aspect of the extremity and is best accessed from the medial surface of the upper arm. The basilic vein is not paired with an artery and is found in the subcutaneous fat of the medial arm where it is not visible or palpable and usually has not been accessed via a landmark technique. For these reasons, the basilic vein is often the best candidate for ultrasound-guided access and is often used for peripherally inserted central catheter (PICC) lines.

PATIENT POSITIONING AND PREPARATION

In the supine position, the patient's extremity should be abducted and externally rotated for easy access to the medial aspect of the arm. If the patient is upright, their arm should be placed on a bedside table for comfort (Fig. 17-6). A tourniquet should then be placed on the upper arm. The area where the needle insertion will occur should be cleaned with an antiseptic wipe.

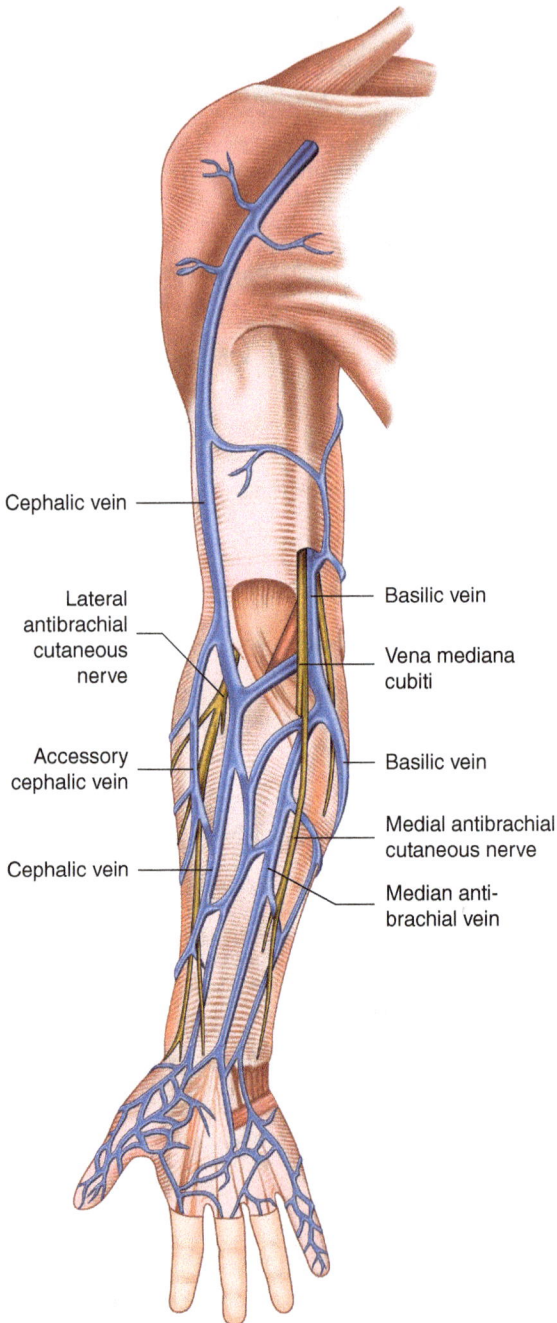

Cephalic vein

Lateral antibrachial cutaneous nerve

Accessory cephalic vein

Cephalic vein

Basilic vein

Vena mediana cubiti

Basilic vein

Medial antibrachial cutaneous nerve

Median anti-brachial vein

FIGURE 17-5 Venous anatomy of the upper extremity.

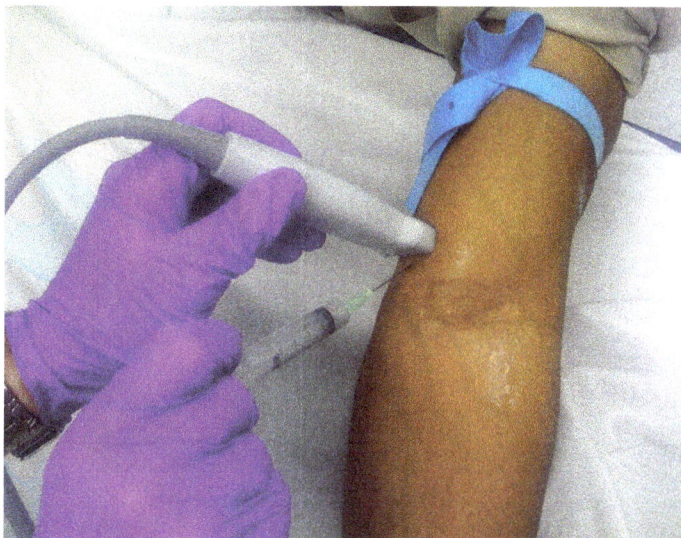

FIGURE 17-6 Correct patient positioning for upper extremity venous access. The ultrasound probe is held in a transverse orientation. The needle is entering the skin at the center of the probe into the medial aspect of the patient's upper arm attempting basilic venous access. Note the patient's arm is abducted and placed on a table for comfort.

ULTRASOUND GUIDANCE

The first step in ultrasound-guided venous access is to identify the target vessel. Gel should be applied to a linear, high-frequency probe. The probe is first oriented in the transverse position, with the marker pointing toward the patient's right side. This orientation will depict the patient's right side on the left side of the ultrasound monitor. It is important to ensure that the probe is held in the correct orientation. This way, if the cannulating needle is redirected to the left or right, the corresponding ultrasound image will be in the proper orientation.

Once the probe is placed on the skin, scanning should take place on the distal portion of the upper arm and the antecubital fossa looking for a vein. The vein that has the largest diameter and is most superficial is the ideal target (Fig. 17-7). Veins will appear anechoic due to their blood-filled lumen. Superficial veins will travel alone, but deep veins, such as the brachial, will appear adjacent to the artery. It is important to distinguish veins from arteries and other surrounding structures. Veins are usually non-pulsatile, have thinner walls, and are compressible. In addition, color-flow Doppler will pick up blood flow inside the vessel and distinguish it from other anatomy such as nerves, tendons, and muscles. The sonographer must make sure that the vein chosen is patent. This can be done by scanning through the vessel looking for internal echoes, which may indicate clot burden (Fig. 17-8), and also making sure the vessel is compressible.

Once the target vein has been identified in its short axis, the probe should be moved either medially or laterally in order to center the vein on the ultrasound screen. It is also helpful to place pressure on the skin at the center of the probe to make sure that the vein wall tents and that the transducer is correctly placed with the vessel centered. To avoid inadvertent arterial puncture, the portion of the vein selected should not overlap with the artery. The sonographer can achieve this by

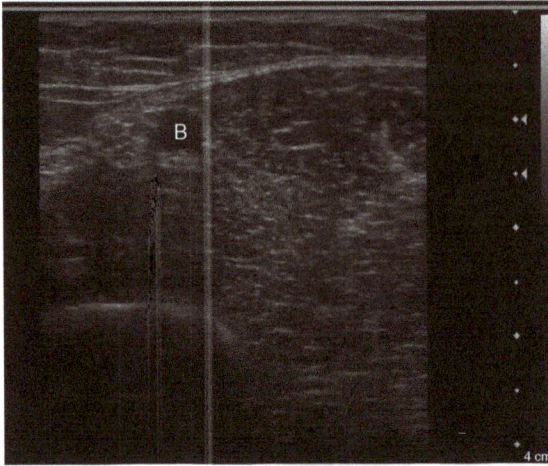

FIGURE 17-7 This image illustrates a superficial target vessel, the basilic vein (B), in its short axis. The distance markers on the right side of the screen estimate its depth at 1 cm from the skin surface. Note the anechoic lumen of the vessel compared to the soft tissue and muscle surrounding it in the upper arm.

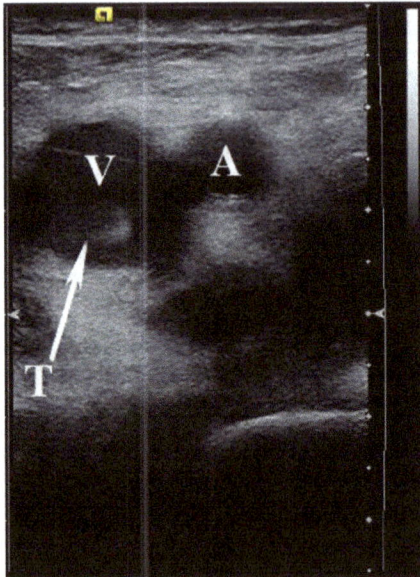

FIGURE 17-8 Hyperechoic area within the lumen of the common femoral vein (V) suggestive of thrombus (T). The probe is placed at the inguinal crease of the patient's left leg in a transverse orientation, depicting a short-axis view of the vein medial to the artery. A: common femoral artery.

slowly scanning up and down the patient's arm to find the place where the vein moves slightly away from the artery and is more accessible. The axis of the vessel relative to the arm should be determined either by scanning proximally and distally in the short axis, keeping the vessel in the middle, or by imaging the vessel in the long axis.

The depth of the vein is determined by using the markings on the side of the ultrasound image. The needle entry site should be at the middle of the probe and is usually the same distance from the probe as the depth of the vein (see Figs. 17-6 and 17-9). The area of entry can then be anesthetized with a small-gauge needle for patient comfort. After anesthetizing the area, the angiocatheter should puncture the skin at a 45° angle, in-line with the axis of the vessel, as determined earlier. The needle will appear as a bright white echogenic structure on the screen. The sonographer should watch the monitor as the needle advances toward the vessel. If the needle is lost on the screen, "jiggling" it may help to relocate it. Also, gentle fanning of the probe in a superior-inferior direction as the needle is advanced will help to follow its course as it approaches the vein. The anterior wall of the vessel will tent inward when the needle touches it. The "target" sign will be visualized, as described earlier, when the needle begins to enter the vein. Sometimes the target sign may be seen prior to actual catheter entry into the vessel lumen, as the tip of the needle tents the endothelial lining of the vein into the lumen. In this case, there will be no flash and the catheter will not advance easily. With experience, a gentle "pop" may be felt as the catheter pierces this lining, and

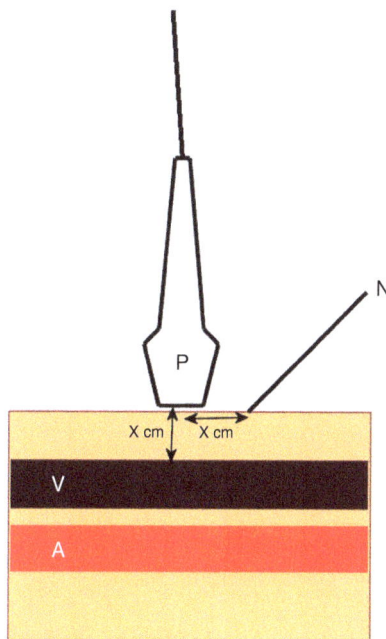

FIGURE 17-9 The image illustrates the correct needle entry site, which should be the same distance from the center of the probe as the depth of the vessel. V: vein, A: artery, N: needle, P: probe.

needle entry into the lumen can be assured by keeping the target sign in view at the tip of the needle and advancing the catheter slightly while flattening it to enter the lumen. Care should be taken not to "backwall" the vein by determining the needle tip location within the lumen, either by fanning through the lumen in the short axis while jiggling the needle or by visualizing the needle tip in the long axis.

Once the needle tip location is confirmed (a flash of blood should also be seen), the catheter should be advanced over the needle. As in standard IV placement, the needle portion of the angiocatheter is removed, adequate blood flow is aspirated to confirm the correct placement within the vein, and a dressing placed to secure the IV. Also, the probe can be placed over the vein proximal to the IV and saline can be injected into the IV and visualized on the screen within the lumen of the vessel to confirm correct placement. When correctly placed, microbubbles (small hyperechoic dots) will be seen to travel through the vein with saline injection.

Dynamic single-user peripheral catheterization is the most reliable way to succeed with this procedure once it has been mastered. However, this is among the most challenging ultrasound-guided procedures in acute care. The small size of the vessel, small size of the catheter (making US visualization more challenging), the need for coordination of imaging and cannulization, peripheral vessels that vary in size and course, and problems with anterior tenting and backwalling the vessel contribute to making this a challenging procedure. It is recommended that the novice begin by performing ultrasound-guided peripheral cannulation on several dozen patients who are well-hydrated and without known vascular access problems prior to expecting to be able to complete this procedure reliably on ill patients with risk factors for difficult cannulation (dehydration, dialysis, IV drug abuse, obesity, sickle cell anemia, pediatric patients, etc).

PERFORMING ULTRASOUND-GUIDED CENTRAL VENOUS ACCESS

EQUIPMENT

- Central line kit
- Sterile gown and gloves
- Face mask and cap
- Sterile drape
- Sterile ultrasound probe cover
- Chlorhexidine applicators
- Additional lidocaine as needed
- Sterile flushes
- Nylon suture
- Sterile dressing kit

INTERNAL JUGULAR VEIN

- *The anatomy:* In the neck, the internal jugular vein (IJV) is generally lateral to the carotid artery but may course anterior to it at certain points. The external landmarks for the superior part of the IJV are the apex of the triangle formed by the clavicle and the sternal and clavicular heads of the sternocleido-mastoid muscle.
- *Patient positioning and preparation:* Place the patient in the Trendelenburg position, helping to distend the vessel and to avoid air entry during cannuliza-tion. Although turning the patient's head 15°–30° to the contralateral side allows greater access to the neck, there is data that suggests that head rotation increases the overlap of the carotid by the IJV. In addition, extreme head rotation

may cause a decrease in the diameter of the IJV, making it a more difficult target. Therefore, a more neutral head position may be favored and the neck should be scanned in both positions to determine the optimal place to insert the needle.

- *Ultrasound guidance:* The neck should be scanned prior to beginning the procedure to locate the vein and its location relative to the carotid as well as looking for scarring, valves, or clots, and to determine the optimal spot for cannulization. This does not need to be performed in a sterile fashion. The probe should be placed on the patient's neck in a transverse orientation and the length of the vessel interrogated along the neck (Fig. 17-10). When standing at the head of the bed, the indicator on the probe should be oriented to the sonographer's left, corresponding to the patient's left and the left side of the screen as it is viewed.

The vein needs to be scanned in a superior to inferior direction, noting its relationship to the carotid artery and finding the location of its largest diameter. It is best to pick a spot where the artery moves slightly medial to the vein as opposed to being posterior to it. This will improve success and limit the possibility of hitting the artery with the needle if it is advanced too far. Scanning the IJV will also ensure its patency by looking for internal echoes and checking for compressibility. If the IJV on one side of the neck is not patent, the other side should be scanned and evaluated.

Once the IJV is located, sterile precautions need to be observed before beginning the procedure. The sonographer needs to wash their hands, put on a cap, facemask, sterile gown, and sterile gloves prior to prepping the patient. The target area is then cleaned using a chlorhexidine applicator usually included in the central line kit. After this, the patient is covered in a full-body drape and all the necessary supplies can be placed on top of it. The ultrasound probe needs to be inserted into a sterile cover and can best be performed with the help of an assistant. There needs to be gel inside the cover, which is not necessarily sterile. Sterile gel is applied to the probe once the cover is in place.

The probe can now be placed back on the patient's neck in the correct position to identify the IJV. The vein should be centered into the middle of the screen and the depth determined using the markings on the side of the ultrasound image (see Fig. 17-10). In the transverse view, the needle insertion point is the same distance

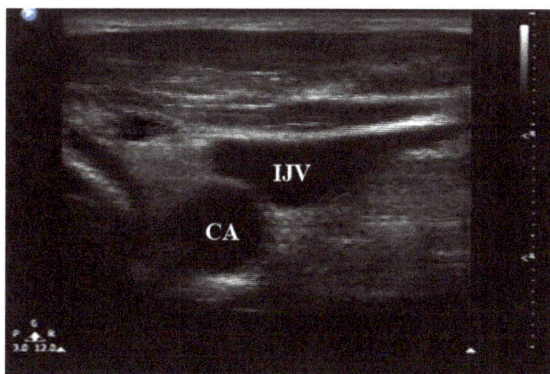

FIGURE 17-10 Short-axis view of the internal jugular vein (IJV) and carotid artery (CA). The probe is placed in a transverse orientation on the patient's left neck depicting the IJV anterior and lateral to the carotid artery. The IJV is approximately 1 cm from the skin surface, according to the markers on the right side of the screen. Note the anterior wall of the IJV tenting with gentle pressure of the probe.

from the middle of the probe as the depth of the vein. An entry site and angle should be chosen so that if the needle is advanced too far, it will not enter the carotid. If the IJV is on top of the carotid, a more lateral approach may accomplish this.

The entry site should be anesthetized using 1% lidocaine from the kit. Visualizing the injection of anesthetic using ultrasound can help the sonographer get an idea of the depth and orientation of the image relative to the IJV. The introducer needle attached to a syringe can then be inserted at a 45°–60° angle to the skin. The needle is at a steeper angle than for peripheral access in order to avoid advancing it too deeply and puncturing the lung. The ultrasound probe may need to be placed on the field in order for the non-dominant hand to stabilize the skin to allow passage of the introducer needle. Once the introducer needle is through the skin, the probe is then picked up and as the needle approaches the vessel, the syringe should be gently aspirated and an indentation of the anterior wall will be visualized on contact.

As in peripheral access, it is crucial to know the location of the needle tip. This can be accomplished in the short axis by fanning along the length of the needle and identifying the target sign in the vessel lumen, making sure that the tip does not travel too deeply. While a transverse approach is excellent for identifying the IJV and ensuring puncture over the middle of the vessel, a long-axis or in-line view of the needle will ensure that the entire needle is visualized up to the tip and is recommended when possible.

When a flashback of blood is obtained in the syringe, the ultrasound probe can be put aside and the remainder of the procedure performed as in a traditional central line placement. The syringe is removed, and the guide-wire is advanced through the introducer needle. The needle is taken out and the puncture hole is dilated by passing a dilator from the kit over the guide-wire and into the skin. The dilator can then be removed and the central line catheter is advanced over the guide-wire. When the guide-wire appears to be coming out of one of the central line ports, it can be pulled out from the skin and the catheter further advanced. Each port of the central line should be tested for patency by aspirating back with a syringe to ensure easy blood flow. The central line should then be secured and stitched into the skin and a dressing placed over it.

SUBCLAVIAN VEIN AND AXILLARY VEIN

The subclavian vein (SCV) is not as easily found on ultrasound due to its location posterior to the clavicle; therefore, this central line is often still performed using the landmark technique.

If it is placed using ultrasound guidance, it needs to be done using a lateral approach through the axillary vein extending up into the SCV.

- *The anatomy*: The axillary vein originates at the lower border of the teres major muscle as a continuation of the brachial vein from the upper arm. It is best located within the axillary fold where it continues up to the lateral border of the first rib and turns into the SCV behind the clavicle.
- *Patient positioning and preparation:* The patient should once again be placed in the Trendelenburg position to increase blood flow to the axillary vein. In order to open up the anatomy, the patient's arm can be abducted 90°.
- *Ultrasound guidance:* The axillary vein should be scanned and located prior to beginning the procedure in a non-sterile fashion. The probe should be placed on the patient's anterior chest in a longitudinal (sagittal) position pointing toward the patient's head. The optimal location is just inferior to the most lateral aspect of the patient's clavicle. This orientation will depict a short-axis

view of the axillary vein and artery. The vein is found inferior to the artery and both vessels will be visualized below the pectoral muscle.

The vein should be evaluated for the presence of internal echoes and checked for compressibility. The axillary vein is deeper than the IJV; therefore, compressibility may be more difficult to assess with probe pressure alone. If the vein on one side is not patent, the other side should be scanned and evaluated.

Once the axillary vein is located, sterile precautions need to be observed, as described earlier, for IJV access. The vein should be centered into the middle of the screen and the depth determined using the markings on the side of the ultrasound image. The needle will be entering from the lateral side of the patient at the middle of the probe. The axillary vessels run close to the lung pleura, and care needs to be taken to not puncture the lung and cause a pneumothorax while advancing the needle. The entry site should be anesthetized and the rest of the procedure carried out similar to the IJV cannulation described earlier.

FEMORAL VEIN

Femoral vein (FV) central lines have the highest rates of catheter-related bloodstream infection and venous thrombosis compared to IJV and SCV lines. They are not favored among critical care physicians and should be placed only in situations where an internal jugular or subclavian line has failed or in patients who have contraindications to receiving a neck or chest line. However, in an acute situation such as a trauma or cardiac arrest, a femoral line may be the only initially feasible approach. While the FV is fairly reliably located by finding the femoral pulse, this can be challenging in the patient in shock. Use of ultrasound for femoral access has been shown to increase first-pass success and decrease arterial puncture and cannulization.

- *The anatomy*: The FV lies within the femoral triangle, which is bordered superiorly by the inguinal ligament, laterally by the sartorius muscle, and medially by the adductor longus muscle. The saphenous vein can be seen to join the common FV medially. The saphenous vein can appear large but is a superficial vein and not paired with an artery and should not be mistaken for the FV. The FV is medial to both the femoral artery and nerve proximally but becomes deeper as it travels distally, diving below the femoral artery (see Fig. 17-8). The vein goes deep to the femoral artery very quickly, and a common mistake of the landmark technique is to approach the FV distally, leading to arterial puncture.
- *Patient positioning and preparation*: The patient should be supine with their hip externally rotated in a "frog-leg" position which will help to keep the vein medial to the artery.
- *Ultrasound guidance*: Prior to creating a sterile field, the patient's inguinal region should be scanned in order to locate the FV, artery, and nerve. The probe should be placed in a transverse position with the indicator pointing toward the patient's right side, just below the inguinal ligament. When scanning the patient's right leg, this orientation will place the FV on the right side of the screen and the artery on the left side. The opposite will be true when scanning the left leg (see Fig. 17-8).

The FV should be followed a short distance inferiorly by sliding the probe down the anterior thigh. This will help to ensure its patency by looking for internal echoes and checking for compressibility (see Fig. 17-8). If the FV on one side of the leg is not patent, the other side should be scanned and evaluated.

Once the FV is located, sterile precautions need to be observed, as described earlier, for IJV access. The vein should be centered into the middle of the screen and the depth determined using the markings on the side of the ultrasound image. The needle will be entering at the middle of the probe, and in a transverse view the insertion point is the same distance from the middle of the probe as the depth of the vein. As the femoral vessels travel down the leg, the artery becomes more anterior to the vein making it more difficult to avoid the artery. Therefore, the optimal entry site is as close to the inguinal ligament as possible. The entry site should be anesthetized and the rest of the procedure carried out similar to the IJV cannulation described earlier.

CONFIRMING CATHETER PLACEMENT

Following either peripheral or central catheter placement, ultrasound may be used to confirm correct placement. A small amount of agitated saline injected will be seen as a "flush" with punctate hyperechoic echoes in the vein proximal to the catheter.

In central line placement, confirmation should be confirmed by aspirating venous blood back through all ports and by the ease of flushing saline into the catheter. While a CXR is still routinely recommended to confirm tip location in an IJV or subclavian catheter, visualization of the right atrium using a subcostal cardiac view should show this flush when a central catheter is correctly placed. Ultrasound may also be used to look for pneumothorax after IJ or subclavian access.

COMMON PITFALLS AND TIPS

FAILURE TO VISUALIZE NEEDLE TIPS

The location of the needle tip may be lost during ultrasound-guided venous access. This makes it difficult for the sonographer to judge how close the needle tip is to the vessel. As a result, the needle tip may be advanced too far through the posterior wall, resulting in an infiltrated vessel. Also, if the needle is not localized, it may cause injury to nearby structures. In the transverse orientation, the needle tip will appear as a bright hyperechoic dot and the "target" sign will be seen when the tip is within the lumen of the vessel (see Fig. 17-2). If the tip is lost, jiggling the syringe may help to relocate it and the needle can then be retracted and redirected toward the vessel. Also, the probe can be moved or gently rocked back and forth to bring the needle tip back into focus. Alternatively, a long-axis approach can be used which visualizes the full length of the needle throughout the procedure, not just the tip.

INJURY TO NEARBY STRUCTURES

One of the most common pitfalls in venous access is inadvertent injury to the adjacent artery. Knowledge of the anatomy is essential in helping to avoid these injuries. The area should always be pre-scanned to locate the anatomy and identify any possible anomalies. Also, the usual differences between arterial and venous anatomy need to be identified, such as pulsatility, compressibility, and wall thickness. The sonographer always needs to watch the monitor as the needle is advanced and make sure it is not heading toward the artery.

Injury to other nearby structures is not as common, but can occur if the sonographer loses sight of the needle. These structures include nerves, lymph nodes, muscles, tendons, and pleural puncture. If there is any uncertainty as to whether a structure is a blood vessel or not, the use of color-flow Doppler is helpful in identifying blood flow. Nerves will be seen paired with deep vessels and need to be avoided. They will appear as "honeycomb"-type structures that are more echoic and heterogeneous than a vessel and will not pick up color flow. In addition, real-time guided ultrasound helps the clinician to direct the needle into the vessel without having to travel through muscle, tendon, or other structures, which may be easily injured using the blind technique.

FAILURE TO ASPIRATE BLOOD FROM VESSEL

Failure to aspirate blood from the vein is usually due to the needle not being in the proper location. The sonographer should pull the needle back slightly and redirect it into the vessel while watching it on the monitor.

"LOSING" THE VEIN

Often times, the vessels will shift off the screen and the vein is missed in an access attempt. This is usually due to the probe not being held in a steady fashion and happens with novice sonographers. When using the one-operator technique, the hand that is holding the probe should be firmly placed on the patient's skin and attempts made to not move it during the procedure. The direct contact of the sonographer's hand with the patient's skin helps to anchor the probe and prevent it from moving around while the introducer needle is inserted.

Also, when scanning a vein, very light pressure should be applied to the skin with the probe. Too much pressure may collapse the vein and make it appear smaller on the screen and more difficult to access. This is especially important in critically ill patients who may be volume depleted hypotensive.

NOT REACHING THE TARGET VEIN

Angiocatheters commonly used for peripheral venous access are 1.25 in (3.175 cm) long. They are adequate for veins that are superficial, but if the vessel is deeper, the catheter may not reach the intended site, or may easily slip out of a cannulated vessel. The sonographer needs to take note of the distance markers on the side of the screen to estimate the depth of the vessel and use the appropriate catheter. A longer angiocatheter (1.88–2.5 in) may be needed for deeper peripheral vessels. Once venous access is obtained, the catheter must be secured appropriately.

INFECTION

Iatrogenic infection from central line placement is a possibility which may be exacerbated in an acute situation. Standard sterile precautions should be used by the clinician performing the procedure, and by any assistant helping with the line placement. In addition, the use of sterile probe covers and gel is essential. Avoiding the placement of femoral lines unless necessary also helps to reduce the incidence of infection.

CONCLUSION

Venous access, both peripheral and central, is a procedure that is performed on a daily basis in most acute care settings. Peripheral venous access is most commonly still performed by palpation and without the use of ultrasound. In cases where gaining IV access is more difficult or impossible using standard methods, ultrasound has been shown to reduce the number of attempts and to decrease patient anxiety and discomfort.

In contrast, ultrasound-guided central venous access is now the standard of care in most acute care settings. Multiple studies have shown that using ultrasound guidance in central line placement has greatly improved success rates and decreased complications. Injury to the artery in central line placement can be a serious complication of the procedure; therefore, if possible, it should be used at all times. Ultrasound helps the clinician to better define patient anatomy as well as to avoid neurovascular structures. Ultrasound-guided line placement has quickly become the preferred method over the blind landmark approaches typically used in the past.

Additional Reading

Feller-Kopman D. Ultrasound-guided internal jugular access: a proposed standardized approach and implications for training and practice. *Chest.* 2007;132(1):302-309.

McGee DC, Gould MK. Preventing complications of central venous catheterization. *N Engl J Med.* 2003;348(12):1123-1133.

Miller AH, Roth BA, Mills TJ, Woody JR, Longmoor CE, Foster B. Ultrasound guidance versus the landmark technique for the placement of central venous catheters in the emergency department. *Acad Emerg Med.* 2002;9(8):800-805.

Milling TJ, Jr., Rose J, Briggs WM, et al. Randomized, controlled clinical trial of point-of-care limited ultrasonography assistance of central venous cannulation: the third sonography outcomes assessment program (SOAP-3) trial. *Crit Care Med.* 2005;33(8):1764-1769.

Mills CN, Liebmann O, Stone MB, Frazee BW. Ultrasonographically guided insertion of a 15-cm catheter into the deep brachial or basilic vein in patients with difficult intravenous access. *Ann Emerg Med.* 2007;50(1):68-72.

18 Ultrasound for Thoracentesis

Richard C. Redman, Scott L. Shofer, and Momen M. Wahidi

BACKGROUND AND INDICATIONS FOR EXAMINATION

Pleural effusion is a commonly encountered condition, which may arise as a consequence of a number of disease states including malignancy, infections, and inflammatory conditions. Patients may develop complaints of shortness of breath, dyspnea on exertion, or pleuritic chest pain as part of their initial presentation. Sampling and drainage of pleural effusions is important to adequately diagnose the patient's condition and to alleviate their respiratory symptoms. Thoracic ultrasound is an invaluable tool for characterizing the quantity and quality of the effusion as well as facilitating safe sampling or drainage of the fluid. Thoracic ultrasound is also useful for the rapid visualization of the parietal and visceral pleural surfaces, evaluation for pneumothorax, and to some extent the evaluation of the lung parenchyma.

A pleural effusion is easily identified using ultrasound owing to the relatively echo-free nature of fluid. Small pockets of fluid can be easily visualized by ultrasound with the patient in the upright position. In contrast, 150 mL of fluid is typically necessary in order to visualize an effusion on a standard upright posteroanterior and lateral chest radiograph. Ultrasound can be particularly useful in differentiating pleural fluid from lung parenchyma, atelectasis, infiltrate, or an elevated hemidiaphragm identified on chest radiograph in the acutely ill patient.

Thoracentesis is typically a safe and relatively simple procedure. However, the incidence of pneumothorax has been reported to be as high as 20%–39%. No randomized controlled clinical trial has compared the use of ultrasound or physical examination alone to guide thoracentesis. However, several studies have shown that ultrasound decreases the complication rate of the procedure.

Bedside ultrasound-guided thoracentesis should be performed in the following patients:

- The diagnostic evaluation of a patient with new pleural effusion

- The patient with a pleural effusion who presents with respiratory compromise or dyspnea

- The patient who presents with a fever, chest pain and/or suspected empyema

PROBE SELECTION AND TECHNICAL CONSIDERATIONS FOR THORACENTESIS

CURVILINEAR PROBE WITH A FREQUENCY OF 3.5–5.0 MHz

A curvilinear probe with a frequency of 3.5–5.0 MHz is best suited for performing a thoracentesis. This allows for better visualization of deeper structures and is more than adequate for visualizing more superficial structures adjacent to the chest wall. A higher-frequency probe between 5.0 and 7.0 MHz is effective for visualizing chest wall structures and the parietal pleura.

DEPTH

The sonographer should initially start off deep and survey the chest, the effusion, and surrounding structures. The depth should then be reduced so that the area where the needle will be introduced takes up most of the screen.

GAIN OR TIME-GAIN COMPENSATION

The total gain can be increased to brighten the image as necessary. In obese patients, where imaging may be more difficult, the far gain can be adjusted in order to compensate for signal attenuation as the ultrasound beam travels to deeper structures.

COLOR-FLOW DOPPLER

Color-flow Doppler can identify surrounding blood vessels. This may help to avoid inadvertent injury to vessels while performing the procedure.

STERILE PRECAUTIONS

Thoracentesis is an invasive procedure and should always be performed with sterile precautions. The sonographer should dress in sterile attire and use a sterile probe cover, gel, and kit.

PERFORMING ULTRASOUND-GUIDED THORACENTESIS

"BLIND" THORACENTESIS—PHYSICAL EXAMINATION ALONE

Performing thoracentesis without ultrasound guidance requires a very careful and thorough physical examination. When a large effusion is present, the trachea may be shifted to the contralateral side. Auscultation can reveal an area of decreased or absent breath sounds corresponding to an effusion. This finding can be confirmed with percussion in the area of decreased auscultation, which should reveal dullness. A decrease in tactile fremitus, however, is the key physical exam finding that distinguishes effusion from consolidation. Except in the case of a complicated and loculated effusion, the area of decreased breath sounds and dullness to percussion should lie in the inferior aspect of the chest and should be dependent on gravity. Pitfalls to performing thoracentesis guided by physical exam alone include the following:

1. Difficulty in accurately locating small effusions.
2. The diaphragm and lung are dynamic and can move into the plane of the effusion being evaluated.
3. Difficulty in distinguishing a pleural effusion from an elevated hemidiaphragm.
4. It cannot assess for loculations.
5. Physical exam is suboptimal in the obese patient, especially if the ribs cannot be palpated and used as landmarks.

DYNAMIC VERSUS STATIC ULTRASOUND GUIDANCE

Ultrasound-guided thoracentesis can be performed by either a static or dynamic technique. Static ultrasound guidance uses the probe to identify the ribs, the intercostal spaces, the pleura, and the effusion itself. It also helps to identify the depth of the effusion, the best angle of entry, and other surrounding structures to be avoided. The skin is marked (based on identifying the best place to drain the effusion), the probe is removed, and the procedure is then carried out in a fashion similar to landmark-based thoracentesis. The main advantage of this technique is that the clinician will have two free hands to perform the procedure. In large effusions, the static technique is usually sufficient as the amount of fluid is easily accessible.

Dynamic ultrasound guidance uses real-time imaging to perform the thoracentesis. The advantage of this technique is being able to visualize the needle entering the intercostal space toward the effusion and the ability to redirect the needle as needed. It is advantageous in smaller effusions that may be more difficult to reach using the static method.

SONOGRAPHIC ANATOMY AND LANDMARKS

The first step in performing an ultrasound-guided thoracentesis is recognizing the normal sonographic anatomy of the ribs, the pleura, and the lung parenchyma. The visceral and parietal pleura can be observed between two ribs and approximately 0.5 cm below the surface. The pleural line, which consists of both the parietal and visceral pleura, is 0.2–0.4 mm thick, and is not differentiated on ultrasound unless a pleural effusion is present separating the two. Therefore, these two structures are in close apposition and will appear as a single bright echogenic line. The normal pleura will exhibit lung sliding, which is viewed as the pleural line between the chest wall and the aerated lung moving up and down in time with respiration. The lung pulse may also be observed, which is described as a subtle shimmering movement of the pleural line in time with the cardiac cycle. The ribs will appear as hyperechoic structures just proximal to the pleural space and will exhibit posterior acoustic shadowing due to an attenuation of the ultrasound beam. The lung parenchyma is visualized as a series of repetitive horizontal lines beneath the pleural line. These are formed by air artifact, and are referred to as "A-lines," which are normal (see Chap. 7).

The boundaries of the thoracic cavity should be carefully determined by examining the diaphragm, the liver, and the spleen. The liver and spleen both appear as isoechoic structures just below the diaphragm and biliary ducts are often seen within the liver structure.

PATIENT POSITIONING

Ideally, the patient should be sitting facing away from the examiner on the side of the bed or examination table. The head and arms can rest on a small bedside table placed in front of the patient at a comfortable height. If a patient is noncompliant, critically ill, or mechanically ventilated, they can be placed in the semi-decubitus position where the patient's hemithorax of interest is rotated upright 30°–45° along the axis of the spine. The ipsilateral arm should be elevated over the patient's head or across the front of their torso and the head of the bed elevated 30°. This position allows for the pooling of pleural fluid at the base of the thorax and gives the sonographer access to the patient's midaxillary line where the fluid may be safely sampled. It is often useful to place a roll of towels below the patient's back to help maintain their position during the procedure.

ULTRASOUND GUIDANCE

Sonographic identification of the pleural effusion should be performed immediately prior to thoracentesis. The probe should be placed on the patient's back, directed cephalad, in a sagittal position (Fig. 18-1). The sonographer should then slide the probe systematically along the superior-inferior axis of the posterior chest surface. Scanning should start at the base of the hemithorax and continue in

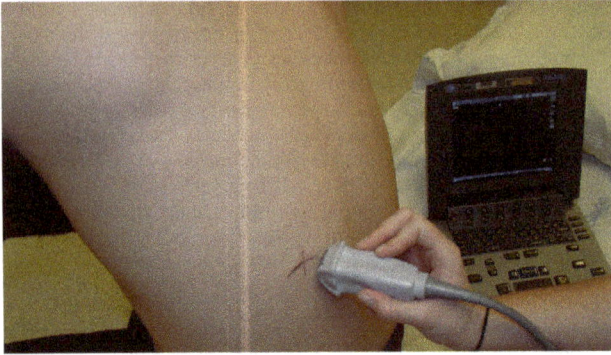

FIGURE 18-1 Correct probe placement for thoracentesis. Note the transducer is placed on the patient's back with the probe marker directed cephalad in a sagittal orientation. The entire pleural space can be examined by moving the probe in horizontal and vertical directions across the posterior and lateral surfaces of the thorax. In this image, the examiner has identified the pleural effusion and has marked a site for needle entry.

a transverse, and a superior-inferior direction across the chest in an effort to visualize the diaphragm, pleura, and surrounding structures.

Most sonographers do not use real-time ultrasound guidance, but instead examine the pleural effusion with bedside ultrasound and place a mark at the intercostal space corresponding to the largest and most inferior collection of fluid just above the inferior rib (see Fig. 18-1). Ultrasound imaging and marking is done prior to the sterile preparation for the procedure. The selected site should be located as dependent as possible while permitting a clear path from the skin surface to the pleural fluid throughout the respiratory cycle. Diaphragmatic excursion can be substantial even with quiet breathing and should be observed through several cycles to ensure the thoracentesis needle will not enter the thorax too close to the diaphragm, potentially resulting in laceration of the liver or spleen. The selected site should be marked using a marker or pen that will not wash off during the sterilization of the area. Alternatively, a blunt instrument may be used to make a "dent" in the skin at the intended entry site.

Once the skin is marked, the area is then prepped and draped as would be done for any sterile invasive procedure. The patient must maintain the same position after placement of the ultrasound-guided mark for thoracentesis or should be sonographically reexamined if a position shift or movement occurs.

SONOGRAPHIC CHARACTERISTICS OF A PLEURAL EFFUSION

In the upright position, pleural effusions will accumulate in the most dependent areas in the hemithorax: between the lower chest wall, the base of the lung, and the diaphragm. However, in the supine patient, the location of an effusion may vary considerably depending on the position of the patient and the degree of elevation of the head of the bed. A large effusion may be visualized laterally in the supine patient, but the patient may need to be rolled onto the contralateral side in order to visualize a smaller effusion adequately. In this position, the fluid will then concentrate in a dependent fashion between the chest wall and the lung. A loculated effusion will be visualized on ultrasound as pockets of fluid separated by various strands and septations (Fig. 18-2).

The first step in examining a pleural effusion is to identify its boundaries. This includes the diaphragm and sub-diaphragmatic organs, the adjacent lung, and the

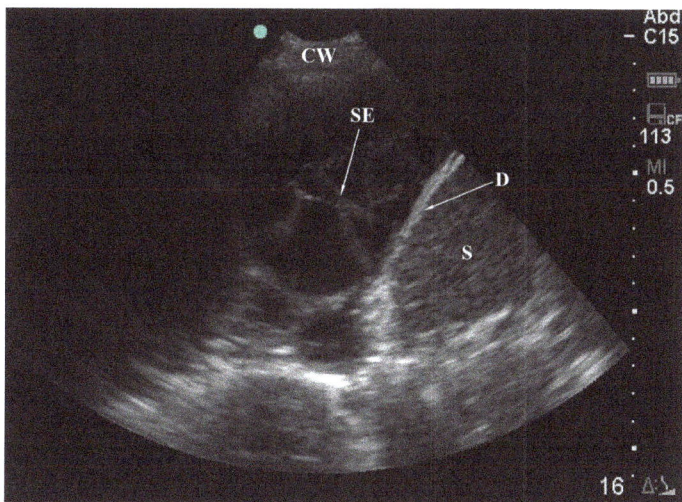

FIGURE 18-2 Loculated left-sided pleural effusion. The pleural effusion is seen as a hypoechoic loculated area with septations (SE) located superior to the hyperechoic diaphragm (D) and isoechoic spleen (S). CW: chest wall.

inner border of the chest wall. The effusion should be relatively echo-free and surrounded by the landmarks discussed earlier. The diaphragm should be a curvilinear structure that moves with respiration and sits atop the liver on the right and the spleen on the left. Rib shadows should be visible within the effusion. The inner aspect of the chest wall is located about 5 mm below the start of the rib shadows. The lung will typically appear as a homogeneous gray and white (hyperechoic) structure owing to aeration of the tissue, but may exhibit less aeration and appear denser if compressed by an adjacent effusion. The compressed lung is often observed undulating within the effusion, a pattern known as "lung flapping" (Fig. 18-3). In addition, debris or fibrous strands may be seen swirling within the effusion as a result of cardiac or respiratory movements.

The volume of the effusion should be qualitatively characterized as small, medium, or large. Some advocate measuring the thickness of the effusion, which has been shown to correlate with volume, but this measurement is dependent on the position of the probe and the dimensions of the thoracic cavity.

The echogenicity of the effusion should also be noted. For instance, the presence of swirling echoes, strands, or septations usually signifies an exudate and that the effusion is likely loculated. These findings are important because it indicates that the effusion may not be completely drainable, that entrapped lung may be present, and that additional procedures (ie, chest tube, thoracoscopy, or thoracotomy) may be necessary to adequately manage the condition.

The depth from the skin to the visceral pleura and the pleural effusion should be measured and noted. A measurement should also be performed from the skin to the center of the effusion and to the lung parenchyma. If these measurements reveal less than 1 cm of pleural fluid between the parietal pleura and diaphragm or lung parenchyma, the thoracentesis should be deferred or performed by an experienced operator, as sampling these small effusions may result in increased risk for procedural complication (Fig. 18-4).

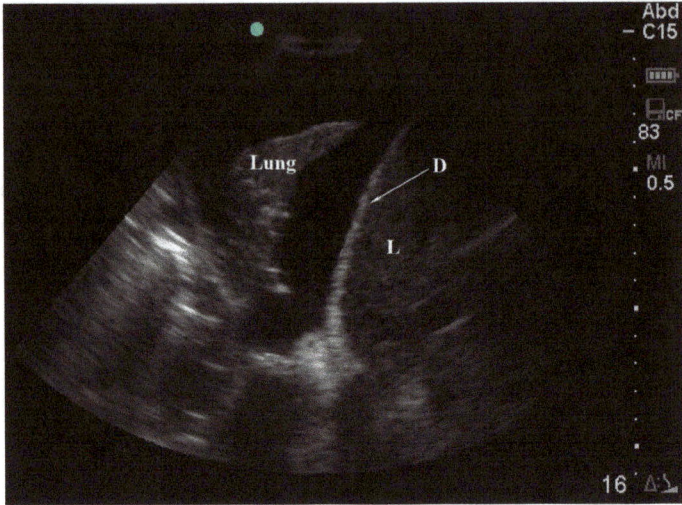

FIGURE 18-3 Moderate-sized right-sided pleural effusion. The pleural effusion is seen as an anechoic area superior to the hyperechoic diaphragm (D). The liver is seen inferior to the diaphragm (L). The "lung flapping" sign is demonstrated within the pleural effusion.

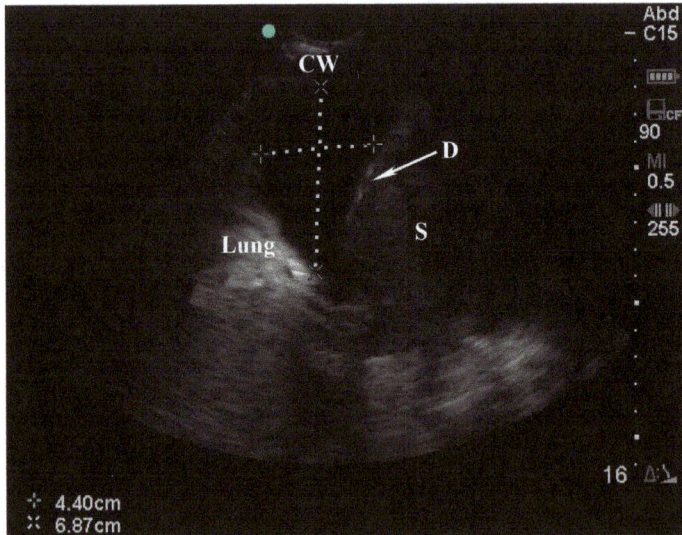

FIGURE 18-4 Moderate-sized left-sided pleural effusion. The pleural effusion is seen as an anechoic area superior to the hyperechoic diaphragm (D) and isoechoic spleen (S). The dotted lines represent the height and depth measurements of the effusion. CW: chest wall.

EQUIPMENT FOR THORACENTESIS

Standard thoracentesis kits are usually available in most acute care settings. The required supplies include the following:

- 1%–2% lidocaine
- A 10-cc syringe and a 25-gauge needle for administering anesthetic
- A slightly longer (ie, 1.5 in) 22-gauge diagnostic needle
- A 6 in, 20-gauge spinal needle for obese patients if needed
- Thoracentesis catheter over an 18-gauge, 7.5 in needle
- A 60-cc syringe
- Tubing
- Sterile collection tubes and a large collection bag or bottle

ANESTHESIA

Local anesthesia should be accomplished with 1%–2% lidocaine at the desired site of entry. The site should be in the intercostal space just superior to a rib in order to avoid hitting the intercostal vessels and nerve. A wheal should be made in the skin with a 25-gauge needle in order to provide superficial anesthesia. A larger-gauge needle can then be advanced through the skin wheal into the subcutaneous tissue to provide deeper anesthesia. The syringe should be aspirated back while advancing the needle to avoid hitting a blood vessel, and then lidocaine can be injected into the pleural space. It is important to note that the parietal pleura is quite sensitive, whereas the visceral pleura lacks sensory fibers.

INSERTING THE CATHETER AND DRAINING THE PLEURAL SPACE

Once appropriate anesthesia is achieved, a small incision should be made in the skin just above and parallel to the inferior rib. The thoracentesis needle and catheter combination should be attached to a small syringe and then advanced through the incision. Gentle aspiration is applied to the syringe until pleural fluid is noted to flow freely into the syringe. The thoracentesis catheter is then completely advanced over the needle into the pleural space. The needle can then be removed, and tubing attached to the thoracentesis catheter for sample collection and drainage. Fluid samples should be collected for cell count and differential, pH, LDH, protein content, Gram stain, cultures, and cytology, if malignancy is suspected. In addition, albumin, amylase, or other studies may be indicated depending on the clinical scenario.

The amount of fluid that should be removed in a therapeutic thoracentesis of a large pleural effusion is a matter of some debate. In general, you would like to drain as much fluid as possible without causing side effects. Manometry can be helpful as a guide to the amount of drainage and can be simply performed by draining fluid until the pleural pressure reaches approximately −20 cm H_2O (see web reference in further reading #2). Reexpansion pulmonary edema is a reported side effect of large-volume thoracentesis, but has been shown to be quite rare (<1% of large-volume thoracenteses). Once the desired amount of fluid is drained, the catheter can be removed, pressure applied, and a dressing placed over the incision site.

Ultrasound-guided thoracentesis has also been shown to be safe and effective for the sampling and drainage of pleural effusion in the mechanically ventilated patient. The procedure must be performed in the supine or semi-decubitus position. The ultrasound can be applied to the midaxillary line or the patient can be rolled onto the contralateral side to facilitate access to a smaller or loculated effusion. The same technique of examining the pleura sonographically, placing a mark, prepping and draping the patient around the entry site, catheter advancement and drainage of fluid, is followed as in the non-intubated patient discussed earlier.

COMMON PITFALLS AND TIPS

THE DIFFICULT PATIENT

As with any procedure, thoracic ultrasound and ultrasound-guided pleural procedures can be made more difficult under certain conditions. It can be difficult to visualize deeper structures in the morbidly obese patient. Using the lowest frequency probe available can help to eliminate this problem. When attempting thoracentesis in this patient population, the effusion may not be accessible with the commonly used short finder needle. A 21-gauge long needle (typically a spinal needle) may be used to reach the deeper location of the pleural fluid. This should only be done after the distance from the skin surface to the effusion and adjacent structures are measured and marked on the needle shaft to avoid inserting the longer needle too deep and injuring lung or other surrounding structures.

MISIDENTIFYING FREE FLUID

When ascites and a pleural effusion coexist, the identification of boundaries is extremely important. Ascites can track above the liver or spleen and can be confused as pleural fluid. Therefore, it is important to identify the liver, spleen, and diaphragm in order to avoid sampling peritoneal fluid or injuring abdominal organs when one is attempting to sample a pleural effusion. In these situations, the diaphragm is visualized as a thin strip of hyperechoic tissue positioned just superior to the liver or spleen between two fluid collections (see Figs. 18-2 and 18-3). In addition, the diaphragm will often be seen to move caudad with inspiration, often forcing the underlying ascitic fluid away from the underlying liver or spleen, aiding in its identification.

ELEVATED HEMIDIAPHRAGM

The presence of an elevated hemidiaphragm can make the identification of a pleural effusion difficult. The sonographer should begin the examination at the apex of the hemithorax and scan down until the liver or spleen is visualized (both are isoechoic and the liver is further characterized by biliary ducts). Moving the probe medially and laterally and repeating the scan from apex to base will help the sonographer to locate or rule out a pleural effusion.

PNEUMOTHORAX

A thoracentesis is an invasive procedure that can inadvertently cause lung damage and pneumothorax. The sonographer can decrease this risk by making sure the needle is not inserted too deeply into the pleural space puncturing the lung. The use of real-time ultrasound guidance is advantageous as the physician can observe the needle enter the pleural space and can stop advancing it once inside the effusion. The use of the static technique helps to avoid a pneumothorax by carefully taking note of appropriate depth measurements and being careful to not insert the needle and catheter beyond this point.

INJURING NEARBY STRUCTURES

There is a risk of injuring surrounding structures while performing a thoracentesis, such as blood vessels, nerves, or other organs. It is important that the sonographer inserts the needle superior to the rib into the space in order to avoid hitting the intercostal nerves and vessels. In addition, color-flow Doppler can be used to highlight blood vessels and help the sonographer in avoiding them when inserting the needle. The course of intercostal arteries is often more tortuous within

4–6 cm of the spine. As such, the optimal entry site will be more lateral along the chest wall. Real-time ultrasound guidance helps to guide the needle in the correct direction preventing the injury to nearby organs, such as the liver, spleen, and diaphragm.

DRY TAP

If the needle is not inserted into the correct place, a dry tap may result. If the static technique is being used, the needle should be removed and a sterile ultrasound probe placed back onto the skin surface to ensure the entry site marked is appropriate. If the real-time technique is being used, the needle can be pulled back and advanced once again while watching it on the monitor until it reaches the correct location and pleural fluid is aspirated.

INFECTION

Although the risk is low, there is always a chance of infection resulting from an invasive procedure. In order to avoid this complication, full sterile precautions need to be observed. In addition, the physician should examine the patient's skin before performing the procedure to make sure there is no overlying infection present.

CONCLUSION

Thoracentesis is an important procedure in the evaluation of pleural effusion. Thoracic ultrasound is a useful tool for quickly and accurately examining the pleural space to diagnose pleural effusions, rule out pneumothorax, and provide guidance when performing pleural-based procedures. Portable sonographic technology is readily available and usable by properly trained physicians at the bedside. Competent use of thoracic ultrasound for pleural-based procedures has been shown to decrease complications and improve diagnostic yield.

Additional Reading

Barnes TW, Morgenthaler TI, Olson EJ, et al. Sonographically guided thoracentesis and rate of pneumothorax. *J Clin Ultrasound*. 2005;33:442-446.

Feller-Kopman D. Ultrasound-guided thoracentesis. *Chest*. 2006;129:1709-1714. http://chestjournal.chestpubs.org/site/misc/videos/diagrams1/index.html

Lichtenstein DA. Ultrasound in the management of thoracic disease. *Crit Care Med*. 2007;35:S250-S261.

Mayo PH, Doelken P. Pleural ultrasonography. *Clin Chest Med*. 2006;27:215-227.

Mayo PH, Goltz HR, Tafreshi M, Doelken P. Safety of ultrasound-guided thoracentesis in patients receiving mechanical ventilation. *Chest*. 2004;125: 1059-1062.

19 Ultrasound for Paracentesis

James Q. Hwang and Calvin Huang

BACKGROUND AND INDICATIONS FOR EXAMINATION

Ascites is the accumulation of free fluid in the peritoneal cavity and is typically caused by portal hypertension due to hepatic failure. Other common causes of ascites include renal failure, congestive heart failure, infection, or malignancy. Ascites may be extremely uncomfortable when large amounts of fluid are present, and may be life threatening if it becomes infected or compromises respiratory efforts or venous return. Physical examination is not sensitive for ascites and cannot reliably determine the optimal location for drainage. Bedside ultrasound can reliably detect ascites and aid in the removal of fluid.

Both critical care and emergency medicine physicians have long performed bedside paracentesis. The traditional blind approach to remove intraperitoneal fluid has been employed until the recent introduction of ultrasound-guided techniques. Ultrasound-guided paracentesis is now the standard of care amongst both critical care and emergency medicine physicians. When compared to the older blind approach, ultrasound-guided paracentesis may increase the success of the procedure and decrease the risk of vascular injury or bowel perforation.

Paracentesis can be diagnostic or therapeutic and sometimes both, depending on the patient's presentation. Diagnostic paracentesis may be required to rule out an infection or malignancy. Ascitic fluid is always at risk for bacterial translocation which can lead to peritonitis. Therapeutic paracentesis can also be performed to relieve abdominal pain or shortness of breath. When massive, ascitic fluid can inhibit excursion of the diaphragm and cause respiratory distress, or compress the inferior vena cava (IVC) impairing right heart filling which lead to hemodynamic instability. In these patients, removal of fluid can relieve cardiopulmonary distress and provide significant symptomatic relief.

DIAGNOSTIC

- Assessment of new onset ascites and/or ascites of unclear etiology
- Concern for spontaneous bacterial peritonitis in a patient with known ascites (may present with abdominal pain, fever, or altered mental status)

THERAPEUTIC

- Relief of symptomatic ascites, particularly if cardiovascular or respiratory compromise is present

PROBE SELECTION AND TECHNICAL CONSIDERATIONS FOR PARACENTESIS

CURVILINEAR PROBE WITH A FREQUENCY OF 3.5–5.0 MHz

The initial probe for detection of fluid should be a large footprint curvilinear probe in the 3.5–5.0 MHz range. This probe is best for identifying large pockets of fluid in the upper and lower quadrants, explained fully in Chap. 9.

LINEAR-ARRAY PROBE WITH A FREQUENCY OF 8–12 MHz

Following the identification of the optimal fluid pocket for aspiration, a higher-frequency linear probe, in the 8–12 MHz range, should be used for actual procedural guidance. This will provide better resolution, improving identification of the inferior epigastric vessels and visualization of the needle entering the fluid pocket.

OTHER EQUIPMENT

The standard equipment required for a sterile procedure, including appropriate local anesthesia (1%–2% lidocaine with or without epinephrine), is needed for a paracentesis. In addition, if available, a packaged "paracentesis kit" or similar supplies are required which include:

- 18–20 gauge needle for fluid withdrawal
- For a diagnostic paracentesis only, a 60-cc syringe can be used to withdraw fluid directly
- For a large-volume paracentesis done for therapeutic purposes:
  - Vacutainer bottles
  - Tubing connected to a luer lock to drain fluid into vacutainer bottles
  - A luer lock to connect tubing to the paracentesis needle
  - An 18-gauge needle to insert into vacutainer bottles

BLIND VERSUS ULTRASOUND-GUIDED PARACENTESIS

The traditional approach to paracentesis relies on the physical examination alone. Ascites accumulates in a gravity-dependent manner within the peritoneum. The classic findings suggestive of ascites include a distended abdomen, presence of a fluid wave, and shifting dullness. Limitations of blind paracentesis are as follows:

- It cannot assess for the adherence of bowel or omentum to the peritoneal lining.
- It cannot determine the distance from the skin surface to the peritoneum or from the peritoneum to underlying bowel or omentum.
- It cannot determine the optimal location for drainage.
- It may not identify the inferior epigastric vessels.

Ultrasound-guided paracentesis helps to eliminate the limitations associated with the blind technique. This method reliably detects fluid and determines the optimal site for needle access and drainage. The focused abdominal ultrasound should include views of both the upper and lower abdominal quadrants, including the pelvis. The inclusion of multiple sites helps to identify the location with the largest pocket of fluid. Ultrasound is very sensitive for fluid when the volume exceeds 500 cc. Bedside ultrasound allows the clinician to directly visualize ascitic fluid deep to the intended insertion site. In addition, it helps to locate adjacent bowel, omentum, and blood vessels that must be avoided by the sonographer in order to prevent perforation, infection, or bleeding. Direct ultrasound visualization is ideal in patients with small pockets of ascitic fluid or when vulnerable structures are near the intended insertion site.

In situations where a patient presents with a large amount of fluid and resultant tense ascites, ultrasound can help to evaluate compartment syndrome by imaging the IVC. These patients will have a baseline compression and pronounced respiratory collapse of their IVC, which indicates the need for more rapid intervention and fluid drainage. In patients with significant cardiorespiratory distress, a bedside echo may also detect impaired right-sided heart filling.

DYNAMIC VERSUS STATIC ULTRASOUND GUIDANCE

Ultrasound-guided paracentesis can be performed as either a static or dynamic procedure. Static guidance uses ultrasound to identify the largest fluid pocket and the optimal site of needle entry by marking the spot on the patient's skin, and noting the angle of approach needed prior to doing the procedure. Dynamic guidance allows the clinician to anesthetize accurately down to the peritoneum, ensures adequate needle entry, and avoids vascular or bowel injury in real time. It may also be used to evaluate why the catheter may have stopped draining during the procedure, and to assess the adequacy of drainage. The single-user approach where the clinician holds the probe in one hand and the needle in the other provides optimal procedural guidance. A two-person approach can also be utilized where an assistant may hold the probe or can help in visualizing the needle entry into the peritoneum on the ultrasound monitor.

PERFORMING ULTRASOUND-GUIDED PARACENTESIS

PATIENT POSITIONING

The most commonly chosen position for paracentesis is a lateral decubitus position. This position shifts peritoneal fluid to the dependent side and increases the distance between the peritoneum and underlying bowel or omentum. If the patient cannot tolerate the decubitus position, the procedure can also be performed with the patient supine and their head slightly elevated in order to drain fluid into the dependent lower quadrants.

EVALUATE FOR THE PRESENCE OF FLUID

A curvilinear probe with a frequency between 3.5 and 5.0 MHz should be used to evaluate for free fluid. The ultrasound examination should include bilateral upper quadrants, bilateral lower quadrants, and the pelvis. The largest pockets of ascitic fluid tend to be found in the lower quadrants or pelvis. The peritoneum lies deep to the abdominal wall musculature and has a characteristic hyperechoic appearance. Ascitic fluid is typically seen as pockets of hypoechoic fluid deep to the peritoneum. It is usually free flowing within the intraperitoneal space and classically takes the shape of its container. As such, ascitic fluid is often seen collecting in gravity-dependent areas, surrounding loops of bowel, and outlining abdominal organs (Fig. 19-1). Once the peritoneum is identified, its distance from the skin surface should be noted by referring to the centimeter depth markers on the side of the screen or by direct measurement using the caliper feature. The sonographer should scan several centimeters in both the cephalad and caudad directions, as well as medially and laterally, looking for peritoneal adhesions. If a midline infraumbilical approach is considered, use bedside ultrasound to identify the bladder and rescan this area post-voiding to ensure adequate decompression.

IDENTIFY THE INFERIOR EPIGASTRIC VESSELS

The inferior epigastric vessels arise from the external iliacs just before they cross the inguinal ligament and course superiorly and medially toward the rectus muscle. Inadvertent injury to the epigastric vessels in a coagulopathic patient can result in significant bleeding. The inferior epigastric vessels can be located by switching to a linear, high-frequency probe (8–12 MHz) and by examining the lower, medial abdominal wall. Their path courses from the external iliac vessels, just above the inguinal ligament, to the lateral border of the rectus muscle. The vessels run along the peritoneum of the anterior abdominal wall and blood flow

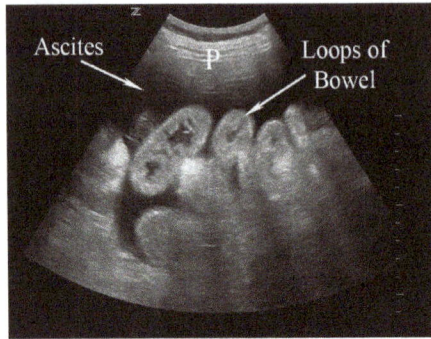

FIGURE 19-1 Lower quadrant view demonstrating ascites and loops of bowel using a curvilinear probe. This is an ideal needle insertion site as the loops of bowel are not located in the near field and not in the projected path of the catheter. P: peritoneum

can be confirmed using color-flow Doppler or pulsed-wave spectral Doppler. They are better visualized in the transverse plane, with the probe pointing toward the patient's right side. They are more difficult to locate when the probe is parallel to the vessels (ie, in a longitudinal or sagittal plane) (Fig. 19-2). Once identified, the location of the vessels can be recorded on the skin with a marking pen.

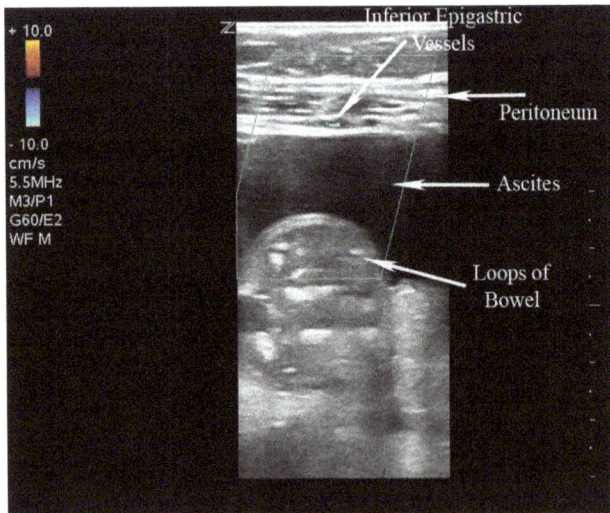

FIGURE 19-2 Transverse view of the inferior epigastric vessels with color-flow Doppler in a patient with ascites using a high-frequency linear probe. These vessels run along the peritoneum of the anterior abdominal wall and should be identified and marked to avoid injury.

CHOOSE THE INSERTION SITE

The abdomen should be scanned for the largest pocket of ascitic fluid. The entry site that is chosen should be lateral to the marked location of the inferior epigastric vessels, unless a midline, infraumbilical approach through the linea alba is chosen. In this case, be sure to identify the bladder and to make certain that it is appropriately decompressed. Patients with ascites can also have hepatomegaly or splenomegaly and care should be taken to scan for the inferior tips of these organs when determining the ideal insertion site. Once the largest pocket of fluid is located, look for any underlying intraperitoneal structures. The presence of abdominal surgical scars should prompt thorough ultrasound interrogation in order to avoid choosing a puncture site with adherent bowel or mesentery.

STANDARD STERILE PROCEDURE PROTOCOL

The ultrasound probe and cord should both be placed in a sterile sheath in order to use the machine for both anesthetizing the peritoneum and in performing real-time guidance. Direct ultrasound visualization can assist with both the delivery of local anesthesia and in guiding the puncture of the needle through the peritoneum.

ANESTHESIA

Local anesthesia may be performed with 1%–2% lidocaine with or without epinephrine. Initially, a small-gauge needle (30–25 G) should be used and the site chosen should be several millimeters distal to the intended puncture site. At this site, approximately 0.5–1 cc of lidocaine should be injected to create a raised wheal on the patient's skin. Next, a medium-gauge needle on a luer lock syringe (22–20 G) should be filled with approximately 5 cc of lidocaine, and inserted through the subcutaneous wheal. The syringe should be aspirated back with negative pressure in order to ensure it is not inside a blood vessel and then the lidocaine should be injected into the abdominal wall soft tissue. Under direct ultrasound visualization, the needle should be advanced to the peritoneum and again, after aspirating back with negative pressure, lidocaine should be injected in order to anesthetize the peritoneal lining. With real-time ultrasound guidance, the lidocaine can be seen leaving the needle tip and collecting in the soft tissue along the peritoneum.

CATHETER INSERTION

A small incision in the skin, at the anesthetized puncture site, should be made with a blade in order to ease advancement of the catheter through the skin and soft tissue. Mild oblique tension should be placed on the skin surface, displacing it laterally by approximately 0.5–1 cm. This tension should be relieved once the needle penetrates the dermis, and will create the so-called "Z-track" upon withdrawal of the catheter, decreasing the likelihood of peritoneal leak. The catheter-loaded needle should then be inserted through the anesthetized soft tissue while maintaining suction and negative pressure on the syringe. Under direct ultrasound visualization, the needle should be seen tenting the skin, penetrating the abdominal wall tissue, and approaching the peritoneum. The sonographer should continue to watch the screen to monitor for any underlying bowel, mesentery, or other intraabdominal structures. Finally, the needle should puncture through the peritoneum. On ultrasound, the ascitic pocket will appear hypoechoic and once the needle enters the fluid, it will appear hyperechoic and produce a characteristic ring-down artifact (Fig. 19-3).

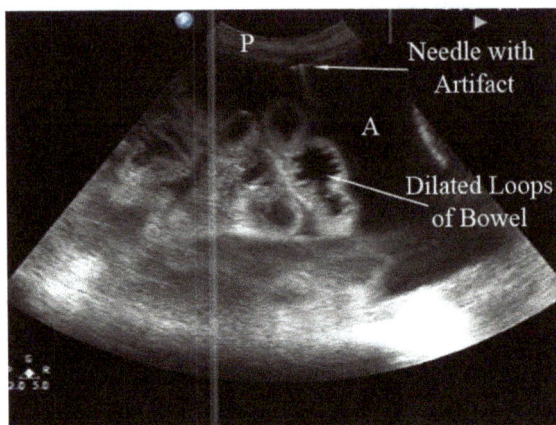

FIGURE 19-3 Lower quadrant view illustrating the paracentesis needle entering the peritoneum into a fluid pocket using a curvilinear probe. Note the hyperechoic appearance of the needle and the ring-down artifact created posteriorly. P: peritoneum, A: ascites.

REMOVING ASCITIC FLUID

Once the needle is visualized within the intraabdominal cavity and peritoneal fluid is aspirated, the ultrasound transducer should be set aside on the field and kept sterile. The needle and syringe should be held steadily at a constant distance from the skin surface and the peritoneal catheter should then be slowly advanced off the needle. The catheter does not need to be advanced all the way to the hub, but enough so that all side-ports are located below the skin surface. This will prevent the creation of a vacuum when aspirating through the catheter. Finally, the needle can be completely withdrawn from the catheter. Ascitic fluid can be withdrawn in the following ways:

- 60-cc luer lock syringe attached to a three-way stopcock
- A one-way valve with syringe and bag
- Directly into a vacutainer bottle

Caution should be used when removing large volumes (>1.5 L) at once, as subsequent fluid shifts may occur. Over the next few hours, equilibration of the patient's fluid spaces will occur with volume from both the intracellular and intravascular spaces moving back into the peritoneum. Patients should be monitored appropriately over this time period. Administration of intravenous albumin (25%, 8 g/L) can be considered when removing volumes of 5 L or greater.

Common laboratory tests to be sent on the ascitic fluid may include cell count with differential, albumin, total protein, Gram stain and culture, and cytology. A neutrophil count of greater than 250 cells/μL may indicate bacterial peritonitis. An elevated serum to ascites albumin gradient (SAAG) (> 1.1 g/dL) suggests that the fluid is transudative in nature due to portal hypertension. A low SAAG (< 1.1 g/dL) is consistent with exudative fluid, most commonly caused by cancer.

ASSESS THE VOLUME REMOVED

Ultrasound can also be used to determine if an adequate amount of fluid has been removed. The upper and lower quadrants, as well as the pelvis, should be rescanned to assess for sufficient drainage. Once the desired volume has been withdrawn, the catheter can be removed. Pressure should be applied over the puncture site to stop any subsequent bleeding that may occur. Finally, there should be an assessment for ascitic fluid leakage, and if none is noted, then the wound can be cleaned and dressed.

COMMON PITFALLS AND TIPS

CHECK LAB VALUES

Many patients with ascites have liver failure and are often coagulopathic or thrombocytopenic. If a patient has an elevated international normalized ratio (>2) or low platelets (<50,000), they may need transfusion of fresh frozen plasma or platelets prior to paracentesis. Ultrasound guidance may be particularly helpful in these patients as it minimizes the risk of vascular injury.

VERIFY FLUID VOLUME

Ultrasound should be used to confirm that there is enough ascitic fluid present before attempting paracentesis. In some instances, repositioning the patient in Trendelenburg, reverse Trendelenburg, or in the lateral decubitus positions may increase a focal collection of fluid, making it more amenable to aspiration. Ultrasound is most helpful when fluid collections are small or when vital structures are nearby.

DRY TAP

The sonographer may not get any fluid back with aspiration after the needle has been placed into the peritoneum. This dry tap usually results from incorrect placement of the needle, the need to further advance the needle, or due to there being only small amounts of ascitic fluid present. The risk of a dry tap is significantly higher with the blind approach or the static (skin marking only) ultrasound technique. If no fluid is aspirated, the sonographer should use ultrasound to verify the correct skin marking or to redirect the needle into a fluid pocket.

TRANSUDATES VERSUS EXUDATES

Depending on its etiology, ascitic fluid can be transudative or exudative. As such, it may not always appear perfectly hypoechoic or free flowing, especially if the patient has had prior surgery, scarring, or infections. This may cause the sonographer to miss intraperitoneal fluid on ultrasound. It is important to know the patient's entire history which may help give clues as to the etiology of the peritoneal fluid and what its likely appearance may be.

MISTAKING OTHER FLUID-FILLED STRUCTURES FOR ASCITES

Occasionally, bowel obstruction can be confused with ascites. It is important not to confuse dilated, fluid-filled loops of bowel with free-flowing ascitic fluid surrounding these loops. Fluid within dilated loops of bowel will clearly be contained inside the walls of the intestine as opposed to free-flowing extraluminal ascitic fluid. In some cases, a distended bladder may be mistaken for free fluid. The sonographer should be careful to identify the bladder prior to performing the procedure. Other fluid-filled structures in the abdomen include pancreatic, renal, or liver cysts, which can be mistaken for ascitic fluid. The sonographer should completely scan all quadrants of the abdomen in order to ensure that the fluid in question is tracking freely and not contained within discrete walls.

FAILURE TO PERFORM PARACENTESIS WITH REAL-TIME ULTRASOUND GUIDANCE

If paracentesis is performed with the static method and not under real-time ultrasound guidance, inadvertent patient repositioning between site marking and puncture can occur. If the static, skin marking-only approach is chosen, the patient should be instructed not to move after the puncture site is marked, prepped, and draped. If the patient does move between ultrasound visualization and skin puncture, the sonographer must keep in mind that intraabdominal structures are mobile and can easily shift to overlie the selected needle track. This can be avoided by ensuring that the patient is initially positioned and supported in the most comfortable manner possible. If the patient does shift positions, the marked puncture site should be reassessed with ultrasound to avoid iatrogenic injury.

DAMAGE TO BLOOD VESSELS

Failure to identify and mark the location of the inferior epigastric vessels can result in puncture and possible hemoperitoneum. This can be dramatic and life threatening in coagulopathic patients with end-stage liver disease. These vessels are usually medial, but anatomy does vary from individual to individual; therefore, it is important to mark their location before starting the procedure.

INFRAUMBILICAL APPROACH

If a midline infraumbilical approach is used, failure to identify and to assess the bladder for decompression can result in injury. The bladder should be identified in a midline position while full, and then visualized by ultrasound after voiding to ensure complete decompression and to decrease the risks of iatrogenic perforation.

INFECTION

As with any invasive procedure, there is always a risk of introducing infection. The physician can limit this risk by making sure the complete procedure is performed using sterile precautions.

CONCLUSION

Paracentesis is commonly performed in the critical care setting for both diagnostic and therapeutic purposes. Ultrasound has a high sensitivity for detecting intraperitoneal free fluid, estimating the total volume present and accurately locating the best point of entry for aspiration. The use of ultrasound-guided paracentesis has been shown to improve success rates while decreasing complications that can result from the procedure. It helps the clinician to better define abdominal and pelvic anatomy, as well as to avoid bowel, vessels, and other intraperitoneal structures. Both the static technique, which simply maps out the site of entry with a skin marker, and the dynamic technique, which observes the needle tip entering the peritoneal cavity, may help improve safety and success of the procedure. As with any other invasive procedure performed in the acute care setting, ultrasound-guided paracentesis has quickly become the preferred method over the more traditional blind approaches.

Additional Reading

Bard C, Lafortune M, Breton G. Ascites: ultrasound guidance or blind paracentesis? *CMAJ.* 1986;135(3):209-210.

Nazeer SR, Dewbre H, Miller AH. Ultrasound assisted paracentesis performed by emergency physicians vs the traditional technique: a prospective, randomized study. *Am J Emerg Med.* 2005;23(3):363-367.

Runyon BA. Paracentesis of ascitic fluid: a safe procedure. *Arch Intern Med.* 1986;146 (11):2259-2261.

20 Ultrasound for Pericardiocentesis and Cardiac Pacing

Michael Osborne

BACKGROUND AND INDICATIONS FOR ULTRASOUND-GUIDED PERICARDIOCENTESIS

Cardiac procedures are typically performed by cardiology or cardiothoracic surgery physicians and though are less common in the emergency or critical care setting, may be life-saving when a patient is in extremis. Two situations where ultrasound guidance may be invaluable for cardiac procedures is in performing pericardiocentesis in a patient with tamponade and in guiding cardiac pacing in a patient with complete heart block or unstable bradycardia unresponsive to medications.

Pericardial effusion can present in very nonspecific ways, with isolated dyspnea, tachycardia, or hypotension. Patients with significant pericardial effusion and signs or symptoms of tamponade may require urgent pericardiocentesis. Ultrasound guidance is used to increase success and decrease complications of pericardiocentesis, and should be considered standard of care when feasible.

Pericardiocentesis is indicated for cardiac tamponade. It is usually performed prior to a pericardial window procedure, as it is quicker and less invasive. Most patients with tamponade can safely go to the cardiac catheterization lab for their procedure. However, there are times when the patient is too unstable and an emergency pericardiocentesis must be performed in the critical care setting. If there is no cardiologist available at the treating facility, then the emergency or critical care physician may need to perform the procedure in an unstable patient.

Tamponade occurs when cardiac filling is compromised due to extrinsic compression of the heart. Cardiac tamponade can occur with either small or large volumes of pericardial fluid. The quicker the fluid accumulates, the faster the rise in pericardial pressure compressing the heart. While true tamponade is a clinical diagnosis (hemodynamic compromise in the setting of pericardial effusion), signs of impending tamponade may be seen on a bedside echocardiography. The left side of the heart is used to higher pressures and has proportionally a larger and thicker muscular structure. Therefore, the thinner-walled right heart, with its lower pressures, will collapse first. Late diastolic collapse of the right atrium is seen first, followed by early diastolic collapse of the right ventricular free wall. A dilated inferior vena cava is typically present, indicating restricted filling. The physical findings of Beck's triad (hypotension, muffled heart sounds, and jugular venous distension) may be present with tamponade, however, they are not sensitive and do not provide much additional information when bedside ultrasound is available.

The first-line treatment of tamponade is to increase preload, typically with intravenous crystalloid. This effectively increases central venous pressure and right-sided heart pressures to compensate for the extrinsic pressure on the heart.

Pericardiocentesis removes extrinsic fluid volume from the pericardial sac, allowing the heart to fill. For example, if you withdraw 50 mL of fluid from the pericardial sac of a patient with tamponade, you have effectively allowed 50 mL more fluid into the heart for each beat. This will increase cardiac output by 3 L/min (50 cc × 100 × 0.6), assuming a heart rate of 100 beats per minute and an ejection fraction of 60%). Normal cardiac output is approximately 3–6 L/min in an adult. Therefore, by removing a relatively small amount of fluid, a normal cardiac output may be restored.

PROBE SELECTION AND TECHNICAL CONSIDERATIONS FOR PERICARDIOCENTESIS

PHASED-ARRAY CARDIAC PROBE WITH A FREQUENCY OF 3.0–5.0 MHz

A phased-array cardiac probe in the cardiac machine setting should be used. A curvilinear abdominal probe with 3.0–5.0 MHz frequency can also be used, particularly if the heart is imaged from the subxiphoid approach.

TISSUE HARMONIC IMAGING

Tissue harmonic imaging (THI) should be used for all cardiac imaging if available. THI helps to brighten the signal returning from the pericardium and to improve the contrast between the anechoic blood-filled chambers and surrounding effusion. This will improve the image and make the procedure easier to perform.

STERILE PRECAUTIONS

Unless it is a code situation, sterile precautions and a sterile probe cover should be used.

EQUIPMENT

Ideally, a pericardiocentesis kit or tray is used that includes proper equipment to introduce a catheter or pigtail using the Seldinger approach. This will allow a drainage catheter to be left in the pericardial sac in case there is reaccumulation of fluid and is also useful in patients transferring facilities. A stopcock with a sterile syringe and a drainage bag attached and taped in place is usually used in these patients. The syringe can be used to pull fluid off which can then be transferred to the bag by changing the position of the stopcock.

If these kits are not available, a spinal needle may be used to remove fluid acutely. It is important to keep in mind that the standard spinal needle is 3.5 in long or 8.9 cm in length (Fig. 20-1). While the pericardium may be as close as 2–3 cm when approached through a parasternal window, the distance may exceed

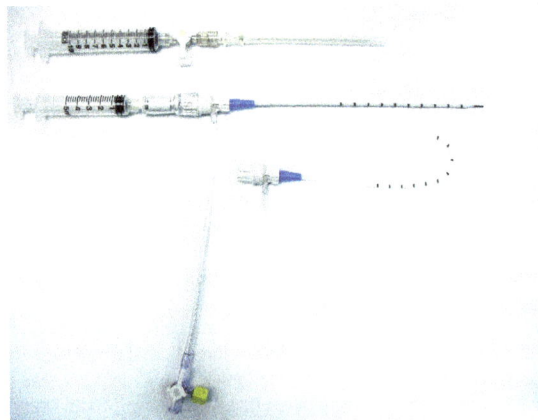

FIGURE 20-1 Top: standard 3.5-in spinal needle with stopcock and syringe. Middle: pigtail catheter attached to a blunt needle with a drainage system. Bottom: pigtail catheter without needle.

the length of the needle from a subxiphoid approach (8–15 cm deep). Therefore, many of the "dry taps" resulting from this approach may be due to the needle being too short. Also, some of the "bloody taps" may be a result of hitting the liver as opposed to aspirating the right ventricle.

PERFORMING ULTRASOUND-GUIDED PERICARDIOCENTESIS

The two main approaches to the pericardium are subxiphoid and transthoracic. The traditional blind method uses a spinal needle attached to a large syringe inserted to the left of the xiphoid process, aiming toward the inferior tip of the left scapula. The success of this method is improved by elevating the head of the bed and dropping the heart down closer to the tip of the needle. This risks a decrease in the hydrostatic blood pressure supplied to the brain, and can be detrimental if performed on an already hypotensive patient.

More recently, the recommended approach used in the catheterization lab is a transthoracic one. This technique allows the pericardial space to be accessed by going through the least amount of tissue and obviates the need to elevate the head of the bed. The pericardium is usually 2–3 cm from the skin surface. The ultrasound transducer is placed on the chest wall and a safe place to insert the needle under direct observation is found. Usually, the needle insertion site will be located somewhere between the parasternal long-axis area and the apex. A spinal needle that is attached to a stopcock is then inserted into the pericardium. The stopcock is attached to a small syringe at a 90° angle to the needle (or tubing attached to a drainage bag), and also a 50-mL syringe that is in-line with the spinal needle. Back pressure is then applied to the larger syringe and the needle is advanced until fluid enters the syringe. In order to confirm that the needle is in the pericardial space, agitated saline can be placed in the smaller syringe and injected under ultrasound guidance. If the needle is in the correct place, the injected saline will appear as a "snowstorm," such as seen in a child's globe toy. Once confirmation is made, the saline can then be aspirated back out.

Ultrasound-guided pericardiocentesis can be either static or dynamic. In the static technique, the spot and the angle where the largest fluid collection may be accessed are noted and marked. The probe is then removed and the procedure performed. In dynamic guidance, the needle can be seen entering the pericardial space in real time. This has the advantage of ensuring the needle tip is in the pericardial space, but it may be technically difficult to place the probe and needle in the same spot. Therefore, this may require that the probe be placed in a different place than the needle (ie, subxiphoid view of a transthoracic pericardiocentesis), which can make visualization and orientation difficult.

In one of the largest series of ultrasound-guided pericardiocentesis, the Mayo Clinic recommends determining the largest collection of fluid accessible in a static technique and then performing the procedure. Using this technique, 85% of procedures were transthoracic. Other groups (particularly in Europe) have found good success with the subcostal approach. In either case, serial ultrasounds can confirm needle or catheter placement and assess the success of drainage.

COMMON PITFALLS AND TIPS

NEEDLE LENGTH TOO SHORT TO REACH THE PERICARDIAL SPACE

This pitfall usually results from using the subxiphoid approach. The obvious solution to this problem is using a longer spinal needle or pigtail catheter that reaches the correct location. The transthoracic approach is useful in these situations as it places the needle closer to the pericardium. In addition, using the dynamic approach helps in order to confirm the needle is actually reaching the pericardial space in real time.

NEEDLE INSERTED INTO THE LIVER

The liver is usually stuck by the needle when using the subxiphoid approach. This once again stresses the advantages of using the dynamic approach in order to view the needle enter the pericardium under ultrasound guidance and to help avoid damaging other structures in the process.

AORTIC DISSECTION

Pericardiocentesis should not be performed on pericardial effusions that are a result of an aortic dissection as this can result in high-pressure arterial fluid exsanguination. If the aortic root measures 4 cm or greater, a proximal aortic dissection should be suspected. Pericardiocentesis should be avoided unless the patient arrests and cardiothoracic surgery should be consulted immediately (Figs. 20-2 and 20-3).

LOCULATED OR COMPLEX PERICARDIAL EFFUSION

Malignant, bloody, or chronic effusions with protein may become loculated. Multiple approaches may be needed to drain enough fluid to allow return of circulation; therefore, the use of ultrasound guidance to direct and assess the heart and pericardial sac is paramount. An urgent pericardial window may be required.

PROCEDURAL COMPLICATIONS

Although ultrasound helps to perform pericardiocentesis safely, there are still complications that can result during the procedure. These include pneumothorax, ventricular laceration, and laceration of the internal mammary artery and epicardial vessels. Pneumothorax is more likely to result from the thoracic approach, but dynamic imaging helps to minimize this risk. Similarly, dynamic imaging aids in the avoidance of cardiac chamber and epicardial vessel lacerations.

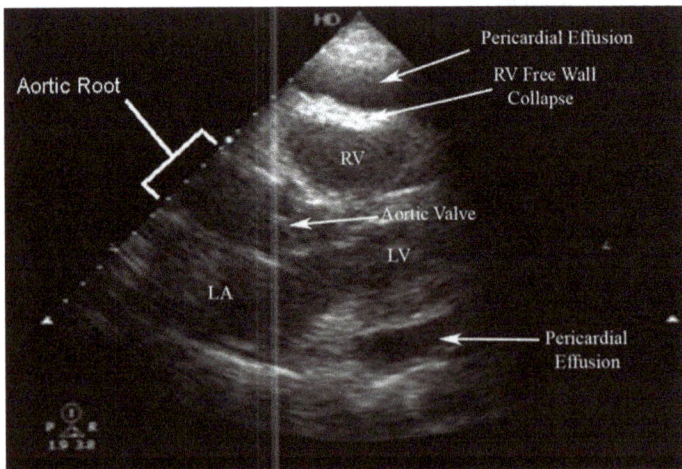

FIGURE 20-2 Parasternal long-axis view of cardiac tamponade with a normal-sized aortic root. Note the effusion both anteriorly and posteriorly. RV: right ventricle, LV: left ventricle, LA: left atrium.

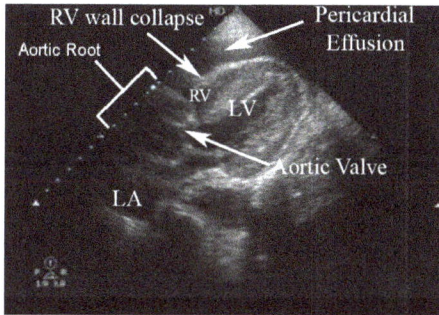

FIGURE 20-3 Cardiac tamponade with an aortic dissection. The aortic root in this image is measured over 4 cm. Pericardiocentesis should be avoided unless there is no alternative. RV: right ventricle, LV: left ventricle, LA: left atrium.

BACKGROUND AND INDICATIONS FOR ULTRASOUND-GUIDED CARDIAC PACING

Sonographic guidance can be helpful in cardiac pacing, typically with symptomatic bradycardia unresponsive to medications. Traditionally, this procedure is performed blindly, but with ultrasound guidance, the correct placement and success of the pacing device is greatly enhanced.

There are two forms of temporary cardiac pacing: transcutaneous (external) and transvenous (internal). Transcutaneous pacing is less invasive and quicker to initiate, but may cause significant discomfort and may not capture as reliably (Table 20-1). Transvenous pacing is more reliable and should be performed when capture with the transcutaneous method is not effective.

TABLE 20-1	INDICATIONS FOR TEMPORARY CARDIAC PACING AS PER THE AMERICAN HEART ASSOCIATION

Class I

• Symptomatic bradycardias unresponsive to atropine. This includes patients with:
  • Hypotension
  • Mental status changes
  • Pulmonary edema
  • Cardiac ischemia

Class IIa
• Bradycardic escape rhythms unresponsive to pharmacologic therapy
• Cardiac arrest with bradycardia or PEA due to overdose, acidosis or electrolyte abnormalities
• Standby pacing in specific MI associated rhythms
  • Symptomatic sinus node dysfunction
  • Mobitz Type II second degree heart block
  • Third degree heart block
  • New LBBB, RBBB, alternating BBB, or bifascicular block
  • Symptomatic Mobitz Type I second degree heart block associated with inferior MI

Class IIb
• Overdrive pacing of SVT or VT refractory to medications or cardioversion
• Early bradyasystolic arrest

PROBE SELECTION AND TECHNICAL CONSIDERATIONS

PHASED-ARRAY CARDIAC PROBE WITH A FREQUENCY OF 3.0–5.0 MHz

A phased-array cardiac probe in the cardiac machine setting should be used. A curvilinear abdominal probe with 3.0–5.0 MHz frequency can also be used, particularly if the heart is imaged from the subxiphoid approach.

TISSUE HARMONIC IMAGING

Tissue harmonic imaging (THI) should be used for all cardiac imaging if available. THI helps to brighten the signal returning from the pericardium. This will improve the image and make the procedure easier to perform.

STERILE PRECAUTIONS

While sterile precautions should be used for ultrasound guided central vascular access, visualization of the heart through transthoracic windows may not require sterile precautions.

EQUIPMENT

External pacer pads are required for transcutaneous pacing. Most critical care and emergency department settings have pacer wire kits that contain all necessary equipment to place a transvenous pacer. The pacer wire kit may include or be separate from a sheath (cordis) introducer catheter, which will need to be inserted prior to the pacing wire, and should be sized appropriately to introduce the wire.

PERFORMING ULTRASOUND-GUIDED CARDIAC PACING

Visualization of the heart for both transcutaneous and transvenous pacing can be achieved using a subxiphoid, a parasternal long axis, or apical four-chamber view.

Transcutaneous pacing is different from transvenous pacing in two major ways. First, the external pacer pads may make it more difficult to find a spot to place the ultrasound probe. The probe should be placed in any orientation where the heart can be visualized best. Second, the electrical shock associated with transcutaneous pacing can be uncomfortable. The stimulus is great enough to cause the chest muscles to contract. Medication for the discomfort, and sometimes the associated anxiety, is necessary.

It is often difficult to discern if the electrocardiogram (ECG) shows capture of the ventricle, as the pacing complex appears wide. Either a subxiphoid cardiac ultrasound view or somewhere between a PSLA and apical four-chamber view will readily demonstrate the cardiac contractility and the heart rate. This should be done in conjunction with a pulse check, but ultrasound may be particularly helpful in determining pacer capture when the blood pressure is low.

Transcutaneous pacing should begin with the pacer set to the asynchronous mode, at a rate of 70. The milliamperes (mAmps) should be gradually increased until one-to-one pacing capture is directly observed on the ultrasound monitor. The patient's clinical status, pulse, and blood pressure should also be followed. When there is adequate capture, the pacemaker can be set to a sensing or synchronous mode where it only paces if the native heart rate falls below the set rate. It can be beneficial to set the pacing rate at 55 or 60 in order to shock the patient less often, resulting in less discomfort (Fig. 20-4).

Transvenous pacing involves cannulization of a vein and insertion of a temporary pacing wire to the right ventricular septum. The vein can be accessed through the pacer wire kit's catheter, or through a Swan–Ganz catheter with sideport. In

Transcutaneous pacing steps

```
┌─────────────────────────────┐
│   Attach pacer pads to chest │
│   electrodes also on patient │
└─────────────────────────────┘
              │
              ▼
┌─────────────────────────────┐
│   Consider sedation and      │
│   analgesia                  │
└─────────────────────────────┘
              │
              ▼
┌─────────────────────────────┐
│   Ultrasound probe to chest  │
│   wall or subxiphoid area    │
└─────────────────────────────┘
              │
              ▼
┌─────────────────────────────┐
│   Asynchronous mode rate 70  │
│   start at low mAmps         │
└─────────────────────────────┘
              │
              ▼
┌─────────────────────────────┐
│   Gradually increase mAmps   │
│   until cardiac capture      │
└─────────────────────────────┘
              │
              ▼
┌─────────────────────────────┐
│   Synchronous mode           │
│   rate 50–60                 │
└─────────────────────────────┘
```

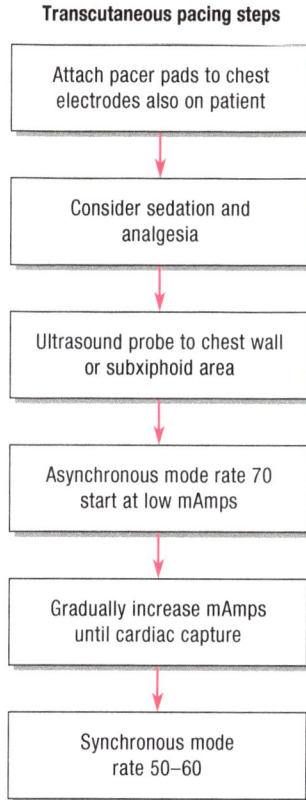

FIGURE 20-4 Transcutaneous pacing flowchart.

either case, a sterile sheath is attached to the introducer so the pacer wire may be adjusted as needed.

The pacer wire is naturally curved which makes it easier to direct it toward the septum. The two easiest approaches are through the right internal jugular (IJ) vein (with the wire's curve pointing toward the patient's left) or the left subclavian vein (SCV) (with the curve pointing toward the patient's feet). The use of ultrasound to find the IJ vein during needle cannulization is helpful, but oftentimes more difficult when using the SCV approach due to the clavicle being in the way.

Ideally, with ultrasound guidance, a pacer wire is first seen entering the right atrium, then traversing the tricuspid valve, and passing through the RV to lodge into the septal wall. If the pacer tip is visualized, the distance to the RV apex may be measured, and the amount of advancement needed can be determined by observing the centimeter marks on the pacer. Pacer wires are easily visualized by ultrasound as they appear hyperechoic within the anechoic blood-filled chamber and often produce ring-down or reverberation artifacts (Fig. 20-5). While the pacer wire should be visualized as it advances into the RV, sometimes the right ventricular windows are not easily obtained on ultrasound. In these cases, mechanical capture

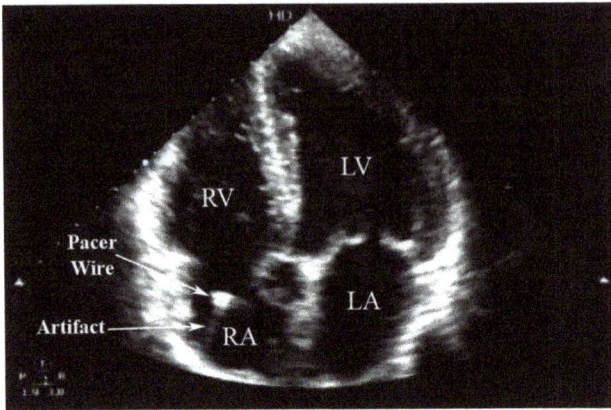

FIGURE 20-5 This image illustrates a pacer wire within the right atrium with resultant reverberation artifact. RV: right ventricle, RA: right atrium, LV: left ventricle, LA: left atrium.

may be seen as ventricular contraction. The sonographer can determine the minimum amperage needed by observing mechanical capture on ultrasound.

A temporary transvenous internal pacer box usually has both atrial and ventricular pacing capabilities (Fig. 20-6). In an emergent setting, ventricular pacing

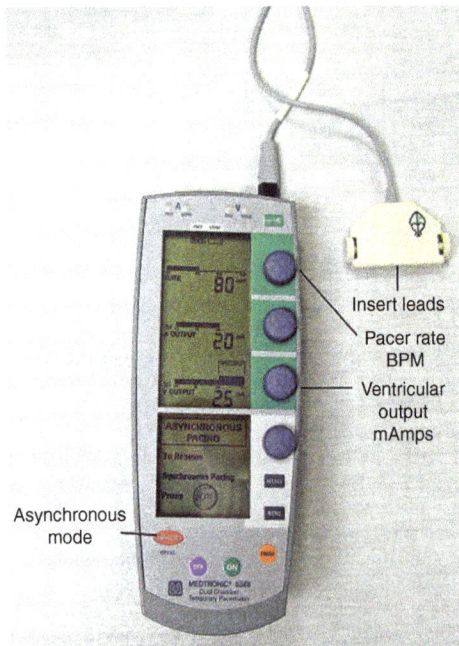

FIGURE 20-6 Transvenous internal pacer box. (*Photograph courtesy of Dr. P. Krochmal, Yale University School of Medicine, Department of Emergency Medicine.*)

is the more important of the two. The electrodes of the pacer wire are inserted into the cable and screwed down tightly to prevent dislodgement.

The ventricular output on the box is set to the maximum of 25 mA, the pacer rate is set to 70 or 80, and the box is then placed in the asynchronous mode. The asynchronous mode results in the pacer pacing all the time and does not sense the patient's native rhythm. The pacer wire is inserted into the RIJ or LSCV and advanced until it is visualized or there is capture. On the ECG monitor, the associated pacer spike will have a wide QRS complex and an associated T wave. The sonographer will be able to show the heart beating at the rate at which the pacer is set by placing the probe in a PSLA prior to inserting the pacer wire and watching the echo on the monitor as it is advanced.

The current should be gradually decreased on the pacer box until the lowest amperage with continuous one-to-one cardiac capture is observed (usually under 5 mA) on the ultrasound monitor and ECG. Once this amperage is found, it should be multiplied by 3, and then the box should be set to this number (ie if

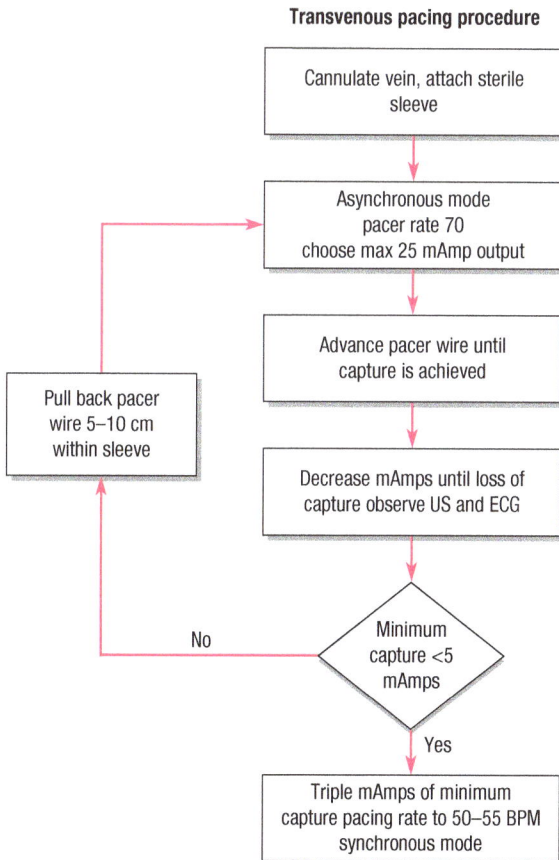

Transvenous pacing procedure

FIGURE 20-7 Transvenous pacing flowchart.

capture is found at 1 mA, the amperage on the box should be set to 3). The machine should now be switched to the synchronous mode in order for the box to sense the patient's native heart rate. If the native heart rate is faster than what the pacemaker box is set at, no spike will be sent from the machine. The pacer should ideally be set at a rate of 50–60, giving the patient's heart a chance to beat on its own.

If the pacer does not achieve capture at fewer than 5 mA, then the wire should be pulled back within the sterile sleeve approximately 5–10 cm, the amperage should be turned back up to 25, and then the wire readvanced to another location. The procedure described earlier should then be repeated in order to determine the minimum amperage level required for capture (Fig. 20-7).

COMMON PITFALLS AND TIPS

MISTAKING A PACING COMPLEX FOR CAPTURE OF THE VENTRICLE

This occurs more commonly with transcutaneous pacing. The pacing complex is large and can look like it may have an associated T wave. Using ultrasound to visualize ventricular contraction at the same rate as the pacer helps to prevent this error.

NOT SWITCHING TO SYNCHRONOUS MODE AFTER CAPTURE

If the pacer is left on the asynchronous mode, the patient is at risk for developing "R on T phenomenon" (a premature ventricular QRS occurring which interferes with the T wave of the previous contraction). This can result in ventricular fibrillation. In order to avoid this, the machine must be switched to the synchronous mode once capture is achieved.

FAILURE TO ENSURE OPTIMAL CAPTURE OF THE VENTRICLE

In the transvenous mode, it is important to make sure that the ventricle is initially captured at less than 5 mA. This number should then be tripled for the proper machine setting. Whether the physician is using transcutaneous or transvenous pacing, there should be frequent monitoring of the patient's mental status, heart rate, and blood pressure in order to ensure adequate capture continues.

CONCLUSION

As the heart is a dynamic structure, ultrasound is particularly useful in assisting the emergency and critical care physician with cardiac procedures. It is a useful modality in both the real-time guidance of these procedures, but also in the monitoring of the patient's condition afterward. The use of bedside echocardiography to assist in the diagnosis and emergent drainage of pericardial effusions can be extremely helpful in an acute situation. In cardiac pacing, ultrasound is now commonly used for venous access wire placement and in the direct observation of ventricular contractions to confirm pacer capture.

Additional Reading

Aguilera PA, Durham BA, Reilly DA. Emergency transvenous cardiac pacing placement using ultrasound guidance. *Ann Emerg Med.* 2000;36(3):224-227.

Francis GS, Williams SV, Achord JL, et al. Clinical competence in insertion of a temporary transvenous ventricular pacemaker. A statement for physicians from the ACP/ACC/AHA Task Force on Clinical Privileges in Cardiology. *Circulation.* 1994;89(4):1913-1916.

Ma OJ, Mateer JR, Ogata M, Kefer MP, Wittmann D, Aprahamian C. Prospective analysis of a rapid trauma ultrasound examination performed by emergency physicians. *J Trauma.* 1995;38(6):879-885.

Teresa SM, Barnes ME, Hayes SN, et al. Clinical and echocardiographic characteristics of significant pericardial effusions following cardiothoracic surgery and outcomes of echo-guided pericardiocentesis for management. *Chest.* 1999;116:322-331.

Tsang TS, Barnes ME, Gersh BJ, Bailey KR, Seward JB. Outcomes of clinically significant idiopathic pericardial effusion requiring intervention. *Am J Cardiol.* 2003;91(6):704-707.

Tsang TS, Seward JB. Letter to the editor pericardiocentesis under echocardiographic guidance. *Eur J Echocardiography.* 2001;2(1):68-69.

21 Ultrasound for Arthrocentesis

Edward Tham

BACKGROUND AND INDICATIONS FOR EXAMINATION

Joint pain and swelling are common complaints in the acute care setting. Diagnostic arthrocentesis may be required to rule out an infectious process or hemarthrosis. Joint aspiration may also relieve joint pain and allow for infusion of medications when appropriate. Much of the technique and equipment for ultrasound-guided arthrocentesis is the same as for a landmark-based approach. The use of ultrasound can determine the presence of a joint effusion and increase the success rate of arthrocentesis while decreasing complications. Ultrasound may also assist in directing a needle into a joint space even when no effusion exists (ie, for injection of dye to determine joint disruption in trauma or for injection of medications).

Bedside ultrasound-guided arthrocentesis should be used for:

- The patient with nontraumatic joint pain
- Large or painful joint effusions
- The diagnosis of traumatic arthrotomy
- The injection of medications into the joint space

PROBE SELECTION AND TECHNICAL CONSIDERATIONS FOR ARTHROCENTESIS

LINEAR-ARRAY PROBE WITH A FREQUENCY OF 5.0–12.0 MHz

A linear-array probe is best suited for arthrocentesis because of its high resolution and linear configuration. A curvilinear abdominal probe with a 3.0–5.0 MHz frequency can also be used for deeper joints such as the hip or in obese patients. A "hockey stick" or pediatric linear probe may be used for smaller joints.

MACHINE PRESET

If available, a superficial or bone preset should be utilized on the machine in order to optimize the image obtained.

FOCUS

The focus should be adjusted so that it is at the level of the joint of interest. This will help to improve the lateral resolution of the image.

DEPTH

The sonographer should initially start off deep and survey the whole joint. The depth should then be reduced so that the area where the needle will be introduced takes up most of the screen.

GAIN OR TIME-GAIN COMPENSATION

The overall gain should be adjusted in order to enhance the brightness of the image as needed. It is often better for the sonographer to increase the far gain of the image only, using time-gain compensation (TGC), in order to improve the quality of the deeper structures. It is important to not use too much gain, which can result in obscuring other important structures within the joint, such as anechoic blood vessels.

STERILE PRECAUTIONS

Arthrocentesis is an invasive procedure, and therefore, sterile precautions with a sterile probe cover and gel should always be used.

DYNAMIC VERSUS STATIC ULTRASOUND GUIDANCE

Like many procedures, ultrasound guidance for arthrocentesis can be performed by either a static or dynamic technique. Static ultrasound guidance involves using the image to identify the synovial space, depth, angle of entry, and vessels/nerves or other obstacles. The sonographer then marks a spot on the skin where success is likely. The procedure is then carried out in a fashion similar to landmark-based arthrocentesis. The main advantage of this technique is that it leaves the clinician with two free hands to complete the procedure.

Dynamic ultrasound guidance uses real-time imaging to perform the arthrocentesis. It has the advantage of visualizing the needle entering the synovial space and the ability to redirect the needle as required. Needles with special echogenic tips may be used to help visualization and guidance into the joint. This technique may initially be more challenging for the novice, but ultimately it is the preferred method. When using dynamic guidance, sterile precautions with probe covers and sterile gel must be used, as in central venous access.

An intermediate technique is a two-person dynamic guidance procedure, where the probe is held by one person and the procedure performed by the other. Either technique may be used depending on operator preference, resources, and time availability, although mastery of the single-operator dynamic approach will result in the most consistent success.

PERFORMING ULTRASOUND-GUIDED ARTHROCENTESIS

KNEE

The knee is the one of most commonly tapped joints in the body. It is often performed successfully using only anatomic landmarks. However, ultrasound may be useful in cases where the anatomy is distorted by soft tissue swelling or bony displacement. The suprapatellar bursa is contiguous with the knee joint; therefore, an effusion of the suprapatellar bursa signifies a knee joint effusion and vice versa (Fig. 21-1). Most often, the medial or lateral recess of this bursa is the site for joint aspiration. The patient should be supine and the knee flexed to 15°–45°. The knee should be scanned on the medial and lateral sides just posterior to the patella in both the transverse and coronal planes (Fig. 21-2). An effusion will appear as an anechoic or hypoechoic area abutting the distal femur (see Fig. 21-1). It may have internal echoes in the case of clotted blood, a septic joint, or a chronic inflammatory process (Fig. 21-3). The needle should be directed toward the largest pocket of fluid. It is important to differentiate the suprapatellar bursa from other bursa and cysts in the region, as these may not communicate directly with the joint space.

SHOULDER

Arthrocentesis of the glenohumeral joint or shoulder can be done with either an anterior or posterior approach. Effusions will usually accumulate posteriorly first, so this approach may be easiest.

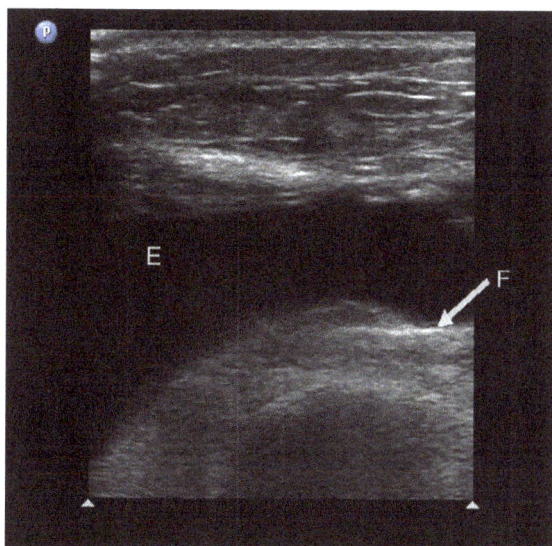

FIGURE 21-1 Longitudinal view of the lateral distal femur. The bony femoral cortex (F) is white-appearing due to its echogenicity. A large suprapatellar effusion (E) is present over the entire distal femur and joint space.

The shoulder joint comprises the glenoid and labrum articulating with the humeral head. This structure is surrounded by a fibrous joint capsule. The joint is also enveloped by a group of muscles with associated tendons collectively known as the rotator cuff. The glenoid and humeral head will be hyperechoic and will produce a shadowing artifact beyond the cortex. The glenoid labrum is a

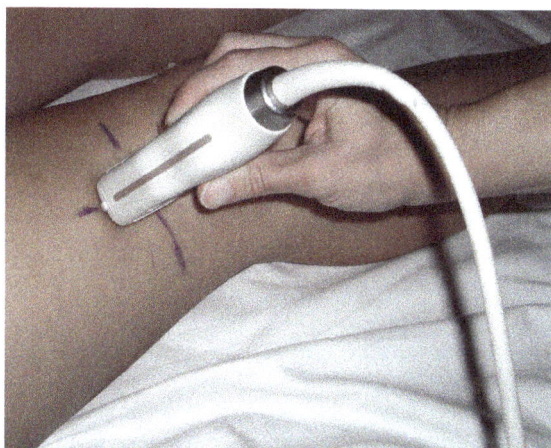

FIGURE 21-2 Patient and probe positioning for aspirating the lateral suprapatellar bursa. In this image, the probe is placed over the distal lateral femur in a longitudinal position.

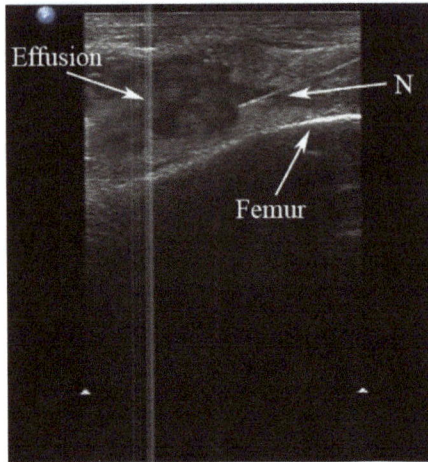

FIGURE 21-3 A longitudinal view of the femur with an overlying complex effusion (containing internal echoes). An echogenic needle (N) can be seen in long axis directed toward the effusion.

hypoechoic stripe closely apposed to the bony glenoid. An effusion will appear as an anechoic space separating the glenoid from the humeral head (Fig 21-4).

The patient should be seated with the shoulder in the neutral position. The elbow should be flexed 90° and can be rested on a stand. The ultrasound should begin in the transverse plane, with respect to the body. The transducer should be placed on the posterior surface of the shoulder, just inferior to the acromion process. It should be fanned superiorly and inferiorly in order to visualize the entire

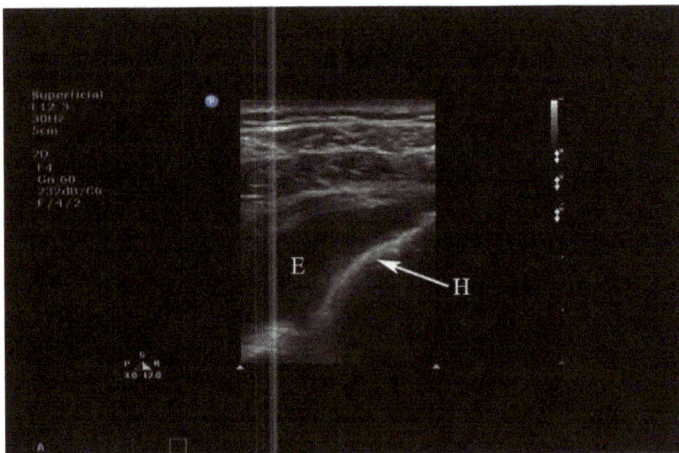

FIGURE 21-4 A view of the shoulder illustrating an anechoic effusion (E) separating the humeral head (H) and the glenoid.

posterior joint surface. The joint should then be scanned in the sagittal plane. The point of maximal joint capsule distention should be noted and this area should be marked on the skin surface if static ultrasound guidance will be used. If dynamic ultrasound guidance is used, sterile precautions should be observed, and the needle should be aimed toward the joint just medial to the humeral head. The sonographer should observe the entry of the needle into the joint space on the monitor in real time.

HIP

The hip is a deep joint with many surrounding neurovascular bundles; therefore, blind hip joint aspiration is rarely done in an acute care setting. Hip joint aspiration is most commonly done with fluoroscopic or ultrasound guidance, which may not be immediately available. Ultrasound guidance at the bedside may safely expedite diagnosis and treatment, particularly for a septic joint.

A high-frequency linear transducer, while providing superior resolution, may not be able to penetrate the deep soft tissue of the hip in some patients. A curved-array probe with a lower frequency of 3.5–5.0 MHz, which provides better penetration, may need to be used in these patients.

The hip is a ball-socket-type joint. The femoral head is almost completely enveloped by the acetabulum, and is a site where effusions commonly occur (Fig. 21-5a and b). The hip is surrounded by a fibrous capsule that extends laterally along a large portion of the femoral neck. In normal joints, there is little synovial fluid and the joint capsule is closely applied to the femoral neck. However, if an effusion is present, the capsule becomes distended and lifts off the femoral neck (Fig. 21-6). The area just lateral and anterior to the femoral head will often accumulate an effusion first. The femoral area also contains important neurovascular structures that must be avoided.

The patient should be supine with the ipsilateral hip slightly extended and abducted. The ultrasound should begin over the femoral neck with the indicator pointing toward the umbilicus (Fig. 21-7). The femoral neck should be imaged in

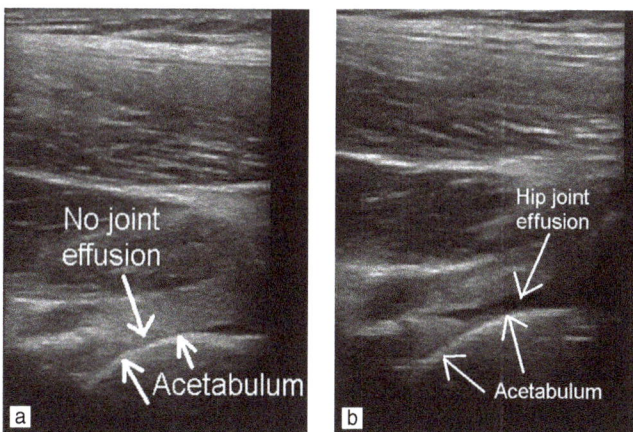

FIGURE 21-5 A transverse view of the femoral head surrounded by the acetabulum depicting a normal hip joint without effusion (*a*). A hip effusion visualized as an anechoic black area surrounding the acetabulum (*b*).

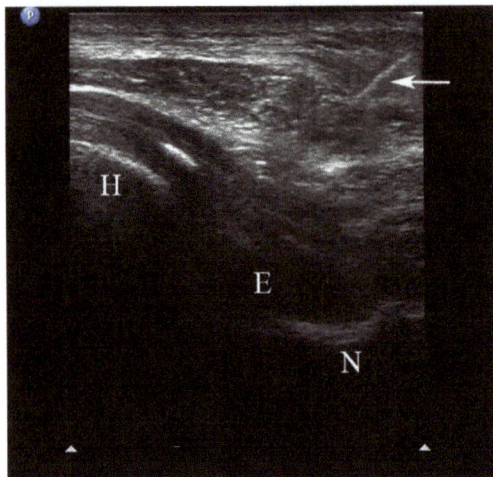

FIGURE 21-6 This is a long-axis view of the anterior femoral neck. The nonarticular portion of the femoral head (H) is visualized on the left side of the image. The femoral neck (N) is seen on the right. The hypoechoic area located in the fossa between the head and neck represents a hip joint effusion (E). A needle (arrow) can be seen in long axis directed toward the effusion.

a long-axis view until the femoral head is seen. Attention must be paid to the femoral vessels and nerve, which course though this area. The area just distal to the femoral head is where an effusion will accumulate first and it often tracks down the femoral neck, producing an anechoic stripe between the neck and overlying soft tissues (see Fig. 21-6). Comparison to the contralateral hip should be routine, and the distance from the femoral neck cortex to the joint capsule should be noted. A difference of greater than 2 mm on the symptomatic side indicates a significant effusion. Due to the depth of the hip and a lack of visible landmarks, arthrocentesis is usually best performed with a real-time dynamic technique using an in-plane approach.

ELBOW

Blind aspiration of the elbow is normally accomplished using a posterolateral approach, with the needle coursing through the space between the radial head and the lateral epicondyle. Linear transducers may be fairly wide and can make posterolateral sonography of the radiohumeral joint difficult due to the small surface area and bony protrusions. Hence, a posterior approach is most often used in ultrasound guided elbow arthrocentesis.

The elbow comprises the radius, ulna, and humerus. Numerous neurovascular structures and tendons course around the elbow to supply the forearm and hand. The ulnar nerve runs just medial to the olecranon and the insertion of the triceps tendon. The puncture site should be just lateral to these structures.

The patient should be seated with the shoulder abducted and the elbow flexed. Resting the forearm on a stand with the elbow hanging over the edge will provide proper positioning. The ultrasound should begin over the posterior humerus in the transverse plane just superior to the olecranon (Fig. 21-8). When the probe is rocked caudally, the olecranon fossa will be visualized as a central depression

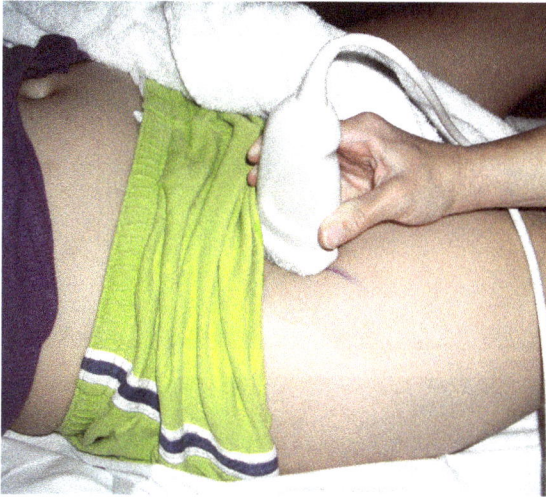

FIGURE 21-7 Patient and probe positioning for aspirating a hip effusion. The sonographer should start with the probe oriented longitudinally, sliding up the femoral neck, until the femoral head is visualized. The probe should then be pointed toward the umbilicus for optimal imaging of the joint.

between the medial and lateral epicondyles. If a joint effusion is present, it will appear as a hypoechoic space within this fossa (Fig. 21-9*a* and *b*).

OTHER JOINTS

In addition to the large joints described earlier, fluid can usually be aspirated using ultrasound guidance in the smaller joints. Joints such as the ankle, wrist, metacarpal, metatarsal, and interphalangeal joints may be amenable to aspiration. In most

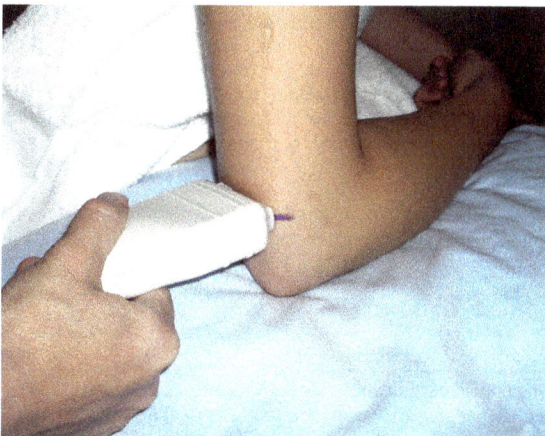

FIGURE 21-8 Patient and probe positioning for aspirating an elbow effusion. The sonographer should start with the probe over the posterior humerus, oriented in a transverse position, just superior to the olecranon.

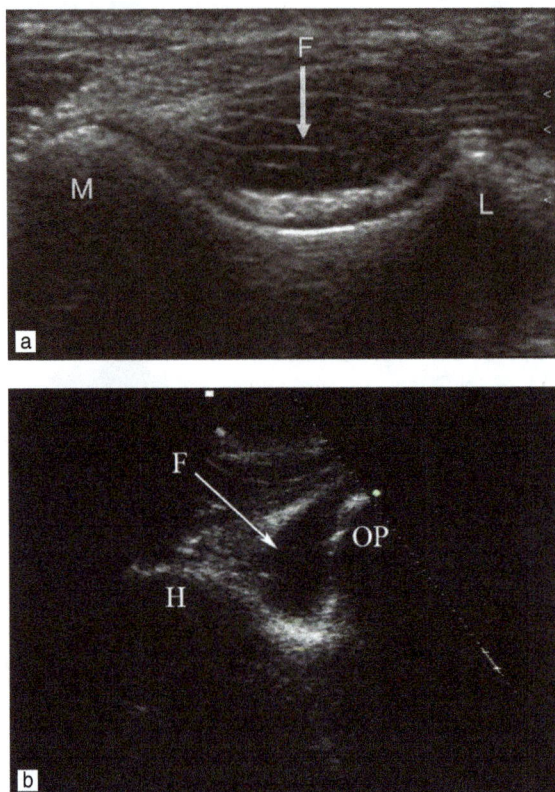

FIGURE 21-9 (*a*) Transverse image of the posterior distal humerus just superior to the olecranon. Both lateral (L) and medial (M) epicondyles are seen. The needle should be directed into the superior portion of the olecranon fossa (F), where fluid often collects. When an effusion is present, the slightly echogenic posterior fat pad within the fossa will be displaced [compare with (*b*)]. (*b*) Longitudinal image of the posterior distal humerus (H) showing an effusion in the olecranon fossa (F). The effusion is displacing the normal posterior fat pad that lies within the fossa. The olecranon process (OP) is visualized on the right side of the image.

cases, dynamic guidance into the largest available pocket will be most effective, with attention paid to avoiding neurovascular structures.

COMMON PITFALLS AND TIPS

FAILURE TO VISUALIZE NEEDLE TIP

When using ultrasound guidance, failure to visualize the needle tip can lead to failure or inadvertent damage to surrounding structures. When using a short-axis technique, the needle tip will appear as a hyperechoic point with reverberation artifact. If only a shadowing artifact is seen, the shaft of the needle is directly under the probe. The needle should be either retracted or the probe should be rocked so as to visualize the needle tip. Alternatively, a long-axis approach can be used. This approach is more difficult and should be attempted by experienced sonographers. If the needle is not directly in the center of the probe or if slightly off angle, the needle will not be visualized. Use of an "echogenic" needle (specially made for ultrasound visualization by providing microabrasions on the bevel) may be helpful.

DRY TAP

Failure to aspirate fluid from a tap could be due to the needle not being in the proper location. If a dynamic ultrasound-guided technique is being used, the sonographer should pull the needle back slightly and redirect it into the joint space while watching the needle on the monitor. If a static technique is being used, the transducer should be placed back over the joint space in order to confirm that the skin marker is accurate.

INFECTION

Although a rare complication, iatrogenic joint infection is a possibility. Standard sterile precautions should be used in addition to sterile probe covers when using ultrasound guidance. If adjustments to the machine need to be made during the procedure, a second non-sterile operator should make these changes. If arthrocentesis on a prosthetic joint is required, orthopedic consultation is advised due to the higher rate of iatrogenic infection.

INJURY TO NEARBY STRUCTURES

Although vessel or nerve injury is a rare complication, a neurovascular exam should be performed prior to and after completion of an arthrocentesis. Color-flow Doppler can be used to help identify blood vessels. Nerves will be seen in cross section as round honeycomb-like structures that are usually paired with deep vessels. Other obstacles that may be encountered are foreign bodies, tendons, or ligaments. Using a real-time ultrasound-guided technique can help the clinician direct the needle into the joint as well as avoiding these obstacles.

FAILURE TO REVIEW SUPPLEMENTAL IMAGING

When preparing to aspirate a joint, taking the time to review supplemental imaging, such as radiographs, before starting the procedure can also help to limit the above pitfalls. This will minimize surprises that may be masked by soft tissue swelling. While ultrasound is superior to plain radiographs for detecting an effusion, a radiograph will be better at identifying fractures, dislocations, and osteomyelitis, and may help to identify the largest effusion pocket. Radiographs and ultrasound should be used as complementary imaging modalities when evaluating musculoskeletal complaints.

MISTAKING A JOINT EFFUSION FOR AN ALTERNATIVE DIAGNOSIS

A soft tissue infection overlying a joint may mimic an effusion clinically. While scanning the joint, the sonographer should look for signs of soft tissue infection, such as abscess or cellulitis, which may appear as cobblestoning. If cobblestoning is present, without a significant joint effusion, the patient probably only has a cellulitis. In this situation, joint aspiration through an overlying skin infection would be contraindicated.

CONCLUSION

Arthrocentesis is one of the most commonly performed procedures in the emergency care setting. Ultrasound has a high sensitivity for detecting joint effusions and has been shown to improve success rates while decreasing complications that can result from the procedure. It helps the clinician to better define bony anatomy as well as to avoid neurovascular structures. Both the static technique, which simply maps out the appropriate anatomy with a skin marker, and the dynamic technique, which observes the needle tip entering the joint space, may help improve safety and success of the procedure. As with any other invasive procedure performed in the acute care setting, ultrasound-guided arthrocentesis has quickly become the preferred method over the more traditional blind approaches.

Additional Reading

Cardinal E, Chhem R, Beauregard C. Ultrasound-guided interventional procedures in the musculoskeletal system. *Radiol Clin North Am.* 1998;36:597-604.

Fessell D, Jacobsen J, Craig J, et al. Using sonography to reveal and aspirate joint effusions. *Am J Roentgenol.* 2000;174:1353-1362.

Fessell D, Van Holsbeeck M. Ultrasound guided musculoskeletal procedures. *Ultrasound Clin.* 2007;2:737-757.

Sofka C, Collins A, Adler R. Use of ultrasonographic guidance in interventional musculoskeletal procedures: a review from a single institution. *J Ultrasound Med.* 2001;20:21-26.

22 Ultrasound for Endotracheal Intubation

William Manson

BACKGROUND AND INDICATIONS FOR EXAM

Endotracheal intubation can be one of the more challenging tasks in emergency medicine and critical care. Misplacement of the tube, most often into the right main stem bronchus or esophagus, has been reported in up to 8% of cases in the literature. Secondary confirmation of tube placement also presents various challenges to the practitioner. Traditionally, direct visualization of the endotracheal tube followed by at least one or more secondary confirmations is required to confirm tube placement. End-tidal colorimetric devices are most frequently used in the acute care setting, as well as auscultation of the thorax and epigastrium. Esophageal bulb detectors, visualization of mist in the endotracheal tube, and bilateral chest rise are also employed. Each of these techniques and devices has specific limitations and pitfalls. Bedside ultrasound may also be used to dynamically observe tube passage into the trachea or esophagus, providing an additional method of confirmation. Following successful intubation, bedside ultrasound may also be used to visualize the presence of bilateral lung sliding and comet-tail artifact, additional indicators of correct placement, and lung expansion post-intubation.

Bedside ultrasound is a rapid and reliable way to confirm proper endotracheal intubation. Sensitivity and specificity are high, especially when compared to end-tidal colorimetry in the acute care setting.

Direct ultrasound visualization of the endotracheal tube passing through the trachea may be particularly helpful for physicians who are supervising a trainee performing an intubation, allowing real-time confirmation of correct placement. Bedside ultrasound gives the senior physician the ability to instantly determine the location of the endotracheal tube, prior to bagging one that is incorrectly placed into the esophagus.

Bedside ultrasound evaluation of endotracheal intubation should be performed in:

- Any patient undergoing intubation, including pediatrics and trauma, if a difficult airway is anticipated
- Training situations, where a physician is supervising a less-experienced performer

PROBE SELECTION AND TECHNICAL CONSIDERATIONS

LINEAR PROBE WITH A FREQUENCY OF 6.0–12.0 MHz

To visualize the trachea and thorax, a linear probe with a high frequency such as 6.0–12.0 MHz should be utilized. A lower frequency, microconvex or curvilinear probe may be helpful in more obese patients.

MACHINE PRESET

The machine should be set to a superficial or small parts setting.

FOCAL ZONE

The focal zone should be placed at the depth of the trachea or pleural line in order to optimize the lateral resolution.

TIME-GAIN COMPENSATION

The far gain or time-gain compensation may need to be adjusted in order to enhance and brighten signals returning to the machine monitor. This will help the sonographer observe the shadow created by the tracheal cartilage and endotracheal tube in the far field.

DEPTH

An image that is either too deep or too shallow can be disorienting. Generally, it is better to start deeper than necessary, and once the appropriate anatomy is identified, the depth should be adjusted so that the pertinent structures are taking up most of the screen.

The trachea originates at the vocal cords and traverses distally. In the neck, the trachea lies posterior to the thyroid gland, which has a homogenous appearance on ultrasound, similar to the liver or spleen. The cartilaginous rings of the trachea create a bright white hyperechoic line just deep to the thyroid gland. In a transverse view of the anterior neck, with the probe indicator pointed toward the patient's right, the ultrasound beam will encounter superficial structures first starting with the skin and subcutaneous tissue, then thyroid tissue, and lastly trachea (Fig. 22-1). The longitudinal or sagittal view may also be viewed, but less experienced sonographers will more easily interpret the transverse view. Due to the cartilaginous composition of the tracheal rings and the inability of the ultrasound beam to pass through them, a shadowing effect will be seen posteriorly (see Fig. 22-1). The esophagus is typically not visualized due to its compressibility with the ultrasound probe unless an endotracheal tube is present within its lumen (Fig. 22-3).

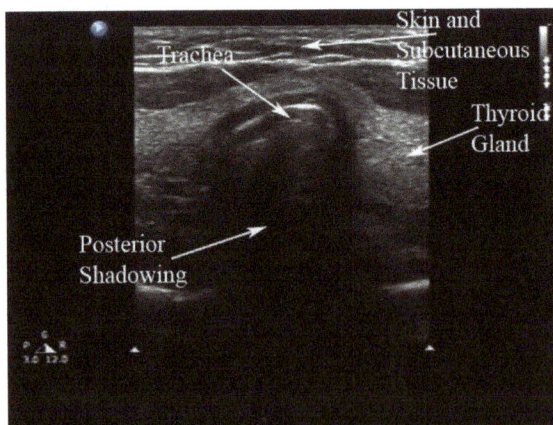

FIGURE 22-1 This image illustrates a transverse view of the trachea with landmarks. The anechoic area posterior to the trachea represents shadowing resulting from an attenuation of the ultrasound beam through the dense cartilage of the rings.

In addition to an ultrasound of the neck, visualization of lung sliding and lung pulse may help to determine that adequate ventilation is occurring. This is described in detail in Chap. 7.

PERFORMING THE PROCEDURE

Because endotracheal intubation is a procedure requiring both hands, ultrasound visualization requires an additional person. While one physician is performing the actual intubation, the other person will perform the bedside ultrasound and visualize the tube placement in real time passing into the trachea. The use of the ultrasound probe may aid in providing cricoid pressure, which may improve visualization for the person performing the intubation and help limit regurgitation of stomach contents.

The ultrasound machine should ideally be positioned on the patient's right side, consistent with other bedside ultrasound exams. The sonographer should also stand at the patient's right side, positioned to see both the viewing screen and the intubating physician. Prior to the actual intubation, the sonographer should scan the patient's neck, identifying important landmarks including the subcutaneous tissue, thyroid tissue, and tracheal cartilage (see Fig. 22-1).

Imaging of the trachea should begin in the transverse orientation, with the probe placed on the patient's neck superior to the suprasternal notch, with the indicator directed toward the patient's right. The probe may be placed in the midline, anywhere between the cricoid membrane and suprasternal notch. If the intubating physician is going to perform a bimanual technique, the ultrasound probe should be placed further down at the base of the neck, just above the suprasternal notch. Only minimal pressure is needed to visualize important anatomy. Too much pressure may displace the trachea laterally, resulting in a more difficult intubation.

During the procedure, the sonographer should observe the passage of the tube into the trachea on the ultrasound screen. This is most easily visualized in real time by observing motion, similar to lung sliding, just distal to the hyperechoic ring in the trachea. There will be subtle changes in the echogenicity distal to the tracheal cartilage as the tube and deflated balloon pass under the beam of the ultrasound (Fig. 22-2). In addition, there is often visualization of two bright echogenic parallel lines, representing the inner and outer walls of the endotracheal tube (see Fig. 22-3). Alternatively, a comet-tail artifact may be seen distal to the tracheal cartilage as the tube passes into the trachea. Some of these changes may initially be quite subtle, and oftentimes, visualization of the tube entering the esophagus in error may be easier to appreciate.

Bedside ultrasound for endotracheal intubation should include complete visualization of the placement of the tube within the trachea and also subsequent visualization of the lung fields bilaterally. One can think of the transverse imaging of the trachea as analogous to confirmation with an end-tidal colorimeter. The second part of the exam, visualizing bilateral lung sliding, is analogous to auscultation with the stethoscope over the right and left lung fields. After tube placement, the sonographer should confirm ventilation of both lung fields by searching for lung sliding. At this point, the patient should be ventilated with the bag valve mask or ventilator. Using the same high-frequency transducer and image preset, the probe should be positioned sagittally over the right chest in the midclavicular line, confirming the presence of lung sliding. The same exam should then be performed on the patient's left side. If adequate lung sliding is present on both sides, endotracheal intubation with appropriate tube positioning has been confirmed.

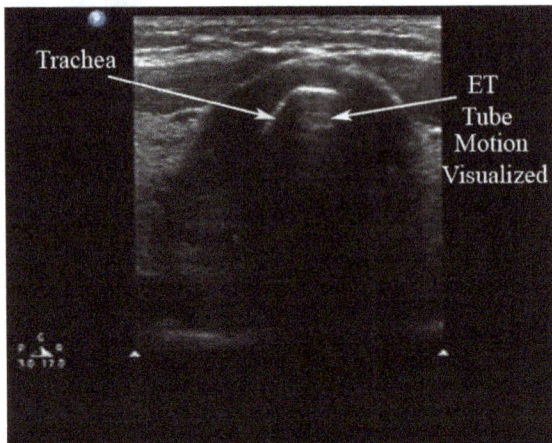

FIGURE 22-2 This image illustrates the trachea during intubation as the tube passes underneath the probe. The arrow points to a subtle area of increased echogenicity just distal to the tracheal cartilage. This area is where movement is most often visualized in real time during an intubation.

In addition to lung sliding, ultrasound may be used to visualize appropriate diaphragmatic excursion. The probe is placed in the flanks in a coronal plane, similar to performing a FAST exam. The diaphragm should move inferiorly with each breath.

The lung pulse sign on ultrasound indicates inadequate ventilation. This occurs when there is an absence of lung sliding, without a pneumothorax being present. This sign results from the heart transmitting a subtle rhythmic pulsation to the pleural line in the absence of true lung sliding. The sonographer will visualize a subtle back-and-forth pulsation of the pleural line. If the lung pulse sign is present on one side, but lung sliding is present on the other, then a main stem bronchus intubation has likely occurred (usually right main stem), though other causes can include lobar atelectasis and airway obstruction from tumor or other etiologies. If the clinician encounters this situation, the tube should be pulled back until bilateral lung sliding is present making sure not to pull the tube out too far.

In normal neck anatomy, the esophagus is more compressible and appears collapsed on ultrasound; therefore, it is not as easily identified as the trachea. Due to these properties, an esophageal intubation is actually easier to visualize than a tracheal one because a tube passing through the esophagus will inflate its lumen and allow it to be visualized in real time. The esophagus is normally situated posterior and lateral to the trachea; therefore, with the probe indicator pointing toward the patient's right side, the trachea will appear lateral and slightly anterior to the esophagus (see Fig. 22-3). In the case of an esophageal intubation, the sonographer will visualize the endotracheal tube lateral to the trachea, and it will appear as a hyperechoic line with distal shadowing (see Fig. 22-3). A small number of esophageal intubations may occur directly posterior to the trachea, making them more difficult to appreciate on ultrasound.

If lung sliding is absent on both sides of the chest after intubation, despite ventilation, then an esophageal intubation has occurred. At this point, the endotracheal tube should be removed and reintubation attempted.

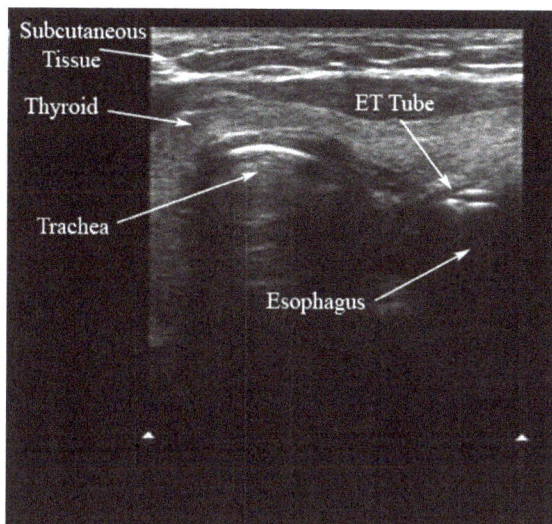

FIGURE 22-3 This image illustrates a transverse view of the trachea and esophagus during an esophageal intubation. Note in this image that the esophagus is visualized posterior and lateral to the trachea. Two parallel echogenic lines are seen in the proximal esophagus representing the inner and outer endotracheal tube walls as it passes through the lumen of the esophagus.

COMMON PITFALLS AND TIPS

PATIENT HABITUS

Patients with short necks and obesity are common causes of difficult intubations. In these patients, a lower-frequency transducer may be used, which provides better penetration, and may improve image quality in individuals with excess soft tissue. In addition, changing the angle of the ultrasound probe may allow the sonographer to visualize the trachea without impeding the ongoing intubation.

NOT PROPERLY IDENTIFYING LANDMARKS

The trachea may be misidentified if the landmarks are not clearly visualized. The trachea and thyroid gland should be visualized in the transverse plane, and depth adjusted so that the image makes up approximately three-fourths of the screen.

INCORRECTLY IDENTIFYING AN ESOPHAGEAL INTUBATION

Passage of the endotracheal tube into the esophagus may be misinterpreted as a tracheal intubation, especially when the esophagus lies immediately posterior to the trachea. As noted earlier, greater than 90% of esophageal intubations will be identified lateral to the trachea (see Fig. 22-3), but a small number of cases will lie immediately posterior, confusing the novice sonographer. This emphasizes the importance of scanning the patient and attempting to become familiar with the anatomy pre-intubation. In addition, it is important to remember that tracheal anatomy will be more easily visualized pre-intubation and esophageal anatomy after esophageal intubation. Therefore, the sonographer must pay close attention to the tube movements on the ultrasound monitor in real time. Finally, esophageal intubations should be suspected when there is a presence of movement in the distal field.

PNEUMOTHORAX

In a patient with a pneumothorax, the absence of lung sliding following intubation may be misinterpreted as a right main stem intubation. As discussed in Chap. 7, a pneumothorax occurs when air separates the visceral and parietal pleura, and no lung sliding is seen. Following a right main stem intubation, lung sliding will also be absent on the left hemithorax. By scanning laterally, into the midaxillary line, the sonographer can distinguish a small pneumothorax from a subtle lung pulse.

TRAUMA

Imaging the airway and lung sliding during a trauma scenario may be especially difficult. The presence of subcutaneous air, secretions, blood, and edema may alter the traditional appearance of the airway. The most experienced sonographer should perform the procedure in these difficult scenarios. Clearly, the presence of a cervical collar will also limit access of the ultrasound probe.

Additional Reading

Blaivas M, Tsung JW. Point-of-care sonographic detection of left endobronchial main stem intubation and obstruction versus endotracheal intubation. *J Ultrasound Med*. 2008;27(5):785-789.

Drescher MJ, Conard FU, Schamban NE. Identification and description of esophageal intubation using ultrasound. *Acad Emerg Med*. 2000;7(6):722-725.

Milling TJ, Jones M, Khan T, et al. Transtracheal 2-D ultrasound for identification of esophageal intubation. *J Emerg Med*. 2007;32(4):409-414.

Raphael DT, Conard FU. Ultrasound confirmation of endotracheal tube placement. *J Clin Ultrasound*. 1987;15(7):459-462.

Werner SL, Smith CE, Goldstein JR, Jones RA, Cydulka RK. Pilot study to evaluate the accuracy of ultrasonography in confirming endotracheal tube placement. *Ann Emerg Med*. 2007;49(1):75-80.

23 Ultrasound-Guided Nerve Blocks

Yiju Teresa Liu

BACKGROUND AND INDICATIONS FOR EXAMINATION

Regional anesthesia provides an alternative to general or local anesthesia, procedural sedation, and parenteral pain management. Conventional anatomic approaches to nerve blocks are imprecise, and success rates vary greatly from one practitioner to another. Electronic nerve stimulation is often used for improved nerve localization, but may not be available outside of surgical suites. In recent years, ultrasound-guided regional anesthesia has gained popularity as an adjunct or alternative to anatomic and nerve stimulation techniques. While simple blocks (eg, a digital block) have long been performed by non-anesthesiologists using the anatomic approach, the more widespread availability of point-of-care ultrasound is providing a safe and effective method to expand the use of nerve blocks in the emergency and critical care setting.

Ultrasound-guided nerve blocks consist of the identification of the target nerve(s), visualization of the surrounding anatomy (such as blood vessels, lymph nodes, and other important structures), and real-time observation of the local anesthetic spread. Direct visualization of the target nerve and deposition of local anesthetic has been shown to improve block success and to decrease some common complications associated with the procedure.

Bedside ultrasound-guided nerve blocks should be performed in:

- The patient undergoing a painful procedure where a regional nerve block will be effective
- Control of pain when parenteral analgesics are not desirable (eg, the elderly patient with hip fracture)
- The patient who has chronic pain due to an underlying medical condition who will gain relief from a regional nerve block

PROBE SELECTION AND TECHNICAL CONSIDERATIONS FOR NERVE BLOCKS

LINEAR ARRAY PROBE WITH A FREQUENCY OF 10–15 MHz

For evaluation of the superficial nerves, such as those in the forearm, the brachial plexus, and femoral nerves, a high-frequency (10–15 MHz) linear transducer is required which provides better resolution. A lower-frequency curvilinear probe (4–7 MHz), which provides better penetration, is recommended for deeper targets such as the sciatic nerve, or for more obese patients. A small footprint "hockey stick" transducer is preferred in pediatric patients where a smaller surface area is being explored.

FOCUS

The focus can be adjusted to the level of the nerve once found. This will further improve the resolution of the image.

DEPTH

The sonographer should initially startoff with a deep field and fully interrogate the area surrounding the nerve. This will help to identify nearby structures that the physician must avoid when inserting the needle and injecting anesthesia. Once the area has been fully explored, the depth can be decreased so that the nerve takes up most of the screen and is better visualized.

GAIN OR TIME-GAIN COMPENSATION

The total gain or far-field gain (TGC) may be increased in order to brighten the signal returning from deeper structures. Most of the nerve blocks done in the acute care setting are superficial; therefore, the gain usually only needs to be increased with deeper targets or in obese patients.

COLOR-FLOW DOPPLER

The use of color-flow Doppler can be helpful when attempting to properly identify the nerve and to avoid surrounding structures, such as lymph nodes and blood vessels. Nerves will not pick up color flow, but nodes and vessels will, which helps to avoid inadvertent injury to these other structures.

PROBE ORIENTATION FOR NERVE VISUALIZATION

Ultrasound-guided nerve blocks are most often done with the nerve visualized in the short axis. The resultant image is the nerve appearing as a circular or elliptical structure with a honeycomb appearance due to hypoechoic fascicles surrounded by a hyperechoic epineurium, consisting of connective tissue (Fig. 23-1a). This technique is the one used most often by physicians and the easiest for the novice to learn, allowing for visualization of vascular structures adjacent to the nerve.

The nerve may also be visualized in a longitudinal (sagittal) plane by orienting the probe along the course of the nerve, again showing a characteristic fibrillar appearance (Fig. 23-1b). This may be a more challenging view, as the plane of the ultrasound needs to be directly in-line with the nerve.

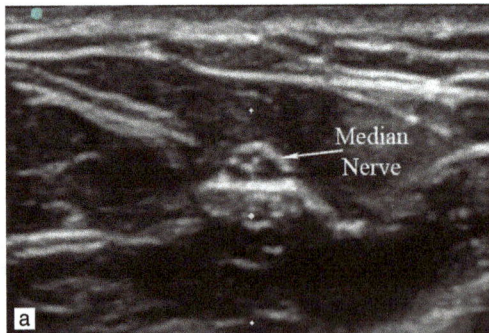

FIGURE 23-1(a) Median nerve (MN) as shown in its short-axis (transverse) at the mid-forearm. The nerve has a "honeycomb" appearance with hypoechoic nerve fascicles surrounded by hyperechoic epineurium. Unlike the ulnar and radial nerve, the median nerve in the forearm is not associated with an artery.

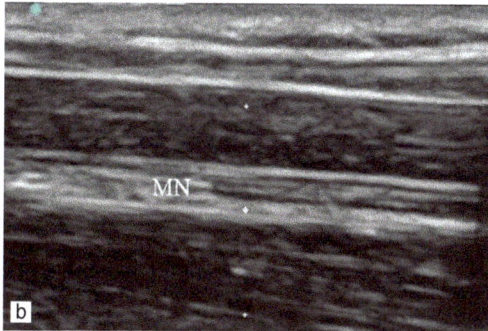

FIGURE 23-1(*b*) Median nerve (MN) as shown in its long-axis (sagittal) at the mid-forearm with a characteristic fibrillar appearance.

PROBE ORIENTATION FOR NEEDLE ENTRY

Once the nerve is located in either plane, the needle may then be inserted and visualized using an "in-plane" or "out-of-plane" technique. In the in-plane technique, the needle enters from the edge of the probe (at the shorter side of the probe footprint) and is visualized entirely in the plane of the ultrasound beam (Fig. 23-2*a*). For ultrasound-guided anesthesia, the in-plane technique is recommended so that the entire length of the needle, not just the tip, is visualized, which helps to ensure precise deposition of anesthetics (Fig. 23-2*b*).

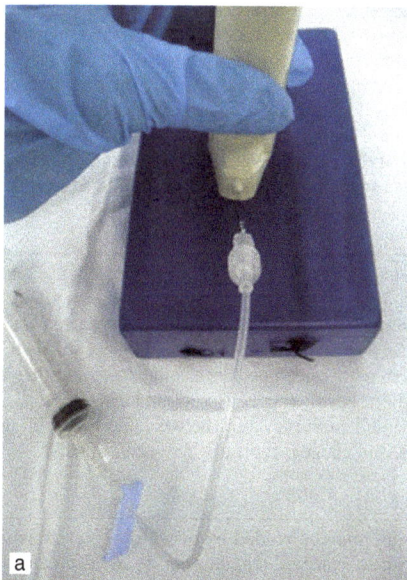

FIGURE 23-2(*a*) Appropriate needle and probe positioning for the "in-plane" technique. The needle is inserted at the shorter side of the probe footprint. Note the use of a spinal needle attached to extension tubing and a syringe.

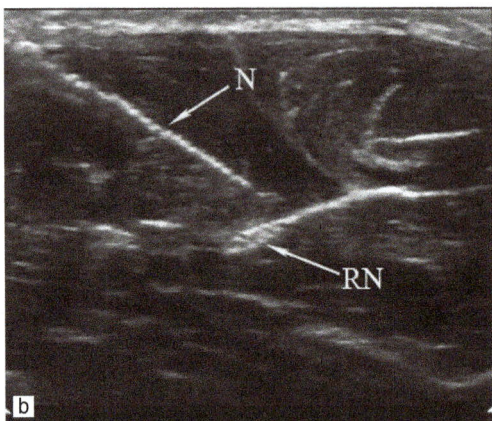

FIGURE 23-2(b) Radial nerve block with the needle visualized in a long axis using an in-plane technique. Note the hyperechoic needle (N) visualized in its full length approaching the radial nerve (RN).

In general, we will be describing the nerve block procedure using short-axis visualization of the nerve with in-plane needle entry. Unlike other ultrasound-guided procedures, the probe is not withdrawn until the termination of the nerve block.

DYNAMIC ULTRASOUND GUIDANCE

Ultrasound-guided nerve block procedures are done using real-time imaging. This technique allows the sonographer to directly visualize the needle approaching the nerve and the injection of anesthesia surrounding it in order to ensure an adequate block. This dynamic imaging also decreases the risks of injuring other surrounding anatomy, such as lymph nodes, blood vessels, or other vital structures. When using dynamic guidance, the sonographer must use sterile precautions including the use of probe covers and sterile gel.

NEEDLE CHOICE

Standard injection needles (found in most emergency departments) tend to have long bevels (steep angle). While there is some controversy over the role of bevel angle in neurovascular injury, most authorities recommend a short bevel needle for more proximal nerve blocks. An alternative that is unlikely to cause injury is a pencil-point needle, with a side port for installation of anesthesia. Spinal needles are typically medium bevel or pencil point and may be appropriate for use in nerve blocks. Needle length may vary between 1.5 and 3 in, depending on the depth of the nerve, and gauge is typically between 22 and 25.

ANESTHETIC CHOICE

Choice of anesthetic may be guided by onset, duration of action, and toxicity. The addition of epinephrine will lengthen action and decrease toxicity. A benefit of ultrasound-guided anesthesia is that typically lower amounts of anesthetic are needed than if the procedure is done blind.

Lidocaine (Xylocaine) is a quick onset, short-acting anesthetic that is appropriate for brief procedures that are unlikely to have significant post-procedure pain. Toxicity occurs at ~4.5 mg/kg without epinephrine and ~7 mg/kg with epinephrine. Lidocaine is typically 1% or 2% (10 or 20 mg/mL). Thus, for a 70-kg adult, 30 cc or less of 1% lidocaine should be used.

Bupivacaine (Marcaine) is a long-acting anesthetic with slow onset of action. It may be mixed with lidocaine for longer-acting post-procedure control. Toxicity occurs at over 2.5 mg/kg, but concentrations of the solution are typically lower (0.25%). Bupivacaine is much more cardiotoxic than lidocaine if injected intravascularly and care should be taken with this agent. Some authorities recommend that a lipid emulsion injection be available for the therapy of the rare complication of cardiac arrest with intraarterial bupivacaine injection.

Mepivacaine (Polocaine, Carbocaine) is a medium-onset, medium-acting anesthetic with a toxicity at 7 mg/kg that is often recommended for regional anesthesia.

PERFORMING ULTRASOUND-GUIDED NERVE BLOCKS

Specific nerve blocks are discussed later. As in any ultrasound-guided procedure, optimal patient positioning is needed in order to gain adequate exposure to the desired anatomical area. The ultrasound machine is positioned so that the monitor faces the operator during the procedure. Sterile precautions are observed, including appropriately cleansing the skin, using a sterile probe cover and gel, and the use of sterile attire by the person performing the procedure.

Once the appropriate nerve(s) are identified, the adjacent area should be interrogated in order to identify the surrounding anatomy. The sonographer should take note of the soft tissue and musculature that the needle may need to puncture through, the location of the vasculature, the position of the rib(s) and lung tissue if performing a brachial plexus block, and the direction that the target nerve travels proximally and distally. This helps to plan the trajectory of the needle and to avoid complications. Once the surrounding area is examined, the nerve should be imaged in a transverse or short-axis plane and centered in the middle of the screen.

The superficial skin may be anesthetized by depositing local anesthetic adjacent to the footprint of the probe, and forming a wheal at the site of anticipated needle puncture, typically using a short 25G or higher needle. In an in-plane approach, the wheal will be adjacent to the shorter side of the footprint. A syringe should be filled with the desired anesthetic medication and connected to short-extension tubing. The amount of anesthetic used will depend on the type and accuracy of block, type of anesthetic, and patient size, but typically ranges from 5 to 30 cc total for an adult patient. Similarly, needle choice will vary in terms of length and gauge, as discussed earlier. A short bevel or non-cutting needle (spinal needle may be used) is preferred (see Fig. 23-2a).

Next, the needle should puncture the skin through the anesthetic wheal. The sonographer needs to focus on the ultrasound monitor while inserting the needle in order to track its course. The entire needle length will be visualized in an in-plane approach (see Fig. 23-2b). As the needle tip enters the desired location adjacent to the target nerve, about 1–2 mL of anesthetic should be slowly delivered as a test dose. The anesthetic spread should be observed as a band of hypoechoic ribbon dissecting out the target nerve from its surrounding soft tissue. The goal is to form a circular spread, or a "donut" around each nerve or nerve bundle, which will improve the visualization of the target nerve. If the spread is too distant from the target, the needle should be pulled back and repositioned and the test dose repeated. If the desired spread is achieved, then the rest of the anesthetic can be slowly injected. If the patient experiences pain during the injection or intraneuronal anesthetic spread is visualized, then the needle should be withdrawn by a few millimeters before further injection. Once the desired amount of medication is given, the needle can be removed completely and the nerve distribution(s) can be checked to ensure complete anesthetic effect.

The choice of anesthetics will depend on the goal of the nerve block. A short-acting medication, such as 1%–2% lidocaine (1.5–3 hours), is adequate for short procedures such as an incision and drainage, or an uncomplicated shoulder dislocation. A long-acting medication, such as 0.25%–0.5% bupivacaine, (10–14 hours) provides longer analgesia for more complex procedures. Also, commonly available is the intermediate-acting 1%–1.5% mepivacaine (4–5 hours).

SPECIFIC BLOCKS

BRACHIAL PLEXUS

The brachial plexus is made of the fifth to eighth cervical nerves, and the major part of the first thoracic nerve. As the nerve roots traverse distally, they form the superior, middle, and inferior trunks that lie between the anterior and middle scalene muscles. The trunks then organize themselves into the lateral, posterior, and medial cords behind the clavicle before becoming terminal nerves that innervate the upper extremity in the axillary crease.

INTERSCALENE BLOCK

The interscalene approach is the most proximal brachial plexus block and is performed on the nerve trunks situated in the groove between the anterior and middle scalene muscles. This approach mostly blocks C5-C7 and is best suited for providing analgesia to the shoulder, clavicle, and upper arm. In the acute care setting, this block is most useful for shoulder reductions or fractures and for injuries of the upper humerus.

It can also block the cervical plexus (C3-C4) in varying degrees. Due to the proximity of the phrenic nerve to the interscalene groove, this approach may cause a transient hemidiaphragmatic paralysis, although the incidence may be lower with ultrasound guidance and smaller amounts of anesthetic. However, respiratory compromise is a contraindication to interscalene block.

The patient should be placed in the supine position with their head turned to the contralateral side. This view can be obtained by scanning the lateral aspect of the neck at the level of the C6 cricoid cartilage. Once the cricoid cartilage is identified, the lateral border of the sternocleidomastoid muscle should be palpated and just lateral to that, the interscalene groove can be identified. The probe should be placed in a transverse oblique orientation over the groove at this level (Fig. 23-3a). The resultant image will show the sternocleidomastoid muscle located superficially and the internal jugular vein and the carotid artery medially. The anterior and middle scalene muscles are visualized laterally. The brachial plexus is lined up vertically within the interscalene groove and is seen as three nerves together in cross section, often described as a "traffic light" appearance (Fig. 23-3b).

Once the anatomy is identified, the needle should be inserted using an "in-plane" posterolateral approach underneath the transducer. It should be advanced anteromedially through the middle scalene muscle toward the nerve trunks where appropriate anesthesia can then be deposited.

AXILLARY BLOCK

The axillary approach is the most distal of the brachial plexus blocks before the terminal nerves appear in the forearm. The plexus at this point divides into its terminal branches. The median, radial, and ulnar nerves all travel closely with the

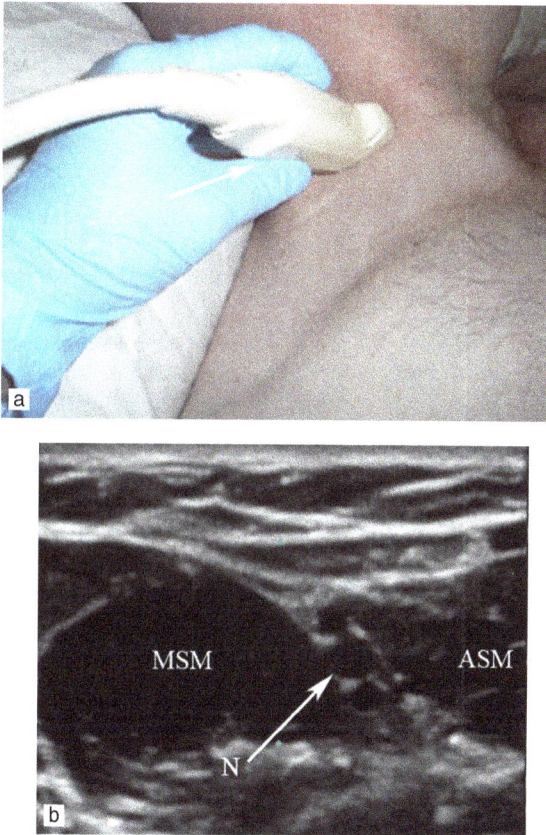

FIGURE 23-3 Proper patient and probe positioning for an interscalene block. The patient is supine with their head turned to the contralateral side. The probe is placed in a transverse oblique (short-axis) orientation over the interscalene groove. The needle is inserted using an in-plane approach from the posterolateral side of the probe advancing anteromedially toward the nerve trunks (see arrow) (*a*). Interscalene nerve block anatomy (*b*). The brachial nerve trunks and roots are seen as three hypoechoic circular structures (N) that are flanked by the middle scalene muscle (MSM) laterally and anterior scalene muscle (ASM) medially. It is in this conformation that the nerves resemble a traffic light.

axillary artery within the axillary sheath, and therefore are easily blocked together at this level. The musculocutaneous nerve (MCN) is more distal from the axillary artery and does not receive adequate anesthesia from this approach. This block is best for analgesia to the forearm and hand, keeping in mind that the area supplied by the MCN (lateral forearm) will not be blocked. This block is best suited for fractures or reductions to the distal forearm or hand, such as a Colles fracture. This is beneficial in the elderly patient who may have comorbidities and limitations to the amount of parenteral analgesia they can receive. This block is also useful in repairing complicated lacerations or draining large abscesses that may involve more than one nerve distribution, such as a palmar laceration of the hand. If large enough, this injury may involve all three terminal branches of the plexus, the ulnar, radial, and median nerves, and therefore a local block may not be effective.

The advantages of this block include the lack of risk for a pneumothorax or respiratory compromise and easier control of bleeding if a peripheral vessel is injured. The disadvantage of this block is the additional anesthesia needed to provide analgesia to the lateral forearm, if needed.

The patient should be placed supine with their arm externally rotated, abducted 90° and flexed 90° at the elbow. The probe should be placed in the axilla at the axillary crease in a sagittal orientation, with the marker pointing toward the patient's head (Fig. 23-4a). This plane will give a short-axis view of the nerves and blood vessels. The crease is located between the pectoralis major and biceps muscles. The axillary artery should be identified with color flow Doppler and used as a landmark as the median, ulnar, and radial nerves surround it at this level. The median nerve is located superficial and cephalad to the artery, the radial nerve is located deep to the artery, and the ulnar nerve is located caudad to the artery (Fig. 23-4b). The needle should be inserted with the in-plane approach at the lateral edge of the transducer toward the axillary artery. Anesthesia should be injected around each nerve when the needle tip is close to the artery, taking care to not inject intravascularly.

MUSCULOCUTANEOUS NERVE BLOCK

The MCN travels separately from the axillary artery within the coracobrachialis muscle, and therefore needs to be blocked separately in order to completely anesthesize the lateral forearm. In addition, an isolated muculocutaneous block can be performed for such things as a laceration to the lateral forearm.

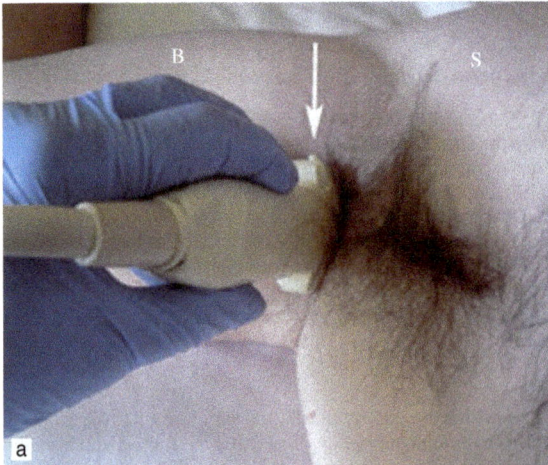

FIGURE 23-4(a) Proper patient and probe positioning for an axillary block. The patient is supine with the arm externally rotated, abducted 90° and flexed 90° at the elbow. The probe is placed in the axilla at the axillary crease in a sagittal orientation. The crease lies between the pectoralis major and biceps muscles. The needle is inserted using an in-plane approach at the lateral edge of the probe advancing medially toward the axillary artery (see arrow). B: biceps, S: shoulder.

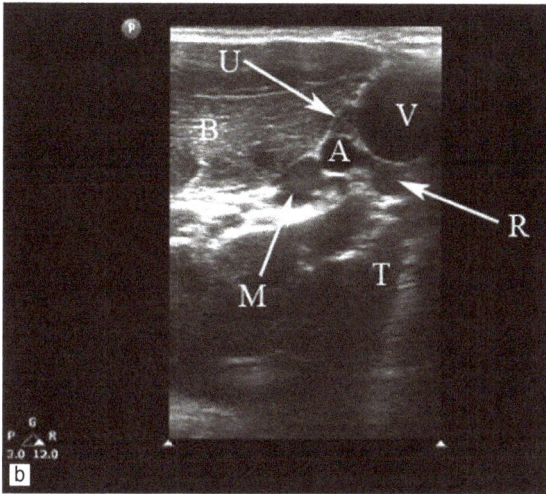

FIGURE 23-4(b) Axillary nerve block anatomy. The median, ulnar, and radial nerves are seen surrounding the axillary artery (A) on top of a fascial plane that separates the arm flexors from the extensors. The median nerve (M) is located cephalad, the ulnar nerve (U) is located caudad, and the radial nerve (R) is located deep to the artery. V: axillary vein, B: biceps, T: triceps.

The patient's arm should remain abducted, externally rotated and flexed at the elbow with the probe placed in a sagittal orientation in between the pectoralis major and biceps muscles. The axillary artery should be identified and the probe should be slowly moved toward the biceps muscle until the MCN comes into view (Fig. 23-5a). The nerve is normally situated between the biceps and coracobrachialis muscles or within the coracobrachialis muscle itself (Fig. 23-5b). Once located, the in-plane technique can be used to deposit anesthesia around the nerve.

TERMINAL BRANCHES OF THE BRACHIAL PLEXUS

The terminal branches of the brachial plexus consist of the radial, median, and ulnar nerves. Blockade of these individual nerves is suitable for minor procedures or injuries that only affect one nerve distribution. It is not difficult to block more than one of these nerves for procedures that affect more than one distribution. These nerves are blocked at the volar aspect of the forearm from the elbow down to the wrist.

At the elbow, the radial nerve lies between the brachialis and brachioradialis muscles, lateral to the biceps tendon. Blockade of this nerve provides analgesia to the dorsolateral aspect of the hand, including the thumb, index finger, middle finger, and the lateral half of the ring finger up to the distal interphalangeal joint. This block is beneficial in fractures, lacerations, or wound explorations to the portion of the hand or digits served by the radial nerve.

The radial nerve is best located distally at the wrist. A linear probe is placed in the transverse plane over the lateral forearm at the wrist. The radial nerve courses with the radial artery which should be used as a landmark (Fig. 23-6). The radial artery can be identified first as a pulsatile circular structure that generates Doppler

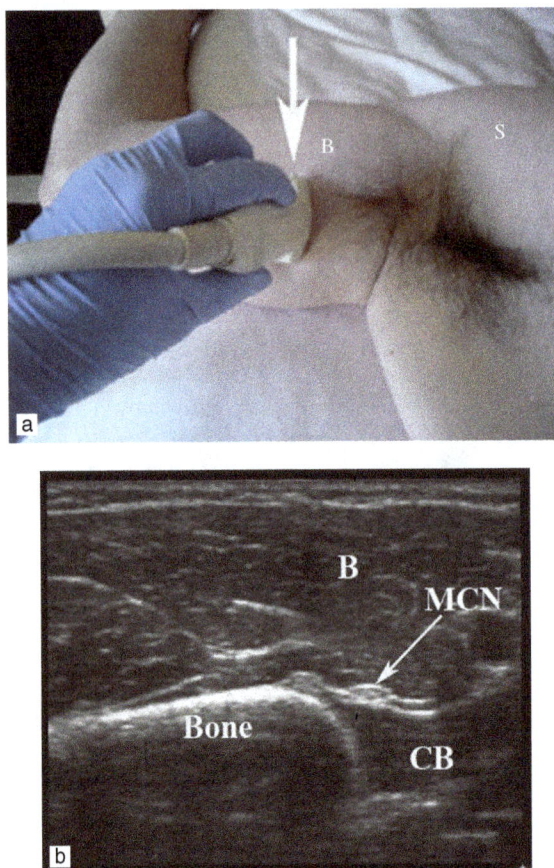

FIGURE 23-5 Proper patient and probe positioning for a musculocutaneous nerve (MCN) block. The patient is supine with his arm externally rotated, abducted 90° and flexed 90° at the elbow. The probe is placed in the axilla at the axillary crease in a sagittal orientation and moved distally down the arm toward the biceps until the nerve comes into view. The needle is inserted using an in-plane technique at the lateral edge of the probe advancing medially toward the nerve (see arrow) (*a*). B: biceps, S: shoulder. Musculocutaneous nerve block anatomy (*b*). The MCN is seen between the biceps (B) and coracobrachialis (CB) muscles.

signals. The radial nerve lies lateral (or radial) to the radial artery. Once the neurovascular bundle is localized, it should be followed proximally toward the elbow at the antecubital fossa where it takes on a more elliptical appearance (see Fig. 23-2*b*). A more proximal blockade provides more effective anesthesia as the radial nerve divides into many small branches in the distal forearm. A block closer to the wrist requires a wide-field infiltration of anesthetics and is typically not done. The probe is kept in a transverse position at the antecubital fossa and the block should be performed using the in-plane technique by

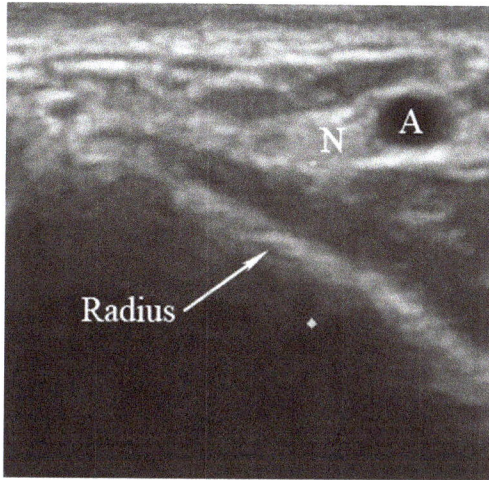

FIGURE 23-6 The radial nerve (N) is seen as a hyperechoic triangular structure lateral (radial) to the radial artery (A) at the level of the mid-forearm.

inserting the needle underneath the lateral edge of the probe and advancing it medially. Once the needle tip is in close proximity to the nerve, anesthetic can be deposited.

Blockade of the ulnar nerve provides analgesia to the medial half of the hand, including the fifth digit and the medial half of the fourth digit. This block is beneficial in fractures, lacerations, or wound explorations to the portion of the hand or digits served by the ulnar nerve. It can be useful in the reduction of a Boxer's fracture of the fifth digit.

The ulnar nerve is best blocked at the wrist area. It is located next to the ulnar artery, which should be used as a landmark. The transducer should be placed in the transverse orientation over the medial surface of the wrist crease (Fig. 23-7). The ulnar artery can be located with the help of color-flow Doppler and the ulnar nerve will appear just medial (or ulnar) to it as a hyperechoic structure. The block should be performed with the in-plane technique inserting the needle underneath the medial surface of the probe and advancing it laterally toward the nerve.

Blockade of the median nerve provides analgesia to the anterolateral surface of the hand, including the thumb through the middle finger. This block is beneficial in fractures, lacerations, or wound explorations to the portion of the hand or digits served by the median nerve.

The median nerve is best blocked at the distal forearm just proximal to the wrist. Unlike the radial and ulnar nerves, the median nerve is not paired with an artery at this level. The probe should be placed in the transverse orientation over the flexor tendons of the wrist (flexor palmaris longus and flexor carpi radialis) (Fig. 23-8). The probe should be slowly advanced proximally until the median nerve emerges as a tightly bundled hyperechoic structure, resembling the appearance of a honeycomb (see Fig. 23-1a). Once this structure comes into view, the needle can be inserted with the in-plane technique at the lateral edge of the transducer, advancing it medially until it is in close proximity to the nerve where anesthesia can be deposited.

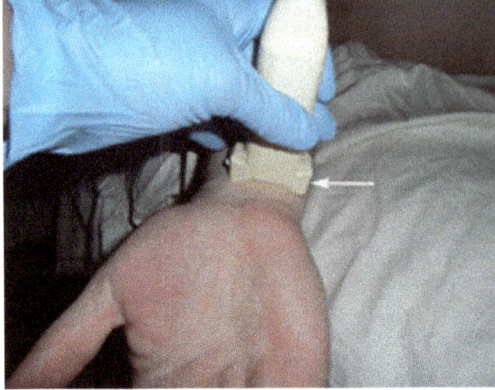

FIGURE 23-7 Proper patient and probe positioning for an ulnar nerve block. The patient's arm should be extended with the anterior surface face-up and the probe placed in a transverse orientation over the medial wrist crease. The ulnar artery serves as the landmark with the nerve appearing just medial to it. The needle is inserted using an in-plane technique at the medial edge of the probe advancing laterally toward the nerve (see arrow).

LOWER EXTREMITY BLOCKS

FEMORAL NERVE BLOCK

The femoral nerve is the largest branch of the lumbar plexus. The nerve and the femoral vessels are both superficially located in the inguinal area enveloped in the neurovascular bundle. Blockade of this nerve anesthesizes the anterior thigh, flexor muscles of the hip and knee, and extensor muscles of the knee. In the acute

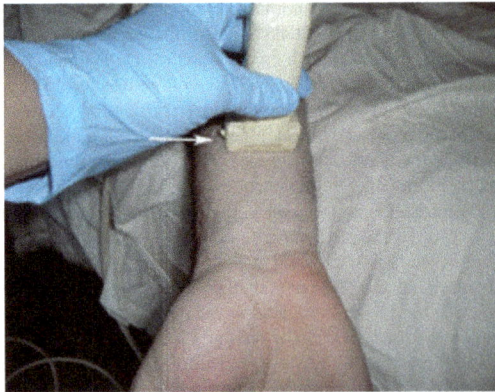

FIGURE 23-8 Proper patient and probe positioning for a median nerve block. The patient's arm should be extended with the anterior surface face-up and the probe placed in a transverse orientation distal to the wrist over the flexor tendons. The needle is inserted using an in-plane technique at the lateral edge of the probe advancing medially toward the nerve (see arrow).

care setting, this block is ideal for both hip and knee reductions, where the patient's pain can be quite significant and the procedure needs to be done as quickly as possible to avoid neurovascular compromise. It is also beneficial in hip fractures, which occur most commonly in elderly patients, in situations where parenteral analgesia is contraindicated. In addition, this block can be used for large complicated lacerations or wounds to the anterior thigh when a local block would not be adequate.

The patient should be placed in the supine position with the leg extended. The transducer should be placed over the inguinal crease in a transverse oblique plane and scanned from medial to lateral to locate the femoral vein, artery, and nerve in sequence enveloped in the femoral sheath (Fig. 23-9). The femoral nerve lies deep to the hyperechoic fascia iliaca, and is separated from the femoral vessels by the ileopectineal fascia. The nerve will be seen just lateral to the femoral artery as a hyperechoic structure. In order to achieve an adequate block, the needle must puncture through the iliopectineal fascia and get as close to the femoral nerve as possible before injecting the anesthesia. This should be confirmed by seeing the fluid collect below the fascial plane as it is being injected.

THREE-IN-ONE BLOCK

The obturator and lateral femoral cutaneous nerves (LFN) branch off the lumbar plexus more proximally and are not typically imaged with ultrasound. The obturator nerve provides sensory innervation to the medial thigh and motor function to the adductor muscles of the lower extremity. The LFN supplies sensory to the lateral thigh. If anesthesia to these additional areas is required, a "three-in-one" block can be performed of the obturator, the LFN, and the femoral

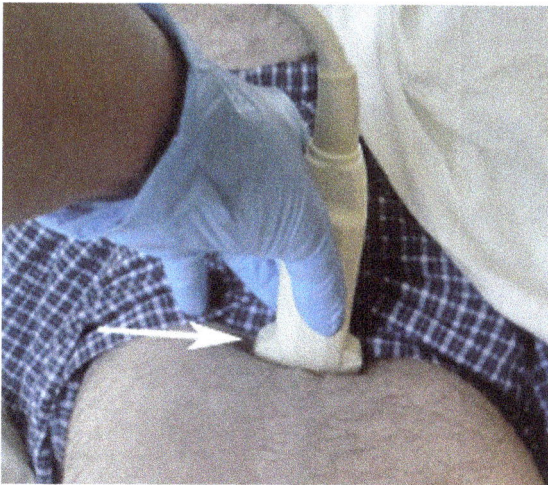

FIGURE 23-9 Proper patient and probe positioning for a femoral nerve block. The patient is supine with the leg extended. The probe is placed over the inguinal crease in a transverse oblique plane and scanned from medial to lateral to locate the femoral vein, artery, and nerve. The nerve will be seen just lateral to the artery as a hyperechoic structure. The needle is inserted using an in-plane technique at the lateral edge of the probe advancing medially toward the nerve (see arrow).

nerve. The three-in-one block may be particularly applicable in the ED setting when elderly patients present with hip fractures. The three-in-one block also has the advantage of not injecting immediately adjacent to vascular structures.

To achieve a "three-in-one" block, the femoral nerve is scanned at or proximal to the inguinal crease. The needle is advanced from a lateral approach approximately 2cm distal to the inguinal ligament. Needle entry should be visualized through the fascial layer and anesthetic agent deposited around the femoral nerve. Pressure should be applied distally to the injection for several minutes to allow the anesthetic to diffuse proximally and effectively block the obturator and lateral femoral cutaneous nerves.

SAPHENOUS NERVE

The saphenous nerve is the only branch of the femoral nerve below the knee. It supplies cutaneous innervation to the medial, anteromedial, and posteromedial lower leg from the knee down to the medial malleolus. Therefore, in order to completely anesthetize the lower leg and ankle, both the sciatic and saphenous nerves must be blocked. The saphenous nerve can be blocked along with the femoral nerve, but it can also be blocked alone, if desired. This block is ideal for wound exploration or laceration repair to the anteromedial leg or medial malleolus. It is also part of a total ankle block.

This procedure is best performed on the medial aspect of the distal one-third of the thigh. The probe should be placed in a transverse orientation on the medial distal thigh, and the sonographer should scan proximally and distally until the superficial femoral artery (SFA) is located (Fig. 23-10a). The saphenous nerve appears as a hyperechoic structure very close to the SFA at this level (Fig. 23-10b). Once the nerve is identified, the needle can be inserted with an in-plane technique from the lateral side of the probe. The needle is advanced medially until it is close to the nerve and anesthetic deposited around it. The saphenous nerve can also be blocked at the level of the ankle, as described later.

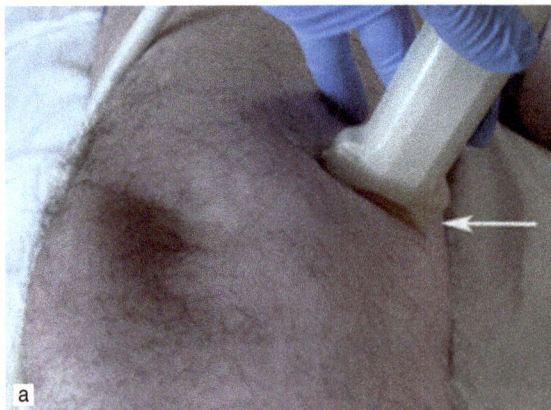

FIGURE 23-10(a) Proper patient and probe positioning for a saphenous nerve block at the distal thigh. The patient is supine with the leg extended. The probe is placed in a transverse orientation at the medial distal thigh. The needle is inserted using an in-plane technique at the lateral edge of the probe advancing medially toward the nerve (see arrow).

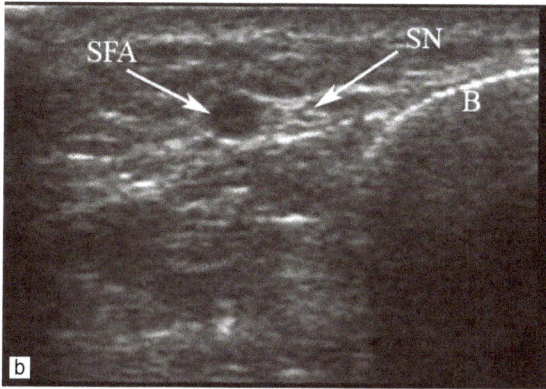

FIGURE 23-10(*b*) Saphenous nerve block anatomy at the distal thigh. The superficial femoral artery (SFA) serves as the landmark and the saphenous nerve (SN) is seen as a hyperechoic structure just adjacent to it. B: bone.

ANKLE BLOCK

In order to completely block the ankle, five nerves need to be anesthetized. These include the saphenous nerve, which is the only branch off the femoral, the tibial, deep peroneal, superficial peroneal, and the sural—all terminal branches of the sciatic. The tibial and deep peroneal nerves supply the deep structures of the ankle and foot, while the other three supply sensory innervation to the skin and are usually blocked more superficially. A complete block at this level is best suited for ankle and foot fractures and reductions, wound explorations, or any other injuries. For these blocks, the patient should be placed in the supine position and the ankle elevated on a pillow.

The saphenous nerve block at the level of the distal thigh is described earlier. This nerve can also be blocked in the distal lower leg or at the level of the ankle where it supplies the area over the medial malleolus. The landmark for the saphenous nerve more distally is the greater saphenous vein, which runs superficially down the medial aspect of the lower leg. The probe is placed in the transverse orientation on the medial lower leg and the greater saphenous vein should be located. The saphenous nerve will appear as a hyperechoic structure adjacent to the vein. The needle can be advanced using the in-plane technique underneath the lateral edge of the probe advancing medially toward the nerve. At the ankle, the probe is placed in the transverse orientation over the anteromedial foot, just above the medial malleolus (Fig. 23-11). The greater saphenous vein once again serves as the landmark. The ideal location to find the vein and nerve is approximately 1–2 cm anterior and superior to the medial malleolus. The needle is then inserted with the in-plane technique underneath the medial edge of the probe advancing laterally toward the nerve. This block is preferentially performed at the distal thigh or mid-leg as it is easier to find the landmarks sonographically, and there is more space to use the probe and maneuver the needle.

The tibial nerve supplies the posterior calf and then dives underneath the heel of the foot. It supplies most of the innervation to the sole of the foot, except for a small area laterally supplied by the sural nerve (SN) and a small area medially supplied by the saphenous nerve. A tibial nerve block at the ankle is ideal for

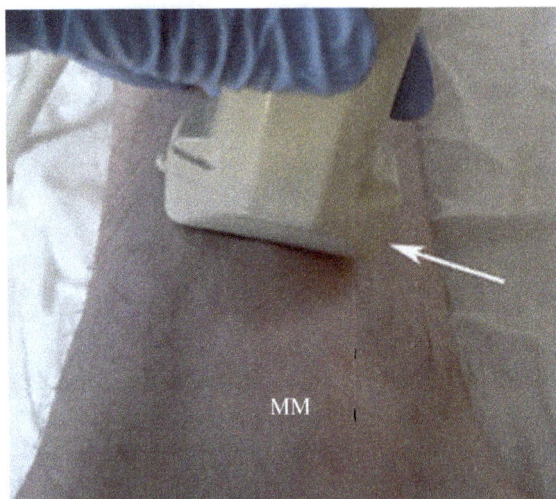

FIGURE 23-11 Proper patient and probe positioning for a saphenous nerve block at the ankle. The patient is supine with the ankle externally rotated. The probe is placed in a transverse orientation over the anteromedial foot, just above the medial malleolus (MM). The needle is inserted using an in-plane technique at the medial edge of the probe advancing laterally toward the nerve (see arrow).

injuries to the sole of the foot, such as volar lacerations, puncture wounds, or foreign-body explorations. The nerve is best approached at the level of the medial malleolus in a more posterior position than described for the saphenous nerve above. The landmark for the tibial nerve is the posterior tibial artery (PTA) which courses down the leg and lies just posterior to the medial malleolus. The probe is placed in a transverse orientation just above the medial malleolus and the PTA is located (Fig. 23-12a). The nerve lies adjacent to the artery in a posterolateral location. The flexor hallucis longus tendon lies lateral and the tendons of the flexor digitorum longus and posterior tibialis lie medial to the tibial nerve at this level (Fig. 23-12b). Once the nerve is located, it should be followed proximally by sliding the probe superiorly up the leg a short distance. The nerve will appear larger at this level and will be easier to anesthetize. The needle is then inserted with the in-plane approach underneath the medial edge of the probe advancing laterally toward the nerve.

The common peroneal nerve travels down the leg through the lateral part of the popliteal fossa and dives deep to the peroneus longus muscle in the lateral lower leg where it then divides into the deep (DPN) and superficial peroneal nerves (SPN). The SPN supplies sensory innervation to most of the dorsum of the foot and the digits except for the first web space. This nerve block is used for any injuries, lacerations, or fractures to the dorsum of the foot and is also helpful in toenail injuries. The SPN is usually not blocked using ultrasound guidance due to its close proximity to the skin surface. Local anesthetic is injected in the skin in between the lateral malleolus and the anterior tibial border.

The DPN supplies innervation to the first web space and the dorsum of the foot just adjacent and proximal to this area. It is best suited for fractures, lacerations, or foreign bodies to this part of the foot or for treatment of chronic pain conditions, such as gouty arthritis. The DPN travels down the dorsum of the foot and is best anesthetized at the level between the medial and lateral malleolus. The probe should

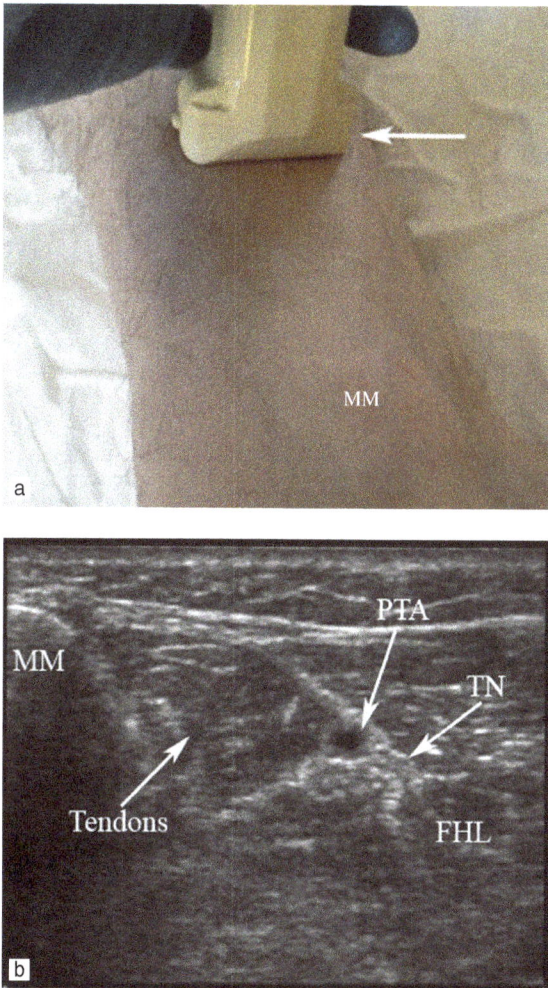

FIGURE 23-12 Proper patient and probe positioning for a tibial nerve block at the ankle. The patient is supine with the ankle externally rotated. The probe is placed in a transverse orientation over the medial foot, just above the medial malleolus (MM). The probe should be moved proximally up the leg a short distance as the tibial nerve will appear larger at this level. The needle is inserted using an in-plane technique at the medial edge of the probe advancing laterally toward the nerve (see arrow) (*a*). Tibial nerve block anatomy at the ankle (*b*). The posterior tibial artery (PTA) serves as the landmark and the tibial nerve (TN) lies in a posterolateral location adjacent to it. The flexor hallucis longus (FHL) tendon lies lateral and the tendons of the flexor digitorum longus and posterior tibialis lie medial to the tibial nerve at this level. MM: medial malleolus.

be placed in a transverse orientation in between the malleoli (Fig. 23-13a). The landmarks for the DPN at this level are the dorsalis pedis artery (DPA) and the extensor hallicus longus tendon, both of which lie medial to the nerve (Fig. 23-13b). The needle should then be inserted with an out-of-plane technique on the anterior ankle surface at the middle of the probe. Anesthetic should then be deposited on each side of the nerve, if visualized.

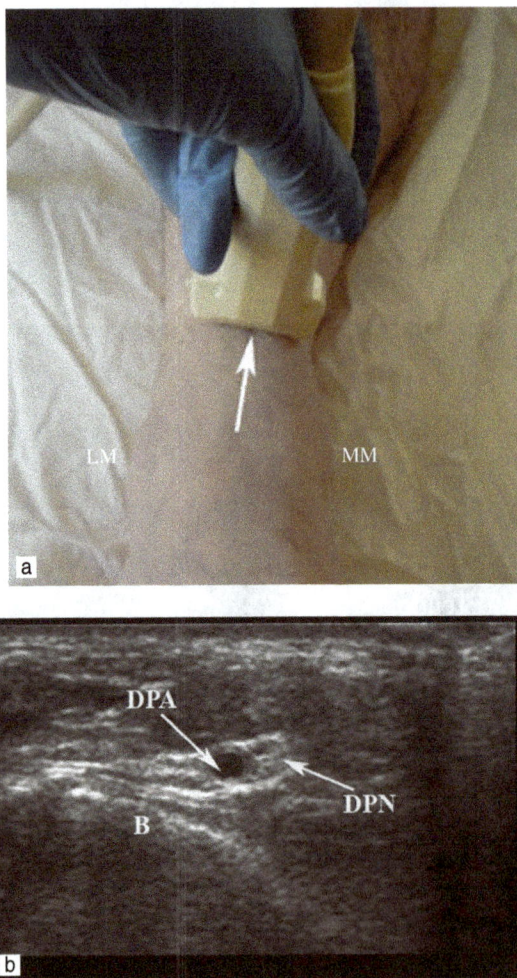

FIGURE 23-13 Proper patient and probe positioning for a deep peroneal nerve (DPN) block at the ankle. The patient is supine and the probe is placed in a transverse orientation over the anterior ankle in between the medial malleolus (MM) and lateral malleolus (LM). The needle is inserted using an out-of-plane technique on the anterior ankle surface at the middle of the probe advancing toward the nerve (see arrow) (a). DPN anatomy at the ankle (b). The dorsalis pedis artery (DPA) and the extensor hallicus longus tendon both serve as landmarks, which lie medial to the DPN. B: bone.

The last nerve needed to complete the ankle block is the SN. The SN supplies sensory innervation to a small area of the dorsolateral surface of the foot, including the fifth digit and the lateral aspect of the heel. It is useful for local injuries, lacerations, or fractures to this part of the foot or the fifth toe. The SN arises in the popiteal fossa and travels superficially down the posterior calf into the foot posterior to the lateral malleolus just deep to the lesser saphenous vein (LSV). The patient is best placed in the prone position (if they can tolerate it) with the ankle externally rotated. The Achilles tendon and the posterior border of the lateral malleolus should be located and the probe placed in a transverse orientation between the two (Fig. 23-14). Once the LSV and SN are identified, the needle is then advanced starting at the lateral border of the Achilles tendon toward the lateral malleolus. Anesthetic injection begins once close enough to the nerve.

COMMON PITFALLS AND TIPS

PROXIMAL BRACHIAL PLEXUS BLOCKADE

The interscalene block can result in an ipsilateral phrenic nerve block with hemidiaphragmatic paralysis. In most healthy patients, this side effect is clinically silent. This block should be avoided in patients with respiratory distress or poor pulmonary reserve. Anesthetic spread can also lead to hoarseness in 10%–20% of patients due to the blockade of the recurrent laryngeal nerve. Horner syndrome may occur when anesthetics diffuse around the anterior scalene muscle and affect the sympathetic cervical ganglion.

INADEQUATE ANESTHESIA

There is always a risk that the nerve block performed may be inadequate. This is usually due to inappropriate needle positioning without penetration of the nerve sheath or not injecting enough anesthetic. The sonographer should use real-time

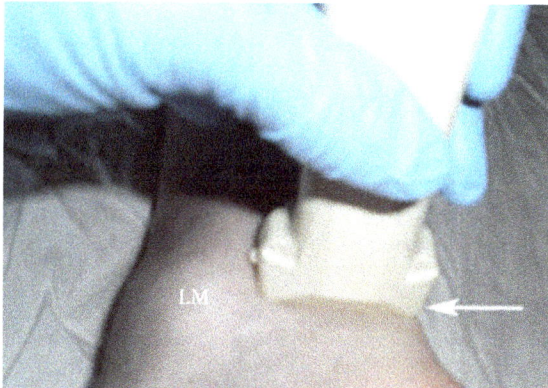

FIGURE 23-14 Proper patient and probe positioning for a SN block at the ankle. The patient is prone with the ankle externally rotated. The probe is placed in a transverse orientation between the Achilles tendon and the posterior border of the lateral malleolus (LM). The LSV serves as the landmark. The needle is inserted using an in-plane technique at the border of the Achilles tendon and advanced toward the lateral malleolus (see arrow).

imaging to locate the needle tip, pull back if necessary, redirect it toward the nerve, and then inject again. A test dose of 1–2 mL of anesthetic should be injected in order to test the patient's response. Once the desired response is achieved, an additional amount can be injected as necessary.

Another common reason for inadequate analgesia is failure to give enough time for the nerve block to take effect. The onset of anesthesia and paralysis depends on the type as well as the quantity of anesthetics used. Patients commonly experience the effect of anesthesia and paralysis 10–30 minutes after the block is performed. Appropriate testing of sensory and motor function of the affected limb should allow time for the medications to work.

ANESTHETIC TOXICITY

This is generally not an issue for adult patients with an appropriate amount of anesthesia, but care should be taken with pediatric patients in particular (see above for toxicity by weight). During installation near the surface, local irritation ("burning") is common due to the acidity of the agents and may be attenuated by buffering with lidocaine. Serious side effects include CNS and cardiac toxicity. Cardiac toxicity has been most widely reported with bupivacaine usage. Cardiac toxicity may be avoided by injecting a lipid emulsion.

INJURY TO NEARBY STRUCTURES

Errant placement of the needle may result in vascular puncture, intravascular injection, pneumothorax, or injury to other structures. These complications may be minimized by adherence to a strict protocol that includes a thorough examination of the patient, recognition of relevant anatomy, precise needle positioning within the nerve diffusion space, and directly observing the slow injection of anesthetic. A complete neurovascular exam should be performed on each patient before anesthetizing the region.

In order to better delineate the anatomy, the image can be optimized by adjusting (increasing) the frequency to maximize the resolution, and also by decreasing the depth to 3 cm or less (except in obese patients where the anatomy is deeper). For a nerve block in a tight anatomical area, such as an ankle block, a hockey stick or a probe with a small footprint can be used to obtain a better image and to leave enough room for needle placement in the skin.

Proper patient positioning, such as turning of the head to the contralateral side, or slight abduction of the hip, can aid in "opening up the anatomy." When performing a proximal brachial plexus block, the sonographer should determine the maximum depth that the needle can be inserted in order to decrease the risk of arterial injury. Blood vessels should be identified to minimize the risk of inadvertent intravascular injection of anesthetics. The use of color-flow Doppler and the compressibility test can help avoid injury to any surrounding vessels.

NEUROPRAXIA

Nerve damage is usually a result of the needle advancing too far and hitting the nerve or anesthetic being injected directly into it. The use of real-time ultrasound visualization as the needle is approaching the nerve before injection greatly reduces this risk. If while performing the procedure, the patient complains of pain or paresthesias, the needle can be withdrawn and redirected in order to avoid intraneuronal injection. In addition, test doses of anesthetic can be used and should always be injected slowly to prevent nerve damage.

CONCLUSION

The use of regional anesthesia has become increasingly popular in the critical care setting with the help of ultrasound-guided assistance. Ultrasound has been shown to increase the success rates of nerve blocks due to the ability of the physician to perform the procedure in real time. Also, the complications that were once feared using the blind method, such as vascular injury or injection, or inadequate analgesia are minimized with the use of ultrasound guidance. In addition, patients receive much more effective analgesia as compared to more traditional local blocks. A thorough understanding and familiarity with ultrasound-guided regional anesthesia can be an extremely useful tool for the busy clinician in the critical care setting. Ultrasound-guided nerve blocks can assist greatly in patient care, time management, and overall improvement of outcomes.

Additional Reading

Christos S, Chiampas D, Offman R, et al. Ultrasound-guided three-in-one nerve block for femur fractures. *Western J Emerg Med.* 2010; 11(4):310-313.

Hadzic A. *Textbook of Regional Anesthesia and Acute Pain Management.* New York, NY: McGraw-Hill Professional; 2006.

Liebmann O, Price D, Mills C, et al. Feasibility of forearm ultrasonography-guided nerve blocks of the radial, ulnar, and median nerves for hand procedures in the emergency department. *Ann Emerg Med.* 2006;48:558-562.

Sandhu N, Manne JS, Medabalmi PK, et al. Sonographically guided infraclavicular brachial plexus block in adults. *J Ultrasound Med.* 2006;25:1555-1561.

24 Ultrasound in Acute Trauma

Nova Panebianco

INTRODUCTION AND BACKGROUND

Traumatic injuries are among the most common presenting complaint to the emergency department (ED). Oftentimes, these patients will arrive unstable and the clinician must quickly and accurately identify the source of injury. Prior to widespread ultrasound and CT scan availability, diagnostic peritoneal lavage (DPL) was used to identify intraperitoneal hemorrhage. The advantages of DPL were that it could be performed rapidly at the bedside obviating the need for transporting the unstable patient out of the department. DPL is now rarely (if ever) performed as it is invasive, insensitive, and nonspecific with consequent risk for iatrogenic injury. Computed tomography (CT) has the advantage of identifying the location and extent of intraabdominal injury, and can evaluate the retroperitoneum. However, it requires the patient to be transported from the resuscitation area and this is not always possible in an unstable situation. It also exposes the patient to ionizing radiation, is expensive, and is not rapidly repeatable.

The focused assessment with sonography for trauma (FAST) exam, utilized primarily by emergency physicians and trauma surgeons, has become a widely accepted screening tool for the blunt trauma patient. Ultrasound for pneumothorax has also been incorporated as part of the extended FAST (E-FAST). The E-FAST exam can be performed quickly at the bedside, is noninvasive, and allows for serial imaging of the injured patient without exposing them to ionizing radiation. Studies have shown that the FAST exam can be learned rapidly by clinicians and is sensitive and specific for intraabdominal and intrathoracic free fluid and pneumothorax. Sonography is particularly helpful in penetrating thoracic trauma. Ultrasound can be used to evaluate a patient's volume status, confirm endotracheal tube placement, and identify fractures. Ultrasound can be used to guide procedures and assess the progress of resuscitation efforts. The E-FAST exam is at the interface between the physical examination and diagnostic imaging, and in the hands of a trained clinician provides a real-time view of patient anatomy, may be used to corroborate clinical findings, and narrows the differential diagnosis.

THE ULTRASOUND APPROACH TO THE ACUTE TRAUMA PATIENT

The ultrasound approach to the acute trauma patient depends on the mechanism of injury and the presenting complaint(s). An algorithmic approach to the trauma patient is outlined in Fig. 24-1.

BLUNT TRAUMA

In any significant blunt trauma, a full E-FAST examination should be performed at the bedside to assess the extent of injuries. The sonographer should begin by evaluating the patient for the presence of free fluid in the abdomen or thorax. This is accomplished by obtaining both right (RUQ) and left upper quadrant (LUQ)

Point-of-care ultrasound in trauma
E-FAST examination (penetrating trauma should start with echo/thorax;
blunt trauma with abdomen)

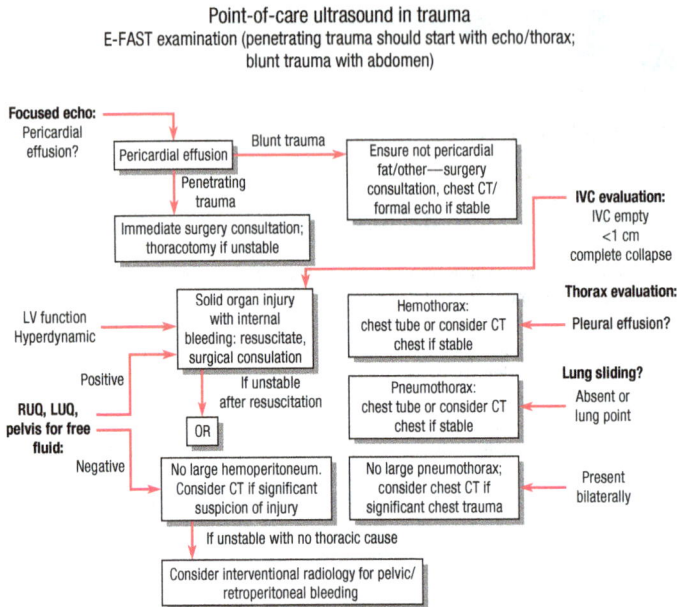

FIGURE 24-1 An algorithmic approach to the acute trauma patient.

views and the pelvis looking for intraperitoneal fluid, indicating a hemoperitoneum. The technique to obtain adequate images is described fully in Chap. 9. In the evaluation of the RUQ and LUQ, a thorough look above the diaphragm should also be performed, looking for pleural fluid, indicating a hemothorax. In the young female patient, the pelvic view should include interrogation of the uterus for obvious pregnancy, which may be visualized prior to hCG results. Ultrasound is also very helpful in the pregnant trauma patient, where radiation from CT is preferably avoided.

If the FAST is positive for free fluid and the patient is stable, it is advantageous to know which organ systems are injured prior to going to the operating room (OR). In this situation, the patient can be sent to CT scan to further delineate any injuries. If the FAST is positive and the patient is unstable, an immediate laparotomy should be performed in the OR and additional studies should be avoided in order to prevent delays in treatment.

Likewise, if a hemothorax is diagnosed in a stable patient, a chest tube may be placed at the bedside. If the patient is unstable, they will need immediate OR treatment. In penetrating trauma, an unstable patient with pericardial effusion or hemothorax may require ED pericardiocentesis or thoracotomy.

In the E-FAST examination, the lungs are evaluated for the presence of pneumothorax. The techniques used to evaluate the lungs are described in Chap. 7. It is important for the sonographer to remember that a lack of lung sliding is sensitive for the presence of a significant pneumothorax, but may not be specific in patients with preexisting pleural disease. The lung point sign is the most specific sign for pneumothorax. If the patient is unstable and there is no sliding present with a lung point sign, then a chest tube should be inserted. If the patient is stable with a lack of sliding, a CXR or CT scan can be performed to better delineate the injury. If the patient is unstable and there is lung sliding present, another cause must be searched for. If the patient is stable and there is lung sliding present, they can be observed and a repeat ultrasound performed later on. If the pleural sliding is equivocal, a CXR or CT scan can be ordered to confirm the diagnosis. Multiple windows looking for lung sliding will improve the sensitivity of ultrasound for small pneumothorax, although a single anterior view will rule out life-threatening ones.

A pericardial view (subxiphoid or parasternal) has typically been included as part of the E-FAST in blunt trauma. However, the utility of a pericardial view in blunt trauma is limited. A significant pericardial effusion as a result of blunt trauma is rare and typically represents an unsurvivable injury. If a pericardial view is included, the epicardial fat pad should not be mistaken for a significant pericardial effusion. The presence of small effusions in blunt trauma is often incidental. In a hemodynamically unstable patient, a cardiac view may be helpful in assessing cardiac function.

If the E-FAST is negative and the patient is stable, the patient may be observed and undergo a repeat ultrasound later on, or the clinician may opt for a CT scan to rule out injuries not detected by ultrasound. If the E-FAST is negative and the patient is unstable, a search for other diagnoses such as a pelvic fracture should be considered. Other possibilities include causes not related to the trauma itself such as an elderly patient who has suffered a fall as a result of sepsis.

PENETRATING TRAUMA

The FAST exam is of limited utility in penetrating abdominal trauma, as these patients typically require operative exploration regardless of the result. However, a positive FAST in penetrating trauma represents a significant organ or vascular injury and should prompt immediate surgical intervention. Ultrasound is very useful in penetrating trauma to the chest. It can quickly diagnose or exclude significant pericardial effusion/tamponade, hemothorax, or pneumothorax. The E-FAST may be invaluable in guiding intervention in an unstable patient with a penetrating chest injury.

CARDIAC FUNCTION

The subxiphoid view of the heart offers an opportunity to assess the patient's overall cardiac function and volume status. Visual estimation of ejection fraction is estimated by the change in ventricular size from diastole versus systole. The sonographer can determine if the ejection fraction (EF) is normal/hyperdynamic (EF>50%), moderately depressed (EF 30%–50%), or severely depressed (EF<30%). If time allows, other echo views can be obtained to better assess the patient's cardiac status.

In most young trauma patients, cardiac function will be preserved. In the unstable patient who has lost a lot of blood leading to hypovolemia and hypotension, the echo will reveal a depleted LV that is hyperdynamic. A hypodynamic LV may indicate cardiac dysfunction as the cause of the patient's instability.

FLUID STATUS

The inferior vena cava (IVC) diameter and respiratory collapsibility can be used in the trauma patient to estimate volume status as described in Chap. 8. While hypotension in a young trauma patient is likely due to hemorrhage and hypovolemia, the presence of normal or increased volume in an elderly patient with hypotension may prompt a search for another cause. In addition to using the IVC and echo findings to determine initial fluid status, serial IVC measurements can help determine if patient resuscitation is proceeding effectively.

CONCLUSION

The E-FAST examination is the best initial imaging modality in any patient with significant trauma. The ultrasound evaluation can be tailored to the mechanism of trauma and the patient's main complaint(s) and obvious injuries. Blunt trauma below the diaphragm should start with an evaluation of the RUQ, LUQ, and pelvis for free fluid. Penetrating trauma above the diaphragm should begin with an evaluation of the lungs and heart for pleural or pericardial effusion and pneumothorax. The examination may be extended as needed from the initial evaluation. The E-FAST examination can be performed at the bedside in only a few minutes while the rest of the primary survey is being completed.

In addition to the benefits of using the ultrasound to diagnose injuries in the trauma patient, it can also be used to determine cardiac function and fluid status and to guide the clinician in the right course of treatment. The echo and IVC assessment can be incorporated into the traditional FAST examination at the bedside and should be included in the algorithm of the trauma patient. These assessments may help determine the need for IVF or blood products and the patient's response to treatment.

Additional Reading

Boulanger BR, McLellan BA, Brenneman FD, Ochoa J, Kirkpatrick AW. Prospective evidence of the superiority of a sonography-based algorithm in the assessment of blunt abdominal injury. *J Trauma*. 1999;47:632-637.

Kirkpatrick AW. Clinician-performed focused sonography for the resuscitation of trauma. *Crit Care Med*. 2007;35(5) (suppl):S162-S172.

Lyon M, Blaivas M, Brannam L. Sonographic measurement of the inferior vena cava as a marker of blood loss. *Am J Emerg Med*. 2005;23(1):45-50.

Ma OJ, Mateer JR, Ogata M, et al. Prospective analysis of a rapid trauma ultrasound examination performed by emergency physicians. *J Trauma*. 1995;38:879-885.

Thomas B, Falcone RE, Vasquez D, et al. Ultrasound evaluation of blunt abdominal trauma: program implementation, initial experience and learning curve. *J Trauma*. March 1997;42(3):384-390.

25 Approach to the Patient with Undifferentiated Hypotension

Paul H. Mayo

INTRODUCTION AND BACKGROUND

Hemodynamic insufficiency, presenting as hypotension and shock, is a common presentation in both the emergency and critical care setting. The etiology of hypotension may be easily identifiable in such cases as massive hemorrhage, profound dehydration, sepsis, or severe cardiac dysrhythmia. More often, there is ambiguity as to the cause of a patient's hypotension, especially when no good history is available and the physical examination and laboratory values are unrevealing. In the patient with hypotension and no identifiable cause, appropriate initial management may be delayed. In this situation, the physician may use bedside ultrasonography to rapidly assess the patient for various causes of shock, possibly leading to immediate life-saving interventions.

The usefulness of bedside ultrasound in the hypotensive patient is based on the principles already discussed in previous chapters. A bedside ultrasound is performed rapidly by the physician taking care of the patient, and interpreted immediately while performing the scan. This allows the treating physician to expedite the patient's diagnosis and definitive care. In addition, a hypotensive patient is usually too hemodynamically unstable to leave the department, and performing an ultrasound at the bedside may help obviate the need for further testing and transport out of the department. Consultant-performed ultrasound is still not always available in every hospital setting and testing may be delayed. This stresses the importance of needing an ultrasound machine available in both the emergency and critical care department and adequately training physicians to use the equipment properly. Along with using ultrasound to search for the cause of a patient's instability, it is useful for procedures needed to treat the condition, such as central line placement. Finally, a bedside ultrasound can be repeated as necessary to assess response to therapy, evolution of disease, and to search for new problems.

CAUSES OF SHOCK AND THE ULTRASOUND APPROACH

The causes of shock can be divided into various categories that help to generate a differential diagnosis for a patient's instability. These categories help to design an ultrasound approach at the bedside tailored to the patient's presenting complaint and most likely diagnosis.

OBSTRUCTIVE SHOCK

Etiologies of obstructive shock are either due to intrinsic or extrinsic factors. Common causes include pericardial tamponade, tension pneumothorax, right ventricular (RV) outflow impedance (ie, pulmonary embolism, high ventilator pressures, auto PEEP), and intraabdominal compartment syndrome. Rare causes of obstructive shock include tamponade from massive pleural effusion and intracardiac obstruction (ie, myxoma or massive valvular vegetation).

Ultrasonography permits rapid assessment for obstructive shock. An echo can be performed to evaluate for pericardial effusion and signs of tamponade, including right ventricular (RV) diastolic collapse. The inferior vena cava (IVC) size can also be evaluated, which will appear plethoric with minimal or no respiratory variability.

An echo can be used to look for evidence of RV outflow impedance, showing a dilated chamber size consistent with acute cor pulmonale and pulmonary embolism. A lower extremity ultrasound can also be used to identify deep venous thrombosis (DVT) along with the echo signs of RV strain in order to confirm the diagnosis.

Although, transthoracic echo (TTE) is not the most sensitive modality to identify valvular vegetations or chamber myxomas, if identified at the bedside it may expedite care.

If a lung etiology is suspected, a right and left upper quadrant abdominal view may identify pleural effusions above the diaphragm leading to an obstructive picture. In addition, a dedicated lung ultrasound may diagnose or exclude a pneumothorax.

HYPOVOLEMIC SHOCK

Hypovolemic shock is due to decreased intravascular volume. This may be related to absolute hypovolemia (blood loss, gastrointestinal fluid loss, third spacing) or relative hypovolemia (loss of vasomotor control function).

Ultrasonography is extremely helpful in identifying possible causes of hypovolemic shock, the correct course of treatment, and in monitoring responses to therapy. The sonographer should begin by searching for signs of free fluid by performing the traditional views of the FAST exam described previously. This examination is always first-line in the trauma patient who presents with hypotension. The patient should be scanned looking for signs of both hemothorax and hemoperitoneum. In addition, searching for free fluid in the elderly patient with risk for a ruptured abdominal aortic aneurysm (AAA) and in the young pregnant patient with abdominal pain at risk for ectopic pregnancy is useful. This examination may also help to diagnose other causes for free fluid in the unstable patient, such as a ruptured hemorrhagic ovarian cyst or ascites in a septic patient with abdominal pain and possible peritonitis.

The specific organ systems that may be contributing to hypovolemic shock should also be examined with ultrasound. The aorta should be evaluated for an AAA in any elderly patient with hypotension and abdominal pain. Although not sensitive for aortic dissection, an intraluminal flap is specific for the diagnosis. The pelvis and adnexa should be scanned, looking for a possible intrauterine or ectopic pregnancy in the pregnant patient with abdominal pain. Although less sensitive for solid organ injury, ultrasound may also help identify the cause of bleeding in a trauma patient.

In patients with suspected dehydration, an assessment of volume status should be performed by looking at the IVC. This helps in identifying the preload sensitive patient, who will have improvement in cardiac output with volume resuscitation. The vessel will often be collapsed in a hypovolemic state. IVC evaluation also monitors the patient's response to therapy, such as intravenous fluids and the need for pressors.

Finally, an echo can also provide important information in a patient with hypovolemia. A heart that appears to not contain a lot of blood that is hyperdynamic implies a hypovolemic cause, whether it is hemorrhage or dehydration, and can convince the physician to start fluids or blood immediately

CARDIOGENIC SHOCK

Common causes of cardiogenic shock include massive myocardial infarction, severe reduction in left ventricular (LV) function by a non-ischemic mechanism, dysrhythmias, and major valve failure [particularly of the aortic valve (AV) or the mitral valve (MV)].

A bedside echo can quickly ascertain if a patient with hypotension is in cardiogenic shock. Most trained physicians can perform an evaluation of the LV and RV for size and function and possible global or segmental hypokinesis. An estimation of ejection fraction can be obtained and compared to previous echo studies. In addition, there may be obvious signs of valvular pathology visualized with the help of color-flow and spectral Doppler. A bedside echo that reveals a blood-filled left ventricle that is hypodynamic combined with a normal IVC is highly indicative of cardiogenic shock.

These echo findings combined with an electrocardiogram and the patient's previous cardiac studies can possibly identify patients who may need pressors or inotropes immediately on arrival.

DISTRIBUTIVE SHOCK

Distributive shock is caused by an interruption in normal vasomotor function. It is most commonly caused by sepsis, anaphylaxis, a transfusion reaction, or a pharmacological effect (therapeutic sedation or drug overdose). Less common causes include cortisol deficiency, poisonings, and spinal shock.

A characteristic feature of distributive shock is vasoplegia, resulting in a low systemic vascular resistance due to peripheral vasodilatation and increased cardiac output, the latter of which can be easily identified by bedside ultrasound. The heart will appear hyperdyanmic in sepsis due to hypovolemia and afterload reduction, and will benefit from volume expansion. If an echo reveals a blood-filled left ventricle that is hyperdynamic, distributive shock is likely. In addition, an assessment of the IVC can estimate the patient's volume status and is often collapsed in this state.

PROCEDURAL APPLICATIONS

In all forms of hypotension and shock, there are often procedures that need to be performed expeditiously at the bedside. Ultrasound helps to improve procedural success, reduce complications and patient discomfort, and expedites the initiation of treatment in the unstable patient. This includes such things as peripheral and central lines or more complicated procedures such as pericardiocentesis or cardiac pacing. These techniques are discussed fully in previous chapters.

SUGGESTED ALGORITHM

Figure 25-1 is an algorithm for the patient who presents with undifferentiated hypotension and shock. The examination can be completed in several minutes at the bedside of the critically ill patient. The bedside ultrasound performed should be focused and goal-directed. For example, if a patient presents after trauma, the abdomen, lungs, and heart should be looked at first for signs of free fluid, effusion, or pneumothorax. If the elderly patient presents with hypotension and abdominal pain, a quick first look at the aorta would be pertinent. The examination can then be expanded as necessary, depending on the clinical scenario.

If a suspected diagnosis is not evident on the patient's arrival, the sonographer can begin with an evaluation of cardiac function in order to categorize the shock state. These results can then be used to develop a management strategy and to guide the next course of action. If a patient has a filled hyperdynamic left

Point-of-care ultrasound in hypotension/shock

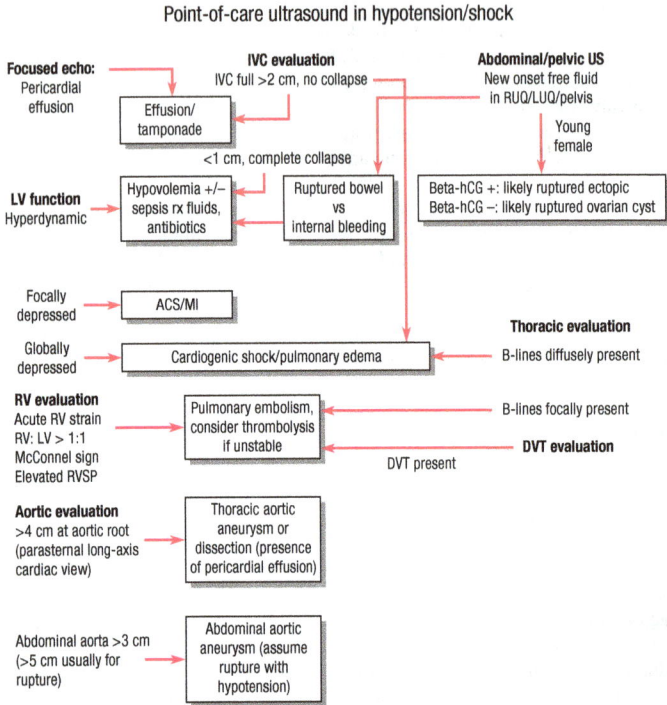

FIGURE 25-1 An algorithm describing how to use ultrasound to approach the patient with undifferentiated hypotension or shock.

ventricle and flat IVC, this is most compatible with sepsis, and IVF with antibiotics should be initiated. If the LV appears filled, but hypodynamic, a cardiac cause is likely and pressors and inotropes would be considered. A hyperdynamic empty LV with a collapsible IVC is seen in hypovolemic states, and the clinical scenario should guide the next step. If the hypovolemia is due to bleeding, free fluid will be visualized in the abdomen or chest. If there is a ruptured AAA present, a large aorta will be seen and possibly free fluid if significant and not confined to the retroperitoneum. If hypovolemia is the suspected cause and no free fluid is seen, dehydration is likely. These findings will influence the physician to start IVF only or to begin a blood transfusion. A large pericardial effusion with right heart collapse and an obstructive picture warrants an immediate pericardiocentesis. An enlarged right ventricle with a dilated IVC is typical for pulmonary embolism, and depending on the stability of the patient, anticoagulation may be started alone or with thrombolytics.

The clinician should remember that several categories of shock may coexist in the same patient both on initial presentation and during the course of critical illness. Many patients have several processes that contribute to hypotension and these may evolve over time. For example, the patient with septic shock may have hypovolemic contribution and coexisting LV failure. During the course of hospitalization, new causes of shock may occur independent of the initial cause, so that the ultrasound examination should be repeated as often as required and in a targeted manner. The clinician must integrate ultrasound results with all the other clinical data in order to develop an effective management plan.

Additional Reading

Atkinson PRT, McAuley DJ, Lewis D, et al. Abdominal and cardiac evaluation with sonography in shock (ACES): an approach by emergency physicians for the use of ultrasound in patients with undifferentiated hypotension. *Emerg Med J.* 2009;26:87-91.

Bahner DP. Trinity: a hypotensive ultrasound protocol. *J Diag Med Sonography.* 2002;18:193-198.

Jones AE, Tayal VS, Sullivan DM, et al. Randomized, controlled trial of immediate versus delayed goal-directed ultrasound to identify the cause of non-traumatic hypotension in emergency department patients. *Crit Care Med.* 2004;32: 1703-1708.

Perera P, Mailhot T, Riley D, Mandavia D. The RUSH exam: rapid ultrasound in shock in the evaluation of the critically ill. *Emerg Med Clin N Am.* 2009;28:29-56.

Weekes AJ, Zapata RJ, Napolitano A. Symptomatic hypotension: ED stabilization and the emerging role of sonography. *EM Pract.* 2007;9:1.

26 Approach to the Patient with Undifferentiated Chest Pain and Dyspnea

Beatrice Hoffmann

INTRODUCTION AND BACKGROUND

Acute chest pain and dyspnea are common complaints amongst emergency department (ED) and intensive care unit (ICU) patients. These complaints account for several million annual ED visits in the United States. The list of potential diagnoses is exhaustive and critically ill patients can appear relatively well, potentially misleading the clinician. Common etiologies are of a cardiac and pulmonary nature, but also the gastrointestinal and musculoskeletal systems are frequently involved.

Physical examination and history taking are often nonspecific and clinical data such as blood pressure, heart rate, and oxygen saturation might not always reflect the true extent of the disease process. Conventional diagnostic tests such as electrocardiogram, chest x-ray, and laboratory data are initiated during the early evaluation phase, but results are not always readily available nor will they always determine the cause of illness. In this challenging situation, the physician's main goal is to distinguish cardiac from pulmonary or other causes and identify a potential life-threatening illness as quickly as possible.

Bedside ultrasound can be indispensible in evaluating patients with unexplained chest pain or dyspnea. It can add vital clinical information in a matter of minutes and is often performed simultaneously with first resuscitation efforts and other medical procedures at the patient's bedside. Ultrasound will often guide medical management and patient disposition.

Common sonographic exams utilized in such patients are pulmonary and cardiac ultrasound as well as point-of-care abdominal and vascular exam techniques. The specific sonographic exam protocols for these applications have already been discussed in previous chapters. This chapter describes an algorithm incorporating bedside ultrasound into the evaluation of ICU and ED patients presenting with acute undifferentiated chest pain or dyspnea.

PULMONARY ETIOLOGIES

Thoracic ultrasound has been shown to be highly efficient in diagnosing diseases such as pneumothorax, hemothorax, pleural effusions, pulmonary edema, pneumonia, and pulmonary embolism. In addition, other advanced applications of lung ultrasound, including acute respiratory distress syndrome (ARDS), pulmonary fibrosis, and carcinoma, although not easily diagnosed at the bedside, are currently being investigated in the critical care setting.

Pneumothorax   Physicians are familiar with the sonographic evaluation of the chest for pneumothorax and hemothorax, as this technique is part of the extended focused assessment with sonography for trauma (E-FAST) protocol. In patients with a clinical suspicion for pneumothorax, physician-performed lung ultrasound is more sensitive and specific than bedside chest x-ray when a cluster of sonographic features are evaluated, such as lung sliding, B lines, and the lung point sign. Furthermore, lung ultrasound has been found to be highly sensitive in the detection of radio-occult pneumothoraces and has been considered an alternative imaging modality to computed tomography in certain instances.

There are no clinical trials evaluating the utility of chest sonography in the diagnosis of tension pneumothorax published to date. The fact that tension pneumothorax is a clinical diagnosis and that physicians initiate needle thoracostomy immediately without reassuring imaging certainly contributes to this fact. However, there is an ongoing debate as to whether lung ultrasound should complement lung auscultation in a cardiac arrest situation, where ambient noise levels at the scene could limit auscultation findings and mask potential reversible causes of pulseless electrical activity arrest such as tension pneumothorax.

Pleural Effusion/Hemothorax

Ultrasound is also an excellent tool to identify fluid collections in the pleural space resulting in dyspnea and chest pain. Pleural effusions result from medical disease or traumatic hemothorax. They most often appear as homogeneously anechoic areas in the pleural space, but can also take on an echogenic pattern or appear as heterogenous septated or nonseptated areas between the two pleural layers. Small pleural effusions, as little as 5 cc, are consistently demonstrated with lung ultrasound, while being missed on chest x-ray.

The detection of the "fluid color sign," a color Doppler signal that appears within a pleural fluid collection during cardiac and respiratory cycles, has been demonstrated to help diagnose very small effusions or loculated fluid collections.

Sonography can also be helpful in distinguishing between pleural transudate and exudate and has been used to accurately estimate pleural fluid volume. Transudates are most often a clear-appearing effusion without echogenicity, while exudates are hyperechoic and can contain mobile particles or septae suggestive of purulent pleurisy or hemothorax. One should remember, however, that exudates can be hypoechoic as well.

Pulmonary Embolism

If there is suspicion for pulmonary embolus, bedside echo can be performed to evaluate for signs of acute right heart strain and acute pulmonary hypertension. Findings such as right ventricular dilatation with thin ventricular walls, right ventricular hypokinesis with apical sparing (McConnell's sign), tricuspid regurgitation, and abnormal septal wall motion support the diagnosis, but it is important to note that these findings can be found in other disease entities. Clearly, visualization of a clot within the vena cava, right heart, or proximal pulmonary artery confirms the diagnosis.

The use of transthoracic sonography to identify peripherally located pulmonary emboli has also been described in the literature. The detection of two or more typical triangular or rounded pleural-based lesions on ultrasound has been reported to have a high specificity for pulmonary embolism.

CHF versus COPD

In addition to the traditional physical exam, bedside ultrasound has been shown to be valuable in distinguishing between patients with an exacerbation of chronic obstructive pulmonary disease (COPD) and pulmonary edema in congestive heart failure (CHF). This clinical distinction can be particularly difficult in certain populations, such as the elderly, where cardiac and respiratory disease often coexist.

The detection of comet tails, also called "B-lines," a sonographic artifact becoming more prominent with increasing interstitial pulmonary edema, can diagnose CHF with high accuracy while virtually ruling out COPD as the cause for acute dyspnea. Bedside echo to assess for overall cardiac function, which would be decreased in the situation of CHF, can also be beneficial in this situation.

Pneumonia

Pulmonary inflammatory changes, such as pneumonia, can be reliably diagnosed using lung ultrasound. Sonography has been found to detect pulmonary consolidation, resulting from pneumonia, when it is located close enough to the chest wall. In addition, other ultrasound findings that occur with consolidation include air and fluid bronchogram patterns. This emphasizes the use of bedside lung ultrasound in patients presenting with fever, productive cough, and dyspnea.

Other Pulmonary Etiologies   Other advanced diagnostic pulmonary evaluations, such as ARDS, pulmonary fibrosis, or lung carcinoma, have been reported in the ICU setting, but their potential impact for the initial ED evaluation has not been evaluated.

CARDIAC ETIOLOGIES

Several life-threatening conditions of the cardiovascular system can be diagnosed with focused transthoracic echocardiography (TTE). The advantages of bedside echo are that it is noninvasive, repeatable, portable, and can be performed with high accuracy by trained physicians without the delay of waiting for a cardiac sonographer. The most common cardiac causes of patients presenting with chest pain and dyspnea include pericardial effusion or tamponade, myocardial ischemia, myocarditis, cardiomyopathy, pericarditis, valvular dysfunction, or vegetations. Although it is not always realistic for a novice sonographer to diagnose all of these conditions at the bedside, a general knowledge of echo can be extremely useful in the acute care setting.

Pericardial Effusion and Tamponade   The detection of pericardial effusion and cardiac tamponade is one of the most common echo applications in critical care ultrasound, especially in the patient who presents with undifferentiated chest pain or dyspnea. Pericardial effusion is characterized by a fluid collection between the parietal and visceral pericardium. It usually appears as an anechoic stripe of fluid between the two layers, but exudative effusions can often appear more echogenic. Bedside echo should not only evaluate for the presence of an effusion, but also for its size and possible hemodynamic complications leading to tamponade. Any patient with signs of tamponade requires immediate resuscitation and emergent pericardiocentesis and cardiothoracic surgical intervention.

Acute Myocardial Ischemia   In patients with chest pain and dyspnea due to acute myocardial ischemia, focal-wall motion abnormalities that follow the distribution of coronary blood perfusion can be detected on bedside echo. This can be an advanced skill for many novice sonographers, and therefore, it is not recommended that emergency or critical care physicians interpret these abnormalities at the bedside to rule out an ischemic event.

However, physicians, with focused sonography training have been shown to correctly estimate overall left ventricular (LV) systolic function. A significant decrease in LV function can be indicative of more severe cardiac disease or injury and is thus helpful information for the clinician. For example, this could be useful when evaluating acute heart failure as the cause of a patient's dyspnea, especially if lung ultrasound shows signs indicative of pulmonary edema.

Myocarditis   Myocarditis, an inflammatory condition of the muscular layers of the heart, can also present with chest pain and dyspnea in the acute care patient. Although a bedside echo may show no acute findings, it can sometimes reveal focal or global hypokinesis and signs of CHF.

Cardiomyopathy   Cardiomyopathy, in the acute care setting, is usually due to a metabolic disorder, a systemic disease, or a post-pregnancy state. A bedside echo in these patients most often reveals decreased LV function or dilatation of the cardiac chambers. An echo in combination with lung ultrasound in these patients, may show findings consistent with pulmonary edema, and suggest the diagnosis of new onset heart failure. Myocarditis and cardiomyopathy can affect many age groups;

therefore, the benefits of performing a bedside echo in a young or postpartum patient presenting with new onset chest pain, dyspnea, or peripheral edema can sometimes provide the diagnosis.

Pericarditis　Pericarditis, an inflammation of the pericardium lining the heart, has a multitude of causes. Similar to both myocarditis and cardiomyopathy, it can affect a wide range of age groups. Echo is usually not diagnostic unless a corresponding pericardial effusion or tamponade is present. This diagnosis should be kept in mind for any patient presenting with the acute onset of chest pain or dyspnea.

Valvular Dysfunction　Acute valvular dysfunction is also not a standard evaluation on bedside echo for emergency or critical care physicians. An acute myocardial infarction can cause papillary muscle dysfunction or rupture with resultant mitral regurgitation and dyspnea. On echo, this may be visualized as a prolapse of the valvular leaflets or abnormal backward color-flow Doppler through the mitral valve.

Vegetations　TTE is not sensitive for diagnosing endocarditis and transesophageal echocardiography (TEE) still remains the gold standard. In addition, evaluating cardiac valves for vegetations is an advanced echo skill. However, the visualization of echogenic or isoechoic irregular-appearing vegetations on or around a cardiac valve on a TTE is suspicious in patients suspected of having infectious endocarditis. In general, these vegetations do not limit valvular motion but valve closure may be inadequate. There are some vegetations that are large enough to be visualized with TTE alone; therefore, a bedside echo in patients presenting with chest pain, or dyspnea and fever, with risk factors for endocarditis, may be useful. All suspected cases should be referred for transesophageal imaging and cardiology consultation.

OTHER ETIOLOGIES

Many patients with noncardiac or nonpulmonary diseases can present with acute chest pain and dyspnea. Several causes can be detected on bedside ultrasound.

Thoracic Aortic Aneurysm or Dissection　Thoracic aortic aneurysms and dissections can both be diagnosed with bedside echo in the parasternal long-axis view discussed in Chap. 5. Although other modalities such as TEE, CT scan, aortography, and MRI are more sensitive in diagnosing these entities, a TTE may identify a dilated aortic root, an intimal flap, or a pericardial effusion.

Abdominal Aortic Aneurysm or Dissection　Patients with aortic abdominal aneurysms (AAA) or dissections can present with a variety of symptoms, including chest pain or dyspnea. Focused ultrasound evaluation for abdominal aortic size can lead to the diagnosis of AAA. Once again, ultrasound is also not sensitive for abdominal dissections, but it is very specific if an intimal flap is visualized in a symptomatic patient.

Viscous Rupture　Patients with acute viscous rupture can present with symptoms such as abdominal or chest pain, syncope, or dyspnea. Free intraabdominal air may be diagnosed on bedside ultrasound. In Boerhaave syndrome, an uncommon cause of acute chest pain, a rupture of the esophageal wall can lead to expulsion of gastric content into the pleural space. This pleural effusion can be diagnosed with thoracic ultrasound.

Biliary or Liver Disease   Acute biliary disease or hepatitis are common causes of ED visits and can present with chest pain. Biliary and hepatic ultrasound is very accurate in identifying a variety of diagnoses, discussed in Chap. 11.

SUGGESTED ALGORITHM

An algorithm for the sonographic approach to patients presenting with undifferentiated chest pain and dyspnea is illustrated in Fig. 26-1. The initial patient encounter is followed by bedside ultrasound performed simultaneously with first resuscitation efforts and other medical diagnostic tests. The sonographic evaluation should begin with either lung or cardiac ultrasound, depending on the most likely differential diagnosis and should be modified or extended during the examination depending on real-time findings.

A thoracic ultrasound should begin by determining if lung sliding and B-line artifacts are present. Specific information about the quantity and quality of these sonographic features could lead to the inclusion or exclusion of certain diagnoses. If no significant pathological findings can be detected, the sonographic exam

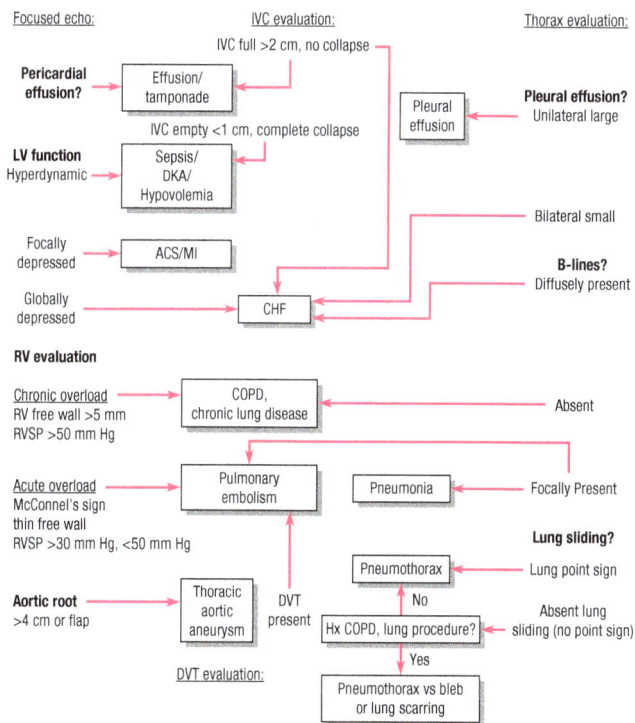

FIGURE 26-1 An algorithm to approach the patient with undifferentiated chest pain and dyspnea.

should be extended to cardiac and abdominal ultrasound, and in the case of suspected pulmonary embolism, a DVT exam needs to be considered.

A primary cardiac exam begins with the evaluation of overall LV function and the pericardium for effusion or tamponade. It can be extended to specific questions, such as localized wall motion and contraction abnormalities, assessment for valvular dysfunction and vegetations, and right-sided heart strain. A pulmonary ultrasound can be complementary or can follow if echo does not offer significant pathology.

If both pulmonary and cardiac sonography do not significantly narrow the differential diagnosis, an extended evaluation for other pathologies needs to be considered. This may include possible abdominal and retroperitoneal causes as well as broadening the differential diagnosis to diseases that are not amenable to bedside ultrasound.

Bedside pulmonary and cardiac ultrasound are extremely useful tools in the evaluation of a patient with unexplained chest pain or dyspnea. A systematic sonographic evaluation, as diagramed in Fig. 26-1, oftentimes can assist the clinician in narrowing the broad differential diagnosis and in sorting out confusing clinical presentations.

Additional Reading

Mathis G, Blank W, Reissig A, et al. Thoracic ultrasound for diagnosing pulmonary embolism: a prospective multicenter study of 352 patients. *Chest.* 2005; 128(3):1531-1538.

Lichtenstein D, Mezière G. A lung ultrasound sign allowing bedside distinction between pulmonary edema and COPD: the comet-tail artifact. *Intensive Care Med.* 1998;24(12):1331-1334.

Lichtenstein DA, Mezière GA. Relevance of lung ultrasound in the diagnosis of acute respiratory failure: the BLUE protocol. *Chest.* 2008 Jul;134(1):117-125.

Meredith EL, Masani ND. Echocardiography in the emergency assessment of acute aortic syndromes. *Eur J Echocardiogr.* 2009;10(1):i31-i39.

Moore CL, Rose GA, Tayal VS, Sullivan DM, Arrowood JA, Kline JA. Determination of left ventricular function by emergency physician echocardiography of hypotensive patients. *Acad Emerg Med.* 2002;9(3):186-193.

27 Approach to the Patient with Undifferentiated Abdominal Pain

Michael Osborne

INTRODUCTION AND BACKGROUND

Abdominal pain is one of the most common complaints encountered in the acute care setting. Undifferentiated abdominal pain can be one of the most challenging conditions that a physician encounters on a daily basis. The decision regarding which labs or radiological tests to order can be frustrating and often unrevealing. Particularly in elderly patients, a difficult history and often inaccurate and changing physical examination can complicate the decision-making process.

There are many conditions that cause abdominal pain, but not all of them are best evaluated with ultrasound. However, there are certain situations in which bedside ultrasound is ideal. In any patient who presents with undifferentiated abdominal pain and is hemodynamically unstable, a quick bedside ultrasound can help to rule out free fluid or possible surgical causes of the pain, such as an abdominal aortic aneurysm. Other etiologies that bedside ultrasound can be useful for are biliary colic or acute cholecystitis, renal colic, bowel obstruction, and appendicitis.

The first distinction that should be made is whether or not the pain is diffuse or focal. This guides the physician in which abdominal areas should be evaluated first. The bedside ultrasound should begin with the evaluation of the most likely organ system to be causing the pain.

DIFFUSE ABDOMINAL PAIN

If the pain is diffuse, it is not always easy to pinpoint which organ system first became affected. Abdominal pain that is generalized is usually of higher concern for the physician as it indicates the progression of the disease. The concerning causes for diffuse abdominal pain include a perforated viscous, a bowel obstruction, the presence of new free fluid from a ruptured structure, or peritonitis in a patient with known ascites.

Perforated Viscous   There are multiple causes of a perforated viscous, including a ruptured appendix, a diverticulitis, a perforated ulcer, a prolonged bowel obstruction, or a ruptured esophagus from excessive vomiting. The presence of fluid in the abdomen in a patient without liver disease or known ascites should raise the suspicion of an abdominal catastrophe, including perforated viscous. Free air is a specific finding for a perforated viscous, and ultrasound may be able to detect free air. When present, free air is best seen at the edge of the liver and will be seen as hyperechoic areas with dirty comet tails that are not within the bowel. Plain radiographs may also detect free air, but a CT scan is much more sensitive than either ultrasound or x-ray.

Free Fluid   If a moderate to large amount of fluid is seen with a cirrhotic-looking liver (shrunken, irregular-shaped), then spontaneous bacterial peritonitis should be considered. Free fluid in a female with abdominal pain should lead to a search for gynecologic origin, such as a ruptured ovarian cyst, ectopic pregnancy with bleeding, or the extension of a pelvic infection. An elderly patient with diffuse abdominal pain and free fluid on their ultrasound should prompt search for a ruptured viscous or bowel obstruction. The abdominal aorta should be evaluated down to its bifurcation into the iliacs for aneurysm or dissection. Ultrasound is not sensitive for aneurysm rupture as this typically occurs retroperitoneally. Its branches should also be evaluated, if possible, including the celiac, splenic, and renal arteries. The spleen should also be evaluated in the presence of free fluid. It may rupture from even mild trauma when enlarged from a viral, congestive, or malignant source.

Small Bowel Obstruction   Small bowel obstruction (SBO) is a common cause of generalized abdominal pain. The most likely cause is previous abdominal surgery, but is also associated with hernias or bowel malignancies. The abdomen can be examined at the bedside, looking for signs of dilated bowel. Small bowel loops greater than 3 cm in diameter on ultrasound is consistent with a SBO. Small bowel can be differentiated from large bowel by the presence of plicae ciculares, folds that extend completely around the inner portion of the bowel, as opposed to haustra, which only partially encircle the interior of the large bowel. In addition to dilated bowel, a bowel obstruction may show a characteristic to-and-fro motion of bowel contents as well as free fluid around the dilated loops. Ultrasound is particularly helpful for detecting bowel obstruction when there is a paucity of air in the bowel on plain radiographs.

FOCAL ABDOMINAL PAIN

Localized abdominal pain should prompt the physician to investigate the organs most likely to be causing the discomfort. The abdomen is divided into quadrants based on the location of different structures.

Right Upper Quadrant Pain   Right upper quadrant (RUQ) pain can have multiple causes. The most common etiologies include biliary tract disease, hepatitis, liver cysts, masses or infections, and renal colic.

The evaluation of RUQ pain should begin with an assessment of the gallbladder and liver. The gallbladder should be interrogated for the presence of stones or sludge and for the additional signs of acute cholecystitis or choledocholithiasis. If gallstones are seen and there is a positive "sonographic Murphy sign" with maximal tenderness over the fundus of the gallbladder, then the pain is most likely biliary in origin. An enlarged common bile duct and hepatic ducts also can be seen on ultrasound and indicate biliary obstruction. The liver should be examined fully looking for cysts, masses, or abscesses. In addition, signs of acute or chronic hepatitis may be identified. The liver may be enlarged and edematous appearing in acute hepatitis, or shrunken and irregular in the chronic state.

The kidneys should also be examined in patients who complain of right-sided abdominal pain. Unilateral hydronephrosis is easily diagnosed on bedside ultrasound and is highly indicative of renal colic. An evaluation for ureteral–bladder jets can also confirm complete obstruction in cases of kidney stones.

Epigastric Pain   Epigastric pain may result from similar causes as the ones listed earlier for the RUQ. More common causes of epigastric pain include peptic ulcer disease (PUD), pancreatitis, AAA, aortic dissection, or an incarcerated or strangulated hernia.

The evaluation of the epigastric area should include the biliary tract and liver, as discussed earlier. In elderly patients, or those with risk factors, such as hypertension, a thorough evaluation of the abdominal aorta should be performed. The vessel should be visualized from its proximal portion down to its bifurcation, looking for a dilatation larger than 3 cm, significant for an aneurysm. Ultrasound is not sensitive for aneurysmal leak, but in patients with an AAA who are not stable, it can be highly suggestive. In patients with a high suspicion for dissection, there should be an evaluation for any intraluminal intimal flaps. Ultrasound is not sensitive for dissection, but is highly specific.

PUD is not readily diagnosed using ultrasound, but advanced disease may be detected by the presence of other signs. A perforated gastric or duodenal ulcer may show free fluid in Morison pouch. In addition, ultrasound may detect a pneumoperitoneum with free air artifacts, obscuring the upper abdomen when the patient is placed in the left lateral decubitus position. Pneumoperitoneum is most often seen in perforated ulcers or colonic diverticula, but can also be seen in perforation of the appendix or gallbladder.

The pancreas is not best visualized using ultrasound, and acute pancreatitis is mostly a clinical diagnosis. When seen, the pancreas is found anterior to the splenic vein on a transverse view of the abdomen. Acute pancreatitis may reveal an enlarged edematous organ, while chronic pancreatitis may show a shrunken calcified structure. Also, ultrasound is sensitive for pancreatic pseudocysts and may be identified as the cause of the patient's pain.

Strangulated or incarcerated hernias may present with epigastric pain. In obese people, hernias can be a challenge to diagnose by palpation alone and ultrasound may help to detect them. If compression over the loop of bowel with the ultrasound probe elicits pain, this points to a hernia as causing the discomfort. Compression may also reduce the hernia while visualizing it.

Left Upper Quadrant Pain

Left upper quadrant (LUQ) pain can be caused by similar entities as RUQ and epigastric pain listed earlier. The most common causes of LUQ pain that can be evaluated by ultrasound include renal colic, hernias, AAA, PUD, or less commonly, splenic rupture. The sonographic evaluation of the LUQ should begin with visualizing the left kidney for hydronephrosis and searching for loops of bowel indicative of a hernia. The signs of advanced PUD, including free fluid and air, can also be searched for. Splenic rupture may occur in nontraumatic situations when splenomegaly is present due to a viral or congestive state. This may present with free fluid in the subphrenic space, splenorenal recess, or in Morison's pouch. It may also be possible to see a splenic laceration or hematoma on bedside ultrasound.

Periumbilical Pain

Periumbilical pain can be as a result of a localized process, such as an umbilical hernia. This area should be scanned looking for an obvious loop of bowel causing the pain. Periumbilical pain can also be a sign of advancement of a focal process that has now become generalized. This includes a SBO, an appendicitis, or diverticulitis with perforation. Appendicitis classically begins with periumbilical pain before it migrates to the right lower quadrant, and therefore, the signs of this entity should be looked for as described later. Urinary retention can also cause periumbilical or suprapubic pain. Any lower abdominal pain in the midline should prompt a look for an unusually large bladder.

Right Lower Quadrant Pain

Right lower quadrant (RLQ) pain is classically associated with an acute appendicitis. Other common causes that can be evaluated with bedside ultrasound include ovarian cyst or torsion, a hernia, and renal colic. In lower abdominal pain, a testicular origin must be considered in the male patient. Likewise, in the female patient, ovarian pathology and ectopic pregnancy must remain high on the differential.

Although ultrasound is not highly sensitive for appendicitis, it can obviate the need for a CT scan if seen at the bedside. It is ideal in the young, thin patient who the physician does not want to expose to unnecessary radiation. The examination should begin by looking for a non-compressible tubular structure greater than 6 mm in diameter in the RLQ. These findings in addition to tenderness ("sonographic McBurney's point") are indicative of appendicitis.

Once again, the kidney should be visualized for signs of hydronephrosis, the small bowel examined for dilatation, the abdomen looked at for possible hernias, and the bladder measured for signs of urinary retention.

In a male patient, a testicular examination should be performed to look for a hernia or testicular pathology causing the pain. If the testicle is swollen or tender, a bedside ultrasound should be used to look for such things as an epididymitis, a hydrocele, a varicocele, an epididymal cyst, hernia, and most importantly for signs of torsion. If there is an enlarged edematous heterogeneous testicle with decreased color flow on ultrasound, urology should be consulted immediately.

In females, ovarian pathology must be entertained, and in women of child-bearing age, a pregnancy test should be performed. Ovarian cysts with rupture, hemorrhage, or torsion can be the etiology of pain. An attempt to visualize the adnexa should be performed to search for an ovarian cyst, mass, or indirect signs of torsion, including a large edematous organ with decreased blood flow. In addition, if a cyst or mass is present, the pelvis and RUQ should be visualized looking for free fluid, indicative of rupture.

If the pregnancy test is positive, then the physician should look at the uterus to determine if there is an intrauterine pregnancy (IUP). If an IUP is not apparent, the adnexa should be searched for any suspicious masses, and once again the pelvis and RUQ should be evaluated for free fluid, signifying a ruptured ectopic. If the adnexa are not clearly visualized, transvaginal ultrasound is indicated.

Left Lower Quadrant Pain   Left lower quadrant (LLQ) pain, in the older patient, is most often caused by diverticulitis. An attempt to visualize inflamed portions of bowel in the LLQ can be made prior to ordering a CT scan. Segments of bowel that have thickened walls with hypoechoic areas are consistent with a diagnosis diverticulitis. This entity is difficult to diagnose using ultrasound, especially for the novice, and therefore is considered an advanced technique.

Additionally, all of the causes of RLQ pain mentioned earlier must be considered in the patient with LLQ pain. The patient should then be evaluated for hydronephrosis, bowel obstruction, hernias, ovarian and testicular pathologies, and urinary retention.

SUGGESTED ALGORITHM

An algorithm for the sonographic approach to patients presenting with undifferentiated abdominal pain is illustrated in Fig. 27-1. The initial patient encounter should be followed by bedside ultrasound performed simultaneously with other medical diagnostic tests. The sonographic evaluation should begin with examining a specific abdominal quadrant based on the patient's history and physical examination and most likely diagnosis. If the pain is generalized, the ultrasound examination will need to be more inclusive and evaluate multiple quadrants. The most likely differential diagnosis may need to be modified or extended during the examination, depending on real-time findings.

Bedside ultrasound is an extremely useful initial tool in the evaluation of a patient with undifferentiated abdominal pain. A systematic sonographic evaluation, as diagrammed in Fig. 27-1, oftentimes can assist the clinician in narrowing the broad differential diagnosis and in expediting patient care and treatment. When ultrasound is nondiagnostic, a CT scan, or other diagnostic modality should be obtained when there is a significant concern for pathology.

Point-of-care ultrasound in undifferentiated abdominal pain

Bowel
Dilated loops >3 cm

RUQ, LUQ, pelvis

Free fluid — History or evidence of liver disease? — Yes — Spontaneous bacterial peritonitis

Bowel obstruction

No

Biliary evaluation
Gallstones
sonographic Murphy
wall thickening
pericholecystic fluid

Dirty comet tails at liver edge

Free air — Perforation or other abdominal catastrophe

Biliary colic/ cholecystitis/ gallstone pancreatitis

>3 cm (>5 cm greater risk for rupture); any flap

Aorta evaluation — Abdominal aortic aneurysm or dissection

Choledocholithiasis/ gallstone pancreatitis — Common bile duct

Genitourinary evaluation — Renal colic

Pelvic evaluation

Ureteral jets

Unilateral — Appendicitis — Ovarian cyst (consider TVUS r/o torsion) — Free fluid / Ovarian cyst

Bilateral

Hydronephrosis — Urinary retention

Blind-ended tubular structure
Noncompressible
Absence of peristalsis
>6 mm
Sonographic McBurney
"target sign"; surrounding edema

Uterus

Bladder volume

Increased

Prostate

Uterine fibroid, metromenorrhagia

Testicular — Hernia, torsion   **Right lower quadrant**

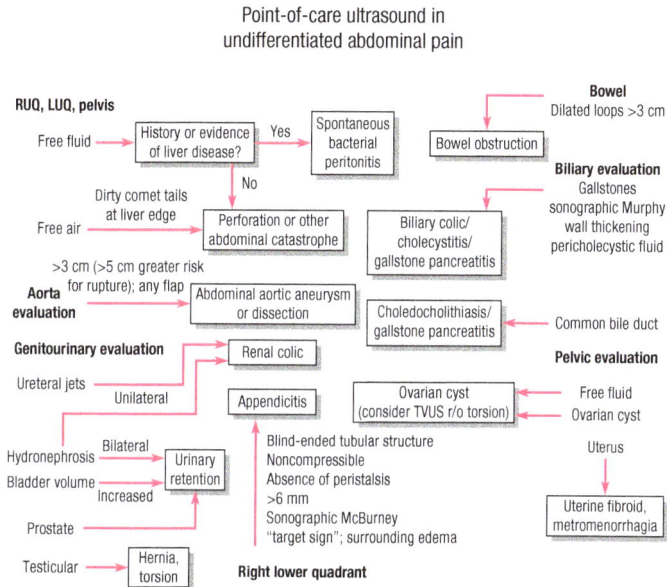

FIGURE 27-1 An algorithm of how to approach the patient who presents with undifferentiated abdominal pain.

Additional Reading

Chaubal N, Dighe M, Shah M, Chaubal J. Sonography of the gastrointestinal tract. *J Ultrasound Med.* 2006;25:87-97.

Glanc P, Maxwell C. Acute abdomen in pregnancy. *J Ultrasound Med.* 2010; 29:1457-1468.

Lameris W, van Randen A, van Es HW, et al. Imaging strategies for detection of urgent conditions in patients with acute abdominal pain: diagnostic accuracy study. *Brit Med J.* 2009;339(b2431):1-8.

Lindelius A, Torngren S, Nilsson L, et al. Randomized clinical trial of bedside ultrasound among patients with abdominal pain in the emergency department: impact on patient satisfaction and health care consumption. *Scand J Trauma Resusc Emerg Med.* 2009;27(17, pt 1):60.

Siegel Y, Grubstein A, Vladislav P, et al. Ultrasonography in patients without trauma in the emergency department: impact on discharge diagnosis. *J Ultrasound Med.* 2005;24:1371-1376.